For Churchill Livingstone

Commissioning Editor: Ellen Green
Project Editor: Dinah Thom
Project Manager: Neil A. Dickson
Project Controller: Nicola S. Haig
Design Direction: Judith Wright
Sales Promotion Executive: Hilary Brown

Toohey's Medicine

A Textbook for Students in the Health Care Professions

Edited by

Stephen R. Bloom MA MD DSc FRCP FRCPath
Deputy Director of Medicine and Professor of Endocrinology, Royal Postgraduate
Medical School, Hammersmith Hospital, London

Nursing Advisor

Helen Steele RGN BSc

FIFTEENTH EDITION

CHURCHILL LIVINGSTONE
EDINBURGH LONDON MADRID MELBOURNE NEW YORK AND TOKYO 1995

CHURCHILL LIVINGSTONE
Medical Division of Longman Group Limited

Distributed in the United States of America by Churchill Livingstone Inc., 650 Avenue of the Americas, New York, N.Y. 10011, and by associated companies, branches and representatives throughout the world.

First edition 1953
Second edition 1955
Third edition 1957
Fourth edition 1959
Fifth edition 1960
Sixth edition 1963
Seventh edition 1965
Eighth edition 1967
Ninth edition 1969
Tenth edition 1971
Eleventh edition 1975
Twelfth edition 1978
Thirteenth edition 1981
Fourteenth edition 1986
Fifteenth edition 1995

ISBN 0 443 04704 9

British Library Cataloguing in Publication Data
A catalogue record for this book is available from the British Library.

Library of Congress Cataloging in Publication Data
A catalog record for this book is available from the Library of Congress.

The publisher's policy is to use paper manufactured from sustainable forests

Produced by Longman Singapore Publishers Pte Ltd
Printed in Singapore

Contents

Contributors

Praveen Anand MA MD MRCP
Senior Lecturer in Neurology,
Royal London Hospital,
Whitechapel, London

William M. Bennet MD MRCP
Senior Registrar, Diabetes Unit, St George's
Hospital, London

Stephen R. Bloom MA MD DSc FRCP FRCPath
Deputy Director of Medicine and Professor of
Endocrinology, Department of Medicine,
Hammersmith Hospital, London

Sarah Bloom
Medical Student, Royal Free Hospital,
Pond Street, London

John Griffiths MD, MRCP
Honorary Senior Registrar, Department of
Medicine, Hammersmith Hospital, London

Peter Hammond MA BM BCh MRCP
Senior Registrar in General Medicine, Diabetics
and Endocrinology, St James's University
Hospital, Leeds

Rohit N. Kulkarni MD
Research Fellow, Department of Medicine,
Hammersmith Hospital, London

Karim Meeran BSc MBBS MRCP
Registrar, Department of Medicine,
Hammersmith Hospital, London

Donal O'Shea MB BCh BAO MRCPI
Wellcome Training Fellow, Department of
Medicine, Hammersmith Hospital, London

John Wilding BM MRCP
Senior Registrar, Department of Medicine,
Hammersmith Hospital, London

Dominic J. Withers BA MRCP
MRC Training Fellow, Department of Medicine,
Hammersmith Hospital, London

Preface

A good grounding in general medicine is essential to all health care professionals. This book is well established and authoritative but has been thoroughly revised in this edition to incorporate the latest concepts and therapy. The text is designed to cover the main diseases in a way which makes them easy to understand and remember. *Toohey's Medicine* is also laid out to make it quick to look things up, and easy to revise when exams loom. Read and enjoy!

A number of active, younger people have advised on particular chapters – nurses, doctors and pharmacists. Thus I would particularly like to thank Helen Steele, Rohit Kulkarni, John Grif-fiths, John Wilding, Dominic Withers, Karim Meeran, Donal O'Shea, William Bennet, Sarah Bloom, Peter Hammond, Praveen Anand and Jo Howells for their unstinting help.

Finally, I must record the sad death of the author of the previous eight editions, Dr Arnold Bloom. Arnold stood for a human approach to health care. Although he applied all the modern advances with the greatest skill, he never forgot that a sick and distressed patient needs reassurance and comfort. He always found the time to give this.

1994   S.R.B.

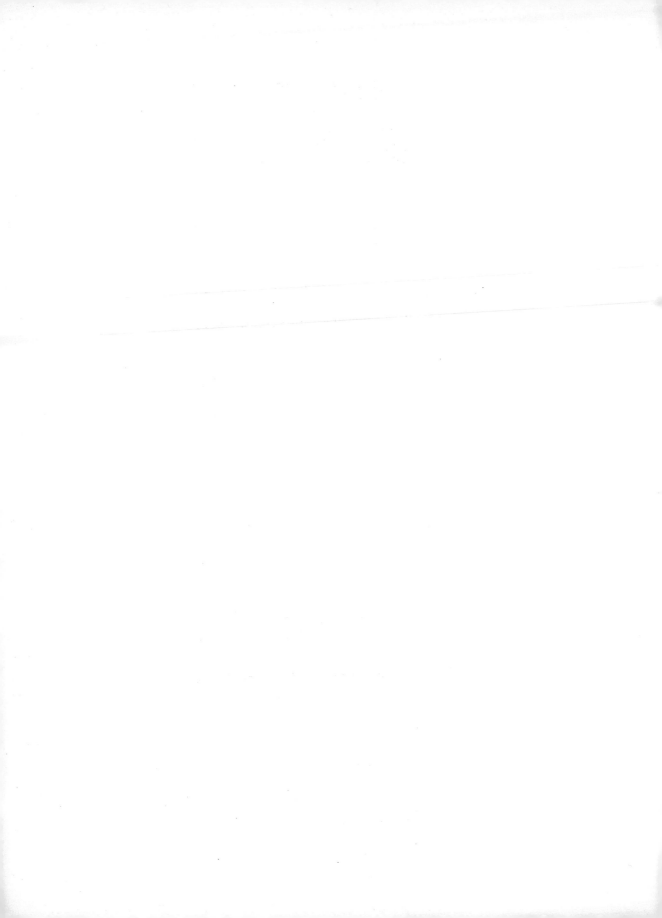

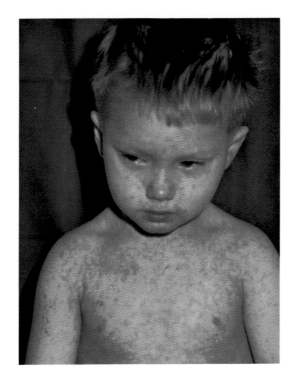

Plate 1 Measles. Note the conjunctivitis.

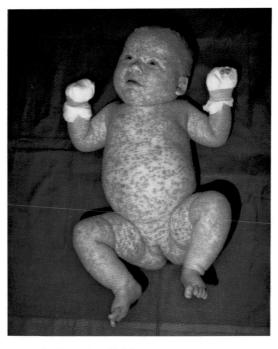

Plate 2 Extensive chickenpox.

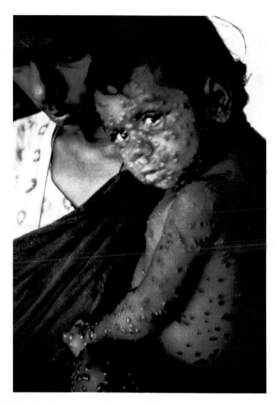

Plate 3 Smallpox, a disease of the past.

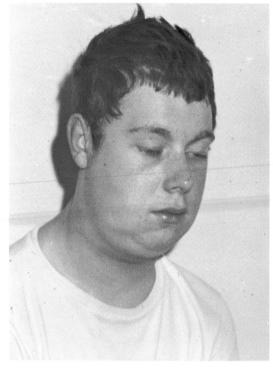

Plate 4 Mumps, showing swelling of the right parotid gland.

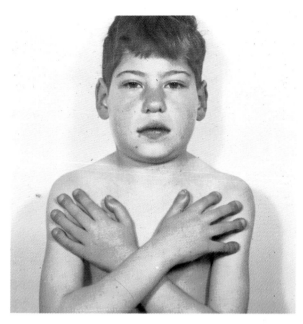

Plate 5 Congenital heart disease. Note the cyanosis and clubbed fingers.

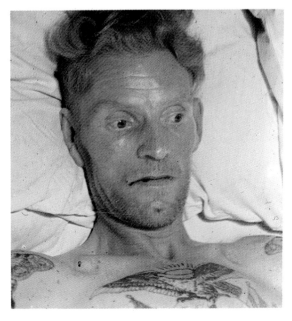

Plate 6 Jaundice

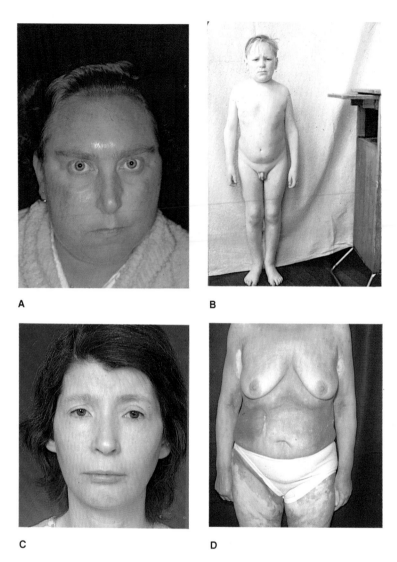

Plate 7   Some endocrine abnormalities.

A.   Cushing's syndrome (obesity, plethora, hypertension)
B.   Pituitary dwarf. (Age 14½ years, height 50 in., no secondary sex changes.)
C.   Simmonds' disease. (Pale smooth skin, hairless trunk, amenorrhoea.)
D.   Addison disease. (Brown pigmentation on trunk and limbs.)

1

Introduction. Clinical observations

The new nurse will make their first real contact with patients in the ward of a hospital and will realize that he or she is part of a team, a team organized with one objective, the welfare of the patient. Many hospitals are large and forbidding, many old and gloomy, some new and impersonal, but all of them depend on the people who work in them. The porters and the clerical staff, the gardeners, the doctors and surgeons, the laundry workers, the telephonists, the electricians and plumbers, the administrative staff, the cooks and the kitchen staff: they all play an important part in the efficient running of a modern hospital and in creating an atmosphere that is friendly and encouraging. Medicine today has become so complex that the physician and nurse alone could not diagnose or treat without the help of their colleagues and the paramedical services. He or she needs the radiologist and the pathologist to reach the diagnosis, and they in turn must depend on their departments with radiographers and pathology technicians to help them provide the answers. In treatment, the physician and nurse will be assisted by the physiotherapist, the chaplain, the occupational therapist, speech therapist, chiropodist, dietitian, pharmacist and social worker. But above all, the medical team depends on the nurse: for it is the nurse who plays the greatest part in providing physical and emotional comfort to the patient in the hour of need, and in supervising the treatment prescribed.

Faced with a ward of patients lying in their beds, it is easy to forget that each is an individual with their family and friends, with anxieties relating to the illness, children, job and future.

The nurse will observe the patient's attitude and response to his illness and surroundings so that he or she can help the patient and communicate their observations to the doctors.

NURSE–PATIENT RELATIONSHIP

Our patients come from all walks of life and with widely differing backgrounds. To a few, the hospital represents a standard of luxury not previously experienced; to some it involves a terrifying loss of personal privacy and an affront to a fastidious nature. Some are frightened by the atmosphere and size of the hospital and by the significance of their illness; others have been in hospital often before and feel a sense of comfort in escaping from the struggle and discomfort of their existence outside. Of course, all patients cannot be treated the same; but in different ways we want to do the best we can to help them all, and this entails an understanding and a perception of the needs of others.

It is easy to be kind and helpful to patients who are pleasant and appreciate our efforts. It is much less easy with patients who are grumpy, aggressive and ungrateful. We have to seek an understanding of these attitudes so that we can help more efficiently and give comfort where it is needed. Sometimes aggression in a patient is a manifestation of fear and anxiety, and sometimes these emotions can be found in the context of his family background, in his uncertainty about the nature of the illness, or about his future. Often a quick talk, with questions directed to the patient's background and his health, will reveal the reason for his attitude and enable help to be offered to restore his self-esteem. Few patients remain hostile when it is made clear that the nurse is genuinely anxious to be helpful.

Explanation and reassurance of the patient as to the nature of his illness is essentially the responsibility of the doctor. The nurse has to be most circumspect in offering medical advice or explanation that might be counter to the doctor's intentions. Certainly the nurse can do much to calm the fears of a patient due for a barium meal or a liver biopsy, for example. She can explain what these routine examinations entail in a reassuring way and so remove the fear of the unknown and the unexpected. The arrival of the porters and the wheelchair to take a patient to X-ray, so commonplace and so routine to those who work in hospital, may be a source of fear and stress to the uninitiated patient.

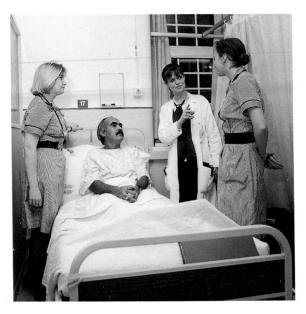

Fig. 1.1 On the ward round.

DIET

In most hospitals today food is prepared in central kitchens and brought to the wards in trollies. In some modern hospitals, the patient states his requirements on a menu card supplied the day before and each individual meal is sent up from the central kitchens in a heated trolley with a compartment for every patient's tray. Very little is now available on the ward itself. The disadvantage of this system is that it lacks flexibility. If a patient unexpectedly falls ill, the food ordered the day before may be totally inappropriate in the changed situation and facilities are not always available to prepare a light meal on the ward. It is important to the patient that meals should be served in as attractive a manner as possible, and that the food should not be lukewarm or served on cold plates. The nurse must observe and record the patient's appetite and particularly whether all the food is eaten or whether most of it is left on the plate. Of course, it is fundamental to assist those whose incapacities make it difficult for them to eat or drink on their own. Hospital catering today has reached a good standard and the nurse can often pass on to the catering staff patients' comments, be they laudatory or critical. Special diets are usually provided under supervision of a dietitian. The nurse will be aware of which patients require a special diet and will keep an eye open for would-be helpful friends and relatives who bring in extras. The diabetic patient should not be offered the temptation of chocolates, for example.

SMOKING

Cigarette smoking is a harmful habit which seriously diminishes the expectation of health and life. Patients on the ward should be discouraged from smoking, particularly when this is to the discomfort of non-smokers, and if possible, areas of the ward should be set aside where smoking is absolutely forbidden. Some hospitals have a total ban on smoking. Similarly, visitors should not be allowed to smoke.

ELDERLY PATIENTS

Partly thanks to better nutrition and better social conditions, and partly thanks to improved medical treatment, the population is getting steadily older. The large majority of retired people lead independent existences, either in their own homes or with their families, but this is the section of the community most likely to need hospital care when ill-health supervenes. 'Geriatrics' is the term used for the special medical and nursing care of old people, and many hospitals today have separate geriatric departments. In practice, these facilities are usually inadequate and most elderly people who require hospital treatment are admitted to an acute medical or surgical ward. Indeed, a high proportion of patients in any general medical ward today are over the age of 65. Many special nursing and medical problems apply to the care of the elderly

apart from those associated with the treatment of the particular disorder which occasioned admission to hospital.

The prime aim of management must be to mobilize and rehabilitate the elderly patient as soon as possible. Lying in bed is potentially dangerous to the old and frail. It promotes the development of incontinence of bladder and bowel, it disposes to pressure sores and it leads to apathy and muscle atrophy increasing frailty.

The admission to hospital of an elderly patient should be regarded as the first step towards returning him back into the community. A proposed date for discharge should be decided as soon as possible after admission so that relatives and friends can plan accordingly. The help of the ancillary services should be sought. The dietitian can advise as to suitable food for a patient who may be without teeth, for example. The physiotherapist may be enlisted to help with mobilisation and exercises. The occupational therapist will assess the ability of patients to perform the daily tasks necessary for an independent existence and, if need be, to retrain patients who have been incapacitated by illnesses such as a stroke. The social workers will have the opportunity to prepare a social report, describing the home background and the facilities available when the patient is ready to leave hospital. In doubtful cases, the patient may be allowed home for a day or a weekend to see how well he can manage, and whether there are unexpected difficulties to be overcome before he is able finally to be discharged from hospital.

Many services are available to help the elderly in their homes, and indeed a team is available, the Primary Care Team, built round the family doctor in this respect. The district nurse (home nurse) can provide a nursing service such as dressings and injections; she can supervize progress and inform the family doctor of any problems; and she can organize the supply of special aids such as walking frames or commodes. The health visitor has specialized knowledge of community facilities available to the elderly and may visit the patient in his home to see if help is needed. The home help, provided by the local authority, is available for the housework and shopping, and may provide company and friendship as well. The Meals-on-Wheels service ensures that elderly people can get a regular hot meal at low cost and helps to keep the elderly in touch with the community. Social workers may visit the elderly in their homes and advise them on such matters as pensions, laundry services, libraries, telephone, old people's clubs and holidays.

CLINICAL OBSERVATIONS

The nurse is responsible for various clinical observations, and much depends on the conscientious recording of the findings.

Temperature

The temperature chart is of prime importance to the physician. In infections, a decline in fever suggests that the treatment is proving effective and the infection is being overcome. A rise of temperature alerts the physician to the possibility of an unexpected bacterial infection.

The thermometer is placed under the tongue with the lips closed, and allowed to remain for at least two minutes. The normal reading is about 36.9°C (98.4°F). A falsely elevated temperature will be obtained if the patient has just taken a hot drink. The temperature is usually slightly higher in the evening than in the morning. In women the temperature is elevated after ovulation in the latter part of the menstrual cycle and indeed this fact is used as a test of ovulation in cases of amenorrhoea. With a comatose or uncooperative patient the temperature can be taken by placing the thermometer in the axilla and holding the patient's arm to his side: the normal temperature taken in this way is less than the mouth temperature, usually 36.7°C (98°F) after two minutes. When a very low temperature is suspected (hypothermia), especially in elderly patients found in unheated rooms in the winter, the thermometer should be inserted in the rectum and allowed to remain for at least two minutes.

A temperature raised above normal is referred to as a *pyrexia* and with some exceptions is associated with a quickened pulse rate (*tachycardia*). Pyrexia without tachycardia suggests the likelihood of a false reading. Neurotic patients sometimes like to draw attention to themselves by surreptitiously warming the thermometer in a cup of tea or hot pipe near the bed, or by other ways, and so falsely appear to have a high temperature.

A sudden rise of temperature may be due to a bacterial invasion into the blood stream and is associated with *rigors*. The patient in a rigor feels intensely cold and shivers violently, often shaking the bed. As the temperature rises, the rigor eases off, the patient sweats profusely and wants to throw off the bedclothes. Rigors are a characteristic feature of septicaemia and are also seen in malaria.

The pulse

The heart is a powerful pump, and each time it contracts it sends a surge of blood through all the arteries. The pressure in the arteries increases with each beat of the heart and falls again when the heart relaxes between contractions. The pulse is the wave of distension in the artery after each heart beat, and it can be felt by the nurse in any large artery that is easily accessible.

The radial artery is the pulse most frequently palpated. It is easily felt at the wrist and is convenient both for the nurse and the patient.

The brachial artery can be felt at the bend of the elbow and should be identified when taking the blood pressure to see where to place the stethoscope.

The carotid pulses can be felt on either side of the neck and may be helpful when the patient is so collapsed that the radial pulse is difficult to find.

The temporal arteries, just in front of the ear, are often used by the anaesthetist during an operation when other pulses are not accessible. The femoral arteries can be felt in the groins, about midway across, and are of great importance as their absence suggests the circulation to the legs is impaired or obstructed. When the femoral artery is partially obstructed, listening over it with a stethoscope may reveal a loud murmur caused by the blood passing through the narrowed lumen.

Two pulses can normally be palpated in the feet. The dorsalis artery is found on the front of the foot and the posterior tibial pulse behind the medial malleolus (ankle).

Taking the pulse is an important observation because it reveals so much about the action of the heart. The rate, the rhythm and volume should all be noted and the rate should be recorded as a routine.

Rate

A rapid heart rate is called *tachycardia*, while a slow heart rate is called *bradycardia*. In most healthy people the heart rate at rest is between 70 and 80 to the minute, but some have a heart rate of only 50 while others have a heart rate of 90. The heart is under the control of the nervous system and responds to the needs of the body, quickening when there is a need for greater effort and slowing at rest. Thus after exercise or an emotional disturbance the heart rate quickens, while during sleep the heart rate slows.

There are many causes of tachycardia (see p. 81) and bradycardia.

Rhythm

The pulse is normally as regular as a clock but in children and young adults the heart rate often quickens with inspiration (breathing in) and slows with expiration (breathing out). Particularly in older people, extra beats of the heart are not uncommon but the basic rhythm is regular. However, in the condition known as *atrial fibrillation* (see p. 81), the pulse rate is totally irregular and, indeed, often the heart beat is so rapid that not all contractions are transmitted to the pulse. Listening with a stethoscope to the heart itself is the only way to determine the heart rate in such cases; the difference between the heart rate and the pulse rate is known as the pulse deficit.

Volume

This describes the strength and character of the pulse, whether it is full and bounding or weak and thready. It gives an indication of the state of the circulation. Thus after a severe haemorrhage or a serious myocardial infarction the pulse volume may be so low that the radial pulse is scarcely palpable.

Respiration

An adult at rest has a respiration rate of about 16 to 20 a minute, and this rate of breathing can be observed and recorded while the temperature is being taken.

The term *dyspnoea* means difficult or painful breathing, such as is seen in pleurisy where every deep breath or cough causes pain; but often the word dyspnoeic is merely used to mean rapid breathing or breathlessness (see p. 119).

Orthopnoea occurs particularly in heart failure and signifies that the patient can only breathe with any comfort when propped up: orthopnoeic patients usually feel easier when sitting up in a high armchair than in bed.

Breathing may be quiet or noisy. In asthma expiration is wheezy. After a stroke the breathing may be stertorous with a snore-like quality. Where there is obstruction to the upper airway tract stridor may be heard – a coarse crowing sound on inspiration.

Blood pressure

The blood pressure is a most important observation and may be difficult to determine, especially in a collapsed patient. Every nurse must practise taking the blood pressure until complete competence is attained.

The blood pressure is measured by an instrument known as the sphygmomanometer. This consists of: (i) an inflatable cuff to be wrapped around the upper arm; (ii) a mercury manometer, attached by a tube to the cuff, which measures the pressure in the cuff.

The arm should be bared to the shoulder so that when the cuff is applied to the upper arm sufficient room is left for the stethoscope to be placed over the brachial pulse.

When the cuff has been securely wrapped round and attached to the manometer, the brachial pulse must be identified, conveniently by the thumb of the right hand. The stethoscope head is now applied over the brachial pulse below the cuff and the cuff is pumped up sufficiently to obliterate the artery pulsation. The pressure in the cuff is now slowly released by turning the screw. When the thumping of the artery can be heard through the stethoscope, the pressure is read on the manometer. This is the *systolic pressure*. The pressure in the cuff is now further reduced until the thumping over the pulse dies away. The reading on the manometer now records the *diastolic pressure*.

The systolic pressure of blood in the artery indicates the peak pressure at the moment the ventricle has contracted. The diastolic pressure is the lowest pressure when the ventricle relaxes before the next beat.

The normal systolic blood pressure in adults at rest is about 110 to 140 mm of mercury (mmHg) on the manometer. The diastolic pressure varies from about 60 to 80 mmHg. Thus, a healthy young adult might have a systolic pressure of 120 mmHg and a diastolic pressure of 70. This would be recorded as 'BP 120/70'. The blood pressure tends to be higher as we get older and the arteries harden. A man of 70 in good health might have a blood pressure of 170/90.

Normally the blood pressure in an individual is lowest when warm and comfortable in mind and body and in the recumbent position. It rises somewhat on sitting up or standing. However, in many patients receiving drugs for the treatment of high blood pressure the blood pressure falls when the patient stands up and rises when he lies down. Hence it is advisable to record the position in which the blood pressure is taken, Lying down, sitting or standing.

Particularly in patients receiving intravenous fluids, it is important to the physician not only to know the blood pressure in the arteries but in the veins as well. The pressure in the veins can be estimated by observation of the jugular veins in the neck. When the patient is lying in the semirecumbent position, with the head and shoulders about 30 degrees above the horizontal, the pulsation of the jugular vein can be seen just above the clavicle. But in congestive heart failure, when the heart is unable completely to sustain the circulation, the right atrium is not emptied at each beat and the pressure in the veins rises accordingly. The veins in the neck are distended and the venous pulsation may be seen well above the clavicle. Precise measurement of venous pressure may be needed in patients when they are receiving fluid intravenously since, if the heart is weak, the circulation may become overloaded. A catheter is introduced into the internal jugular vein and attached to a water manometer reading up to 10 cm of water. The reading on the manometer is called the central venous pressure and will help determine the rate and volume of administered fluid that the heart can tolerate.

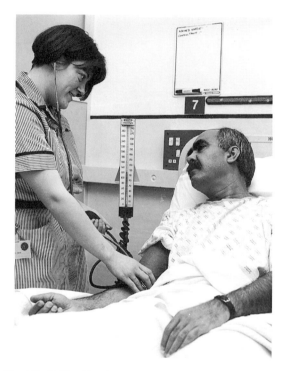

Fig. 1.2 Taking blood pressure.

Cough and sputum

A cough is a reflex mechanism to expel irritants, foreign material and secretion from the respiratory tract. It is a protective mechanism. Elderly or debilitated patients with bronchopneumonia may be too feeble to cough adequately and the smaller bronchioles become clogged with thick secretions, which they are unable to expel; physiotherapy and suction by a pump may be required to clear the airway. On the other hand, a cough may be due to irritation of the mucous membrane lining the upper respiratory tract and serves no useful purpose since there is nothing to cough up. A dry cough of this sort may keep the patient awake and cause needless distress; a cough suppressant medicine may be prescribed in such cases.

A productive cough is one in which sputum is brought up. Waxed cartons with screw tops are provided for the collection of sputum by the bedside. These cartons, which are easily destroyed by burning, allow inspection of the sputum and this provides valuable information as to the nature of the respiratory illness. The nature and the amount of sputum coughed up should be noted. When infection is minimal, the sputum is usually mucoid: it is clear, viscid and not profuse. When infection is present, the sputum becomes purulent: it may be very profuse and foetid (foul smelling), as occurs in bronchiectasis or lung abscess: or it may form round blobs, the so-called nummular sputum of pulmonary tuberculosis. The extent to which the sputum is profuse and purulent offers the physician a guide to progress and treatment.

Coughing up blood is called *haemoptysis* and is seen particularly in pulmonary tuberculosis and in bronchial carcinoma, due to the rupture of small vessels in the affected area. More common than pure blood is sputum with streaks of blood in it due to inflammation of the bronchial wall and sometimes to the strain of coughing (see p. 118).

Sputum may be sent to the laboratory for two important investigations. (1) It will be examined and cultured for bacteria so that the nature of the infection can be determined and, if need be, appropriate antibiotic prescribed. (2) It can be examined microscopically to see whether malignant cells are present as a test for bronchial carcinoma.

Urine

Examination of the urine is a most important routine which is always undertaken for each new patient. It is easy to do and may give valuable information.

Volume

The amount of urine passed is modified by the amount of fluid drunk and the amount lost in perspiration, in the breath and from the bowel. An average daily output of urine for a normal adult is about 1200 ml but it can vary from as little as 400 ml to as much as 3000 ml according to circumstances. A significantly increased output of urine is described as polyuria, a diminished output as oliguria and a complete absence of urine as anuria.

Especially in severely ill patients or in those receiving intravenous fluids, an intake and output chart must be kept. This records all the fluid taken by mouth or drip over 24 hours and all the fluid lost by urine, vomit or bowel over the same time. Normally fluid intake will exceed output by about 500 ml because no record can be kept of fluid lost in the breath or in perspiration.

Reaction

The urine is normally slightly acid and turns blue litmus paper red. If excess alkalis have been taken or if the urine is infected or has been allowed to stand, the reaction becomes alkaline and red litmus paper turns blue.

Specific gravity

The specific gravity of urine depends on the weight of substances dissolved in it compared with water. The specific gravity of water is 1000 and that of urine usually 1012 to 1024 as measured by a hydrometer: this partially floats in urine and the depth to which it sinks is calibrated to give the reading. After a large intake of fluid, the urine is dilute with a low specific gravity. When fluid intake is restricted, the urine should be concentrated with a high specific gravity if the kidneys are healthy. In diabetes, although a lot of urine is passed, the presence of sugar in the urine leads to a high specific gravity.

Normal deposits

Healthy urine may often show a deposit on

standing. This may be due to mucous secretion or to urates or phosphates from certain foods; it disappears on adding acid.

Protein (albumin)

Occasionally protein (albumin) appears in the urine in healthy young adults after exercise or prolonged standing and this is known as orthostatic proteinuria. However, usually the glomerular filter (see p. 261) is too fine to allow molecules of protein to pass through into the urine and the presence of albumin in the urine suggests kidney disease. Since the urine test may provide the first indication of a renal disorder, the test is of great importance. Commercial urine test sticks offer a simple, rapid and reliable test for protein in the urine. The test end of the strip is dipped in the urine, and the colour compared with the colour strip provided on the tin. The greater the amount of protein, the deeper is the green on the strip.

Sugar (glucose)

The presence of any appreciable amount of sugar (glucose) in the urine suggests that diabetes may be present. In many cases of diabetes developing in older people there may be no symptoms of the disorder and the diagnosis is only suspected after finding sugar on routine testing of the urine. Commercial urine test sticks provide a specific test for glucose. The test end of the strip is dipped in the urine and if sugar is present, the moistened end changes colour in about 10 seconds. If the strip remains unchanged, sugar is absent. The test is valuable for demonstrating the presence or absence of glucose but is not very reliable as a quantitative guide as to how much sugar is present. After 30 seconds the amount of sugar can be gauged by comparing the colour with the chart on the bottle.

Ketone bodies (acetone)

Acetone is derived from the abnormal or rapid burning up of fat and it appears in the urine when it is produced in excess. This happens after starvation (perhaps to reduce weight) or after persistent vomiting. It also occurs in diabetics when the diabetes is poorly controlled as in diabetic ketoacidosis (see p. 311). Again a commercial urine test strip is used to show whether ketones are present, the depth of the colour depending on the degree of ketosis.

Other tests

Tests are also available for blood, bile and pus and these are dealt with in the appropriate chapters. The compound urine test strips combine more than one test in the same strip.

Faeces

Inspection of the stools may provide valuable information as to the condition of the bowel.

In severe constipation the bowel may only be evacuated after a suppository or an enema and the stool may consist of small hard balls of faeces known as *scybalae*. Sometimes impaction of scybalae in the rectum occurs in elderly dehydrated patients and only manual evacuation by doctor or nurse can relieve the patient of his misery.

Diarrhoea means frequent loose stools. When this is due to an intestinal infection, the stools are watery. In the malabsorption syndrome (see p. 173), the motions are large, bulky, and pale. In thyrotoxicosis (see p. 322) although the motions are very frequent, they are usually small but normally formed.

Melaena is the term applied to blood in the motions. When the bleeding occurs in the stomach or duodenum, the blood is altered in its passage through the bowel making the motions black and sticky, the so-called tarry stool. There may be a characteristic smell of blood. It should not be forgotten that iron preparations taken for anaemia also colour the stools black and this can be confused for melaena. When bleeding occurs in the lower bowel, perhaps from a carcinoma in the rectum or from haemorrhoids, the blood is bright red and often appears as streaks of blood in the faeces.

In ulcerative colitis, diarrhoea may be very severe, the motions may be loose or watery and may contain blood and mucus. The normal brown colour of the motion is due to the presence of stercobilin, a derivative of bile. Hence in conditions in which the flow of bile into the intestine is obstructed, as occurs in gallstones or severe hepatitis, the stools may be pale or clay-coloured.

The stools should also be inspected for the presence of worms. Threadworms, roundworms or tapeworms may be seen (see p. 175).

2

Causes of disease

GENERAL CAUSES OF DISEASE

The cause of a disease is referred to as its *aetiology*. Sometimes the aetiology of a disorder is environmental and induced by factors outside the body. For example, infected food can cause enteritis, or intense cold can lead to frostbite. In other cases, however, the disease is due to the inheritance of a genetic disorder, sometimes manifesting itself in childhood, sometimes not until late in life. Some ailments are partly environmental and partly inherited. Thus, although a tendency to diabetes may be inherited, in many cases the disease will become manifest after a long period of overeating. Indeed, there is always an interplay between the environment and the bodily constitution. Many environmental and social factors may play a role in the development of disease; for example an elderly man in a state of poor nutrition, with poor housing and inadequate heating is more prone to bacterial infection than someone young and living in relative comfort. Air pollution may contribute to respiratory disease, particularly asthma and bronchitis. Furthermore, the body is endowed with a complex system to counter and overcome noxious agents which invade and threaten it. This is called the *immune system* and disease can occur when this immune system functions improperly. A simplified classification of disease follows:

1. Hereditary disorders
2. Physical and chemical agents:
   (a) drugs, including cigarettes and alcohol
   (b) excess of heat or cold

(c) electricity and radioactive substances
(d) physical injury
3. Uncontrolled growth resulting in cancer
4. Living organisms (microbes) (Ch. 3)
   (a) bacteria
   (b) viruses
   (c) fungi
   (d) parasites (protozoa and helminths)
5. Disorders of the immune system
6. Metabolic diseases
   (a) hormonal
   (b) malnutrition and vitamin deficiencies (Ch. 12).

HEREDITY

Parents transmit certain characteristics to their children, so that a child inherits qualities from each parent. These phenotypic (physical) and genotypic (genetic) characteristics are transmitted by the germ cells following fusion of the male sperm and the female ovum. Each sperm and each ovum contains 23 chromosomes.

Chromosomes and genes

Chromosomes lie within the nucleus of every human cell. They are threads of basic material known as DNA (deoxyribonucleic acid). Sited along the length of each chromosome are a series of genes, which are responsible for the phenotypic and genetic characteristics of the offspring. A faulty gene results in a *genetic disorder*.

The fertilized ovum contains 46 chromosomes, i.e. two sets of 23 chromosomes, one set from the sperm and one already in the ovum. This fertilized ovum, containing chromosomes and genes from both parents, is the blueprint from which all cells in the growing fetus will be derived.

Of the 23 chromosomes, the ovum has one special sex chromosome, designated X. The sperm also has a sex chromosome which may either be X, similar to the ovum, or a smaller chromosome designated Y. The sex of the offspring will depend on whether the union yields XX or XY:

Sperm X + ovum X yields female XX
Sperm Y + ovum X yields male XY

Occasionally abnormalities of the sex chromosomes may occur. The ovum may contain an extra sex chromosome XX. If junction occurs with a sperm having a sex chromosome Y, this yields XXY. Males born with this abnormality are sterile with small genitalia and may be mentally retarded.

Chromosomes other than sex chromosomes are known as *autosomes* and these have been identified and enumerated by special radioactive and staining techniques. It is now known that certain diseases in man are associated with abnormalities of the autosomes. Thus, *Down's syndrome* (Trisomy 21, see p. 223) is due to an extra autosome. At the time of conception the ovum has 47 chromosomes instead of 46. As a result, every cell produced in the growing fetus carries this abnormality and a mentally subnormal child is born with characteristic physical defects.

Many different types of metabolic and blood disorders are due to abnormalities of various genes. Genes control the way in which proteins are formed from basic amino acids. For example, normal blood clotting requires the presence of a particular protein known as factor VIII. In haemophilia, this protein is not formed because of an inherited genetic defect. Consequently, this person has excessive bleeding from a minor injury and this can be fatal unless the missing factor VIII is administered.

There are many other genetic disorders, some common, some rare but all of them inherited to a lesser or greater degree. An abnormal gene may be passed on from a single parent or from both parents. This defect may continue to be transmitted through generations. These hereditary defects are more likely to be seen when there is inbreeding in a family, as when cousins marry. The reason for this is that many of the defects passed on to the future generation are recessive (quiescent or dormant). Such a gene may only cause disease if it links up with a similar recessive gene, one from each parent. The mating of two recessive defects is much more likely to occur following conception between people with the same parents or grandparents. Other hereditary genes are called dominant since a single copy of the gene result in disorders affecting siblings irre-

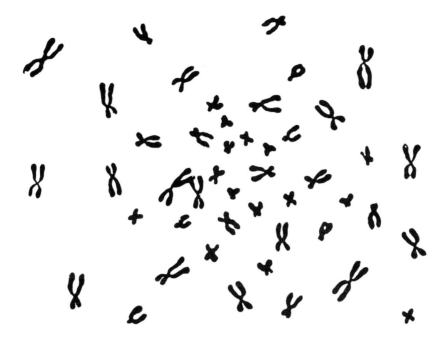

Fig. 2.1 Chromosomes spread out and photographed under a high-power microscope.

spective of the presence or absence of a second recessive gene.

Some common diseases appear to have a genetic factor as part of the aetiology. These ailments are more common in some families. Diabetes mellitus, hypertension and peptic ulcer are examples of diseases in which heredity plays a considerable part in the aetiology. When both parents have diabetes their children are more likely to develop diabetes than the children of parents without diabetes. However, even when both parents have diabetes, only about a quarter of their children develop the disease, suggesting a significant role for other factors.

PHYSICAL AND CHEMICAL AGENTS

Drugs

Drugs are prescribed:

1. for the treatment or prevention of illnesses and infections
2. for the alleviation of pain and discomfort, relief of anxiety, depression and sleeplessness.

Other preparations, sometimes included under the heading of drugs, replace substances normally present in food, such as vitamins, or are normally produced within the body, such as hormones. Although vitamins and hormones may be prescribed as replacement therapy where these are deficient, they may also be used in the treatment of other unrelated disorders.

Drugs are widely prescribed and, indeed, many people have such faith in drugs that they feel cheated if they are not given tablets after a visit to the doctor. It is important to educate and explain to patients the reasons for not prescribing medication if it is not required. For example in the case of the common cold many people expect to be given antibiotics. It should be explained that these will not help the patient as the condition is caused by a virus, and the condition will improve anyway in a few days.

Properly prescribed and properly taken, drugs play an important role in the treatment of ill-health and the alleviation of suffering. However, it must be realized that different people react differently to the same drug and that drugs exert effects on the body other than those for which they have been prescribed (side-effects). Furthermore, since drugs of all sorts are readily available, deliberate or accidental overdosage is a common cause of admission to the hospital. Consequently, although drug treatment can be a powerful aid to better health, drugs can also be a frequent cause of illness.

Before any new drug is released for general prescription it has to undergo stringent trials, initially on animals. When no untoward effects are found, large clinical trials are then undertaken, usually on patients suffering from the disorder which the drug is designed to cure. Finally, if these trials show the drug to be safe and effective, it has to be approved by the Committee on Safety of Drugs before it can be released for general use.

Drug-induced illness is sometimes described as *iatrogenic* and may be due to different causes.

Drug sensitivity

Not all patients react similarly to the same drug. Most people tolerate penicillin but some people react to it by developing skin rashes. This sort of sensitivity is common and liable to be more serious when the drug is given a second time. Hence, if a patient has had a reaction to a particular drug, he should be warned to avoid this preparation in future and the fact recorded, preferably on the front of the case notes in a hospital patient.

Perhaps one of the most dangerous types of drug sensitivity is that which affects the blood cells. Many drugs can be toxic to the bone marrow where blood cells are produced. Aplastic anaemia refers to complete suppression of all blood cell production and becomes fatal unless the bone marrow recovers. Agranulocytosis is the suppression of just the white cells and this predisposes to infection. Many drugs in current use can cause these blood disorders. The justification for prescribing them is that they are effective in treating serious diseases and the incidence of this sensitivity reaction is rare. The onus is on the physician to weigh the advantage of using the drug as against the possible danger of a reaction. Having prescribed the drug, however, the physician needs to be cautious. For

instance, sodium aurothiomalate, a gold preparation used in the treatment of rheumatoid arthritis, occasionally leads to kidney damage. The urine must therefore be tested for protein before each administration; if protein is present no further therapy should be given.

Side-effects

No drug has a single pharmacological action. It may be prescribed effectively for a specific purpose but it may have other undesirable effects as well. Aspirin may be effective in relieving pain but it sometimes results in the development of stomach ulcers. Some diuretics, while successfully relieving oedema, also deplete the system of potassium. Cortisone relieves inflammation but leads to obesity, infections and thin bones (osteoporosis) over long-term treatment. Consequently, in prescribing drugs for a specific purpose, the physician has to consider the possible side-effects and adequate measures to minimize them.

Drug overdose

Accidental Very few households today do not have drugs available, sometimes carefully kept in a closed cupboard for emergencies, more often lying around in bottles, half-full and forgotten. These tablets are an attraction and dangerous to small children. Children are admitted to hospital frequently, having taken a dangerous dose of their parent's tablets; the nurse therefore has a duty to remind parents of their responsibility. Bottles containing drugs should be firmly closed and kept out of the reach of small children.

Apart from mistakes in prescribing the wrong strength or dose of tablets, a potent cause of overdosage occurs in elderly people who are becoming forgetful. Having taken a sleeping tablet, they may well forget and take a repeat dose. If an elderly person is on regular daily tablets, it is advisable to leave out the day's dosage each morning.

Deliberate overdosage (acute poisoning) with dangerous drugs is common, especially in teenagers. Hypnotics and tranquillizers are freely

Maintain clear airway

When — Normal breathing
— Good colour
— Cough reflex
are present

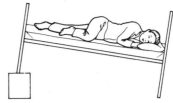

Left lateral position

When cough reflex is absent

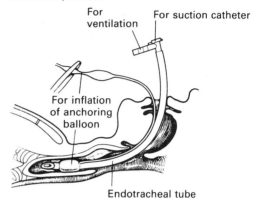

For ventilation

For suction catheter

For inflation of anchoring balloon

Endotracheal tube

Seek information to identify drug

Gastric lavage

Especially when a dangerous amount has been swallowed within the previous 4 hours

1st washing — 500 ml
Then repeated until clear fluid recovered

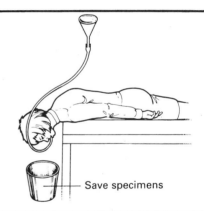

Save specimens

Intravenous fluids and forced diuresis
in some cases
(especially in salicylate poisoning)

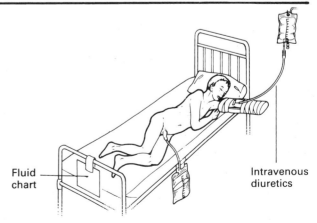

Fluid chart

Intravenous diuretics

Fig. 2.2 The treatment of drug overdosage.

prescribed to those who are anxious, harassed or depressed and this is the typical patient most likely to attempt suicide. Not all cases of deliberate drug overdosage mean to commit suicide. More often the taking of the tablets is a gesture to demonstrate to others the depth of misery or despair that is being experienced. The tablets most commonly taken are aspirins, barbiturates and various tranquillizers, all easily available on prescription or, in the case of aspirin, at any chemist's shop. However, almost any drug prescribed may be taken in large quantities with the intention of self-destruction. Any substance thought to be harmful may be consumed by the desperate or the deluded, including paraffin, bleach, cosmetic preparations or weedkiller. Combinations of drugs are frequently taken, and often with alcohol.

Carbon monoxide poisoning Coal gas contains carbon monoxide and was a common cause of poisoning, either accidental or deliberate, when coal gas was used for heating and cooking. Since coal gas has been replaced for domestic purposes by natural gas, the risks in this respect have been greatly reduced. However, it can still be a danger in badly ventilated garages since the exhausts of motor cars contain carbon monoxide. Carbon monoxide combines with haemoglobin in the blood to form carboxyhaemoglobin and prevents the blood carrying oxygen.

General management of acute poisoning and drug overdosage

1. Urgent information must be sought from relatives or friends as to the nature of the drugs that have been taken. Often the ambulance men will bring in any empty bottles lying by the bedside, although the labels on the bottles may be misleading.

2. The airway must be kept clear. Dentures are removed and the mouth cleared of phlegm or vomit. If the complexion is not bluish (cyanosed) and the breathing is unimpaired, the patient can be kept in the left lateral position with the foot of the bed elevated to avoid the risk of inhaling mucus or vomit. If the breathing sounds obstructed or laboured or if the patient is too unconscious to clear the chest by coughing, it will be necessary to insert an endotracheal tube into the trachea. Oxygen can be administered through this tube or suction can be applied to clear it of secretions.

3. Gastric lavage. The stomach should be emptied as soon as possible to prevent further absorption of ingested tablets or other poisonous material.

Gastric lavage can be undertaken to recover tablets not yet absorbed. A Jacques tube (30 English gauge) is lubricated with liquid paraffin and passed gently but firmly into the stomach; in an adult this is a distance of about 50 cm. Warm water (500 ml) is introduced into the stomach via the tube and then immediately siphoned out by inverting and lowering the funnel attached to the end of the tube. The first washout is likely to contain the maximum amount of drug or poison and should be set aside and kept separate from all subsequent washings. The washout is then continued using 300 ml water at a time, until 2 or 3

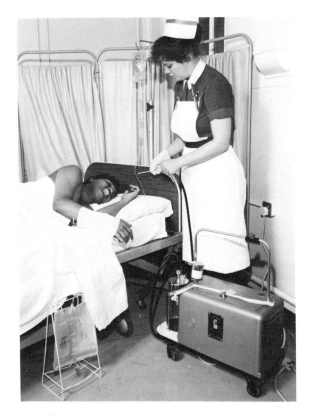

Fig. 2.3 Maintenance of the airway in an unconscious patient.

litres have been used.

All stomach washings, with the first washing kept separately, must be labelled with the name of the patient, date and time and sent to the laboratory for analysis.

4. Activated charcoal. This is effective at absorbing some drugs such as tricyclic antidepressants.

5. Forced diuresis. Especially in barbiturate and salicylate poisoning, acceleration of renal excretion of the drug from the blood stream can be achieved by forced diuresis. Alkaline fluids are given intravenously with a diuretic; this leads to a large output of urine from the kidneys. The rate of the infusion can be controlled by watching the central venous pressure (if it rises too high the rate must be reduced) and by the urinary volume. Some drugs commonly taken in overdose cases include:

1. Salicylates (aspirin). The main features are nausea, vomiting, tinnitus (ringing in the ear), over breathing and sweating. Blood should be taken for salicylate levels.

2. Paracetamol. Particularly dangerous since a small dose can cause irreversible liver damage.

3. Carbon monoxide. The patient is often pale and cyanosed with respiratory depression. Examination of the blood will reveal the presence of carboxyhaemoglobin.

4. Tranquillizers. Mental confusion followed by deep sleep and coma.

5. Morphine. Pinpoint pupils, slow pulse, shallow breathing, cyanosis and hypotension.

Cigarette smoking

This is a harmful habit which reduces the expectation of good health and shortens life. Cigarette smokers absorb into the lungs:

1. Nicotine. This is a habit-forming drug with a mild stimulatory effect. It causes constriction of small blood vessels and a rise in blood pressure.

2. Carcinogenic tars. These tars isolated from cigarette smoke have been shown to cause cancer in experimental animals.

3. Carbon monoxide. Cigarette smokers have raised blood levels of carboxyhaemoglobin. If the mother smokes during pregnancy, carboxyhaemoglobin passes through into the fetal circulation.

The following conditions are prone to occur in cigarette smokers:

Cancer of the lung. Heavy cigarette smokers are 30 times as liable to develop cancer of the lung as are non-smokers. There is overwhelming evidence that lung cancer is caused by cigarette smoking.

Bronchitis and emphysema. Prolonged cigarette smoking commonly leads to progressive cough and breathlessness, ultimately leading to respiratory incapacity and failure.

Coronary thrombosis (p. 93) and intermittent claudication (see p. 111) are more prone to occur in those who smoke cigarettes.

Gastric and duodenal ulcers take longer to heal in cigarette smokers.

Pregnant women who smoke cigarettes have smaller babies than do non-smokers, with a higher incidence of fetal abnormalities.

Alcohol

Alcohol is the basis of wine, beer and spirits. Taken in moderation, with a meal, or socially, it can be regarded as one of the niceties of life. It may even reduce the risk of heart disease if taken in moderate amounts (particularly red wine). However, as with any drug, there are dangers as well as advantages associated with alcohol.

How much alcohol is safe? Alcohol can be measured in units, one unit of alcohol being equivalent to half a pint of beer or lager, one small glass of wine or a single measure of spirits. The currently recommended upper safe limits are 20 units per week for men and 15 units per week for women.

Alcohol is rapidly absorbed from the stomach and intestine and soon appears in the blood. As the blood circulates through the lungs, alcohol diffuses into the air in the alveoli. The higher the concentration of alcohol in the blood, the higher the concentration in the breath. This is the basis of the breathalyser test used by the police on motorists suspected of driving while under the influence of drink. Alcohol can also be measured

In Britain

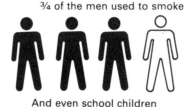

¾ of the men used to smoke   and   ½ the women

And even school children

**But heavy smoking
reduces life expectation**

In general under the age of 65, heavy smokers are twice as liable to die as non-smokers

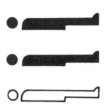

In particular, heavy cigarette smokers are 30 times more liable to die of lung cancer than non-smokers

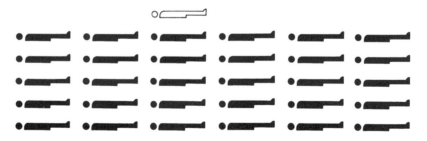

**Cigarette smokers
are much more
prone to**

Chronic
bronchitis

Coronary
thrombosis

Delayed healing of gastric and duodenal ulcers

Fig. 2.4 Dangers of smoking.

in the blood. It is metabolized (broken down) by the liver at a rate of approximately one unit per hour.

Apart from the pleasures to the palate, one of the social reasons for drinking is removal of shyness and restraint. However, judgement is diminished, as are technical skills demanding accuracy and co-ordination. This is particularly dangerous when driving a car, and it has been abundantly demonstrated that even a moderate intake of alcohol can diminish critically the driver's ability to deal with the unexpected.

Many men and women are ill-equipped to cope with the stringencies of life. Alcohol offers a temporary escape and an easement of depression and stress. However, alcohol is unfortunately an addictive drug and more and more has to be taken to achieve the same effect. The term alcoholic is used to describe a person who has become dependent on alcohol. Alcoholism has become a serious health problem. Its onset is gradual and leads to a disintegration of the personality and of physical health.

Delirium tremens in the alcoholic can be induced by a sustained high intake of spirits or by sudden deprivation of alcohol. It is characterized by a delusional state, often of a terrifying nature, by restlessness and by tremor; the behaviour may become aggressive and violent.

In the long term alcoholism can lead to:

1. *Korsakoff's psychosis.* This develops gradually with disordered behaviour, confabulation (telling plausible accounts of imaginary events), disorientation (unsure of place or time), hallucinations and emotional disturbances.
2. *Polyneuritis.*
3. *Cirrhosis of the liver* (see p. 186).

The treatment of alcoholism is difficult and demands the willingness of the patient to cooperate. Hospital treatment is often necessary during the period of alcohol withdrawal since tranquillizing drugs are necessary to suppress intolerable symptoms. Supportive treatment by a psychiatrist or trained social worker is necessary on leaving hospital, and the organization 'Alcoholics Anonymous' can play an important role in restoring confidence and self-esteem.

Drug addiction

Many commonly prescribed drugs, if taken regularly and for long periods, may lead to drug dependence or addiction. The list includes sedatives, tranquillizers, weight reducers, stimulants, pain relievers and hypnotics, so that, when prescribing such helpful medicaments, great care must be taken that the patient is not allowed to take them indefinitely unless under medical supervision and for good purpose. When a patient becomes addicted to a drug he feels an overwhelming need to continue to take the drug and will make any excuse to get further supplies. He becomes physically and psychologically dependent on it, so that if the drug is not available he will suffer symptoms of withdrawal. Often the dose of the drug has to be steadily increased to make life bearable, and this leads to changes detrimental to physical and mental health. Doctors, dentists and nurses are at particular risk of drug addiction because such drugs may be more easily accessible to them.

Unfortunately, the problem of addiction has increased alarmingly in recent years, not as a result of medical treatment but as a result of obtaining drugs from illicit sources for self-indulgent purposes. Alcohol and tobacco are two habit-forming drugs widely used and socially acceptable, though carrying serious hazards to health. Many other drugs are taken illegally, often by young people and with tragic results. These include:

1. *Morphine, heroin and cocaine.* These are known as narcotics or 'hard drugs' and form the core of the addiction problem. Opium is a mixture of compounds obtained from poppy seeds, from which morphine is obtained. Heroin, or diamorphine, is itself a derivative of morphine. Used as a powerful pain reliever, it induces a drowsy sensation which may be pleasurable to some people, though not all. Dependence on the drug soon follows regular administration. Intolerable symptoms occur when the drug is withdrawn; these symptoms include shivering, watering of the eyes and nose, stomach contractions, violent vomiting, diarrhoea, twitching and complete physical and mental collapse. Prolonged usage leads to organic brain damage and disintegration of personality, so that the addict becomes untrustworthy and obsessed with the need to obtain the next dose. Hard-drug addicts usually die young. Cocaine is derived from the leaves of the coca plant and is a stimulant. It is usually injected by addicts together with heroin, at first subcutaneously and later intravenously. Since no precautions are taken to ensure sterility, infection

is liable to follow. It can also be inhaled (crack).

2. *Cannabis indica*, also known as hashish, is obtained from the flowering top of the Indian hemp plant which grows wild in many countries. It is usually smoked in cigarette form, the so-called 'reefers', and its sale is illegal. It induces a sense of excitement and unreality. It is less likely to lead to addiction than are the hard drugs and is much less harmful to health. The danger lies in the fact that since it can be obtained only from illegal sources, access is also available to more serious narcotics. Many heroin addicts have started with cannabis.

3. *Amphetamine* groups, including 'purple hearts', are taken because they lead to an elevation of the mood with a sense of being able to think and act more quickly, though in reality this does not occur. When under the influence of amphetamines, behaviour becomes erratic and irresponsible. Emotional dependence on the drug develops after a time, and larger doses may be needed to achieve the desired effect.

4. *Lysergic acid or LSD* produces hallucinogenic effects so that those under its effect develop a heightened and distorted sense of their surroundings, which seem to attain unusual significance. The experience, which is not uniform in its effect, may last several hours and may lead to self-inflicted harm.

Treatment

Many or most drug addicts have unstable personalities and take to drugs because they are unable to resolve or accept the problems and pressures of life. Often they are unwilling to be treated, requesting only a regular supply of drugs. If these drugs are not supplied through legal channels, illicit sale of narcotics is encouraged by a network of unscrupulous 'pushers' who sell drugs for profit. Hospital centres are available for the treatment and supervision of drug addicts, who must be registered in order to obtain treatment of drugs.

Treatment is two-fold. First, the drug of addiction is slowly withdrawn, often by weaning the addict onto an alternative drug, such as the synthetic narcotic methadone which is taken as a drink and which is an easier drug to control.

Secondly, an attempt must be made at mental rehabilitation, perhaps by group psychotherapy, and at social rehabilitation, for a place in society. Unfortunately, the success rate of methods currently employed is not high and there is an urgent need for more knowledge and research before the problem can be tackled more successfully.

Effects of heat or cold

Extremes of heat or cold, if prolonged, can lead to serious metabolic and electrolyte disturbances.

Heat stroke

This is most likely to occur in individuals subjected to high temperatures to which they are unacclimatized. It may be provoked by prolonged exercise or by heavy clothing which prevents evaporation of sweat.

The patient may become restless and confused and sometimes convulsions occur. The skin is hot and dry. The oral temperature exceeds 41°C (106°F) and the pulse is rapid with a poor volume.

Effective cooling is essential, usually by spraying the exposed body with cold water and by using fans to promote active air movement. Intravenous saline fluids may be given to replace salt loss from perspiration.

Hypothermia

Serious lowering of the body temperature is now recognized as a common cause of stupor or coma, particularly in elderly patients during the winter months. The ordinary clinical thermometer does not record temperatures below 35°C (95°F), and every ward should now possess a special low-reading thermometer for recording the rectal temperature in suspected cases. In elderly people, particularly those living on their own, various circumstances dispose to hypothermia:

1. inadequate room heating, a meagre food intake, unsuitable clothing, and cold weather
2. immobilization, due to a fracture or a stroke,

for example, which prevents the summoning of help

3. overdosage with drugs or alcohol and falling asleep in an unheated room without adequate covering; the unconscious patient loses heat very quickly

4. Myxoedema (see p. 323).

In the early stages of exposure to cold, the skin goes white, the extremities are cold, and shivering occurs. This is followed by stiffness of the muscles, the shivering ceases and a stuporous state supervenes. The breathing becomes slow and shallow and the blood pressure falls. At this stage the rectal temperature may be less than 30°C (86°F). With further lowering of the temperature, the patient loses consciousness and coma ensues.

Prevention

Poverty, poor housing and insufficient heating are not easily eradicated but awareness by local authorities and social workers of this problem may do much to help. Regular visiting, meals-on-wheels and advice as to forms of heating may all be necessary. Special grants may be made available to help with heating bills during particularly cold weather.

Treatment

No attempt should be made to heat the patient rapidly, since this causes the skin vessels to dilate. Fluid is then lost from the general circulation. It is best to wrap the patient in a heat reflective sheet and blankets in a warm room or hospital ward and ensure that the rectal temperature is recorded regularly. Since dehydration is often present, a slow drip of warmed 5% dextrose may be given intravenously.

Electricity

Most cases of electric shock occur in the home or at work due to faulty electrical apparatus, inadequately earthed. The passage of electricity through the body causes burning of the skin, and if the current is large enough it may lead to cardiac arrest.

Radiation

Natural radiation exists in small amounts in the atmosphere, some in the form of cosmic rays from the sun and the stars, some from radioactive materials in the earth. Man-made radiation comes from the products of nuclear energy, from the use of X-rays and in radiotherapy.

Excess radiation can do irreparable damage to various tissues of the body, particularly the skin, hair, blood and reproductive organs and can predispose to cancer. Hence, those working or visiting X-ray departments must be protected by stringent safety regulations to avoid any possible long-term dangers. Techniques are adopted to minimize the patients' exposure to radiation, particularly since some investigations, such as a barium meal, involve lengthy exposure and may have to be repeated on several occasions. The adoption of safety standards is routine in all X-ray departments. Radiotherapy can be used to control the spread of certain malignant growths. The cells of the growing tumour are particularly vulnerable to the burning effect of deep X-rays directed on them while the healthy surrounding tissues are largely unaffected. Superficial X-ray therapy can be used for malignant skin disorders.

Radioactive forms of normal elements are also used in the treatment of various disorders. Radioactive iodine, for example, when given orally is taken up by the thyroid gland. It suppresses the metabolism of overactive thyroid cells and so can be used in the treatment of disorders of the thyroid (see p. 321).

TUMOUR FORMATION

The various organs and tissues of the body grow and are maintained in an orderly and regulated manner. A tumour is an abnormal growth of tissue which has no useful function.

Some tumours are called *benign* because their growth is restricted and local: they may compress surrounding structures, but they do not invade them. Examples of benign tumours are warts, lipomas under the skin, papillomata in the nose or bowel and fibroids in the uterus. In contrast, malignant tumours continue to grow in size and invade and destroy neighbouring tissues; cells from this growth enter the lymphatics and the blood vessels and so are carried to the lymph nodes and to other organs. These cells which spread to other organs form similar malignant growths and are called *secondary deposits* or *metastases.* Malignant tumors are commonly referred to as *cancer.* A malignant tumour of epithelial cells is called a *carcinoma* and a malignant tumour of connective tissue, such as bone or muscle, is called *sarcoma.* Thus we talk of a carcinoma of the bronchus or a sarcoma of the femur. The malignant process is referred to as *neoplasia,* and a cancer is often referred to as a *neoplasm* (which means new growth). The study of management of malignant growth is known as *oncology* and the physician who specializes in this subject is an *oncologist.* The cause of neoplasia is unknown in many cases. However some forms of cancer can be brought about by:

1. radiation (see above)
2. various industrial chemicals and tars, including cigarettes
3. certain viruses can probably cause cancer in animals and possibly in man

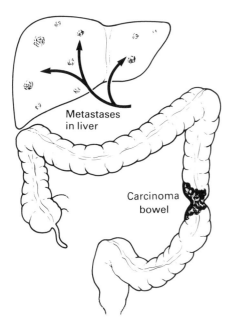

Fig. 2.5 Carcinoma of bowel with secondaries in liver.

4. the tendency to some cancers is inherited (for example in multiple endocrine neoplasia).

Malignant growths cause harm in different ways:

1. They invade and destroy neighbouring tissues, including blood vessels and nerves.
2. They spread to more remote organs and tissues. Malignant cells enter the blood vessels and lymphatics and settle in other areas. These secondary deposits (metastases) also begin to grow and invade local structures. Thus, a carcinoma of the bronchus can cause metastases in the liver and brain.
3. They produce toxic substances which can damage the function of the nervous system, including the brain and the peripheral nerves.
4. They can produce hormones such as ACTH (see p. 315) which lead to symptoms due to excess hormonal effect.
5. They lead to metabolic disorders and a general malaise, wasting and exhaustion known as cachexia.

Management of malignancy

The successful treatment of most cases of carcinoma and sarcoma depends on early diagnosis and surgical treatment, either by operative removal or by radiotherapy. However, particularly when surgical treatment has failed to prevent the spread of carcinoma, administration of drugs (chemotherapy) may be considered. Drugs used for this purpose are called cytotoxic drugs: malignant cells are sensitive to their destructive action and healthy tissues are not seriously affected. Some forms of neoplasm often respond very well to chemotherapy – for example, Hodgkin's disease, and acute leukaemia in children. Cytotoxic drugs act by interfering with the growth processes of the malignant cells. Since they may also exert harmful effects on healthy tissue, particularly the bone marrow, they have to be administered with great care. Usually combinations of different types of cytotoxic drug are administered, sometimes intravenously and in intermittent courses. Close supervision is obligatory where this form of treatment is used. Particularly in the treatment of leukaemia, steroids

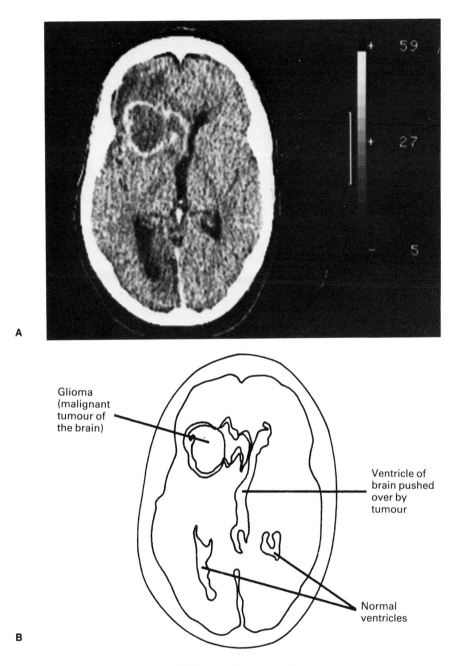

Fig. 2.6 A, B. Computerized axial tomography (CAT scan) of brain revealing a malignant tumour.

(see p. 329) may be given in addition to the cytotoxic drugs to help reduce complications of the treatment on healthy blood cells. In carcinoma of the prostate, and in some forms of breast cancer, the malignant cells seem to be influenced by hormones; thus, for example, anti-androgens in the form of stilboesterol can be effective in suppressing the growth and spread of prostatic cancer, and anti-oestrogens can be effective in breast cancer.

3

Infection, immunity and chemotherapy

INFECTIONS

Many types of living organism can invade and damage the human body:

1. *Bacteria.* These are single-celled forms of life, visible under the microscope. They exist all around us, in the atmosphere, food, on our skin, in the mouth and in the bowel. They are mostly not harmful or disease-producing (*pathogenic*) and, indeed, may be beneficial. Bacteria normally present in the bowel many prevent the growth of pathogenic organisms and help to produce vitamins.

2. *Viruses.* Viruses are too small to be seen under the microscope. They can only survive inside living cells since they depend on the nutriment of the cell for their growth and replication. Viruses are resistant to the action of antibiotics.

3. *Fungi* (mycoses). Numerous fungi or moulds exist in the soil, in decaying vegetation and in the excreta of birds. Fungi can be regarded as a form of vegetation and sometimes are antagonistic to the growth of bacteria; penicillin is derived from one such mould. Other fungi, known as mycoses, can infect the skin, the mouth (commonly known as candida or thrush), and the lungs.

4. *Protozoa.* These are single-celled parasites, bigger than bacteria and changing form during their life cycle. Malaria and amoebic dysentery are two widespread tropical diseases caused by protozoa.

5. *Metazoa.* These are many-celled organisms, the majority visible to the naked eye. They include parasites such as lice, scabies and intestinal worms (see p. 175).

Bacteria

There are a large number of different types of bacteria, some of more importance than others in both the seriousness and the frequency with which they cause disease. Only the most common and important bacteria will be discussed here.

Bacteria are usually divided by appearance into different groups known as cocci, bacilli and spirochaetes.

Cocci

These are round organisms and, depending on the manner in which they grow, they are subdivided into different families. When they grow in clusters they are termed staphylococci. If they form chains they are called streptococci, and if they grow in pairs they are termed diplococci.

These subgroups are further divided into classes according to various factors. For example, certain streptococci, when grown on media containing blood cause the red blood cells to be destroyed or haemolysed and hence are called haemolytic streptococci, to distinguish them from other forms which do not cause haemolysis.

Some cocci are named after the disease they cause in the body. The common disease of the lungs known as pneumonia is usually due to a group of cocci known as pneumococci. Some cocci and bacilli cause inflammation with pus formation, and hence are often classed together as pyogenic organisms. Important pyogenic organisms include staphylococci, streptococci, pneumococci, meningococci and the coliform bacilli.

Table 3.1 gives the names, types of lesions or pathological changes, and the most common diseases caused by important cocci.

Bacilli

Bacilli, instead of being round-bodied, are rod-shaped and are classified mainly according to the type of disease they cause.

Table 3.2 lists the common bacilli and the diseases they cause.

Spirochaetes

The third important group of bacteria is the spirochaetal group. These organisms are larger than either cocci or bacilli and have helically shaped bodies. Fewer diseases are caused by spirochaetes than by the two preceding groups. One of the important diseases in man due to a spirochaete is syphilis.

Table 3.3 lists the few well-known diseases caused by the spirochaetes.

Table 3.1 The cocci

Name	Pathological effects	Diseases
Staphylococci	Acute inflammation with pus formation; lesions tend to remain localized with the development of abscesses	Skin conditions; boils, carbuncles, impetigo, bone lesions: osteomyelitis. Otitis media, meningitis, pneumonia, acute bacterial endocarditis, septicaemia
Streptococci (a) haemolytic	Acute inflammation with pus; lesions usually spread	Skin conditions: cellulitis, erysipelas and impetigo; acute tonsillitis, scarlet fever, otitis media, meningitis, pneumonia, acute bacterial endocarditis, septicaemia
(b) non-haemolytic	Subacute inflammation	Subacute bacterial endocarditis
Pneumococci	Acute inflammation with pus	Broncho- and lobar pneumonia; otitis media, meningitis, peritonitis
Meningococci	Acute inflammation with pus	Meningitis (cerebrospinal fever)
Gonococci	Acute and chronic inflammation with pus formation	Gonorrhoea causing acute urethritis, epididymo-orchitis, and prostatitis in the male, acute urethritis, vaginitis and salpingitis in the female; ophthalmia in the newborn; arthritis

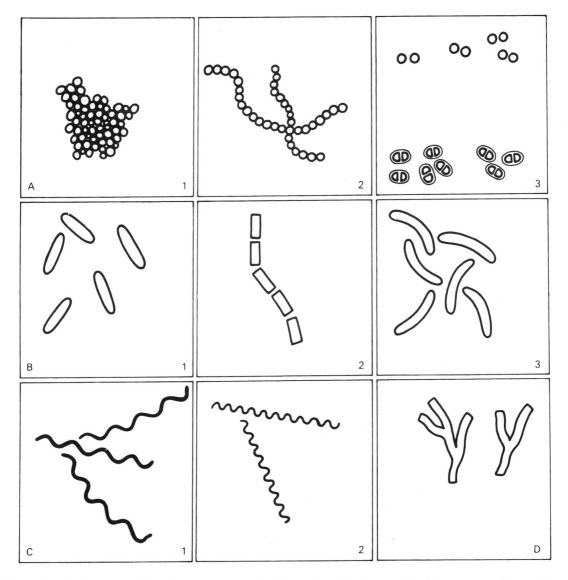

Fig. 3.1 Classification of bacteria by shape. **A.** Cocci (spherical bacteria) 1. Staphylococci. 2. Streptococci. 3. Diplococci. **B.** (1–3) Bacilli. **C.** (1, 2) Spirochaetes. **D.** Actinomyces.

Viruses

Viruses are responsible for widespread ailments such as influenza and the common cold. Many acute infectious fevers, which include measles, rubella, mumps and chickenpox are due to viruses. More serious viral infections include poliomyelitis, encephalitis and viral pneumonia.

Unlike infections due to bacteria, viral infections do not respond to antibiotics or sulphonamides so there is no effective treatment to overcome these ailments. Fortunately, in most viral infections the body's immune system overcomes the virus. However, occasionally very severe strains of virus become rampant, as occurred in the influenza epidemic in 1918, with resultant high fatalities.

The acquired immunodeficiency syndrome (AIDS), first recognized in USA in 1981, is caused by the human immunodeficiency virus (HIV),

Table 3.2 The bacilli

Name	Pathological effects	Diseases
Tubercle bacilli	Specific type of subacute and chronic inflammation; tubercles form and may break down to a cheesy material (caseation); ulceration with cavity formation; healing by fibrosis	Tuberculosis – affects many organs and tissues; particularly important are: pulmonary tuberculosis, tuberculous meningitis, glandular tuberculosis, tuberculosis of the bones (especially the spine), joints, kidneys and skin
Coliform bacilli	Acute and chronic inflammation with pus	Pyelitis, cystitis, peritonitis, cholecystitis, meningitis, puerperal sepsis
Pertussis bacilli	Specific acute infectious fever mainly involving the lungs	Whooping cough
Diphtheria bacilli	Specific localized lesion – the diphtheritic membrane – and a powerful toxin with widespread effects	Diphtheria, with the membrane in the throat, nose or larynx; toxin causes albuminuria, acute myocarditis and neuritis
Typhoid and paratyphoid bacilli	Specific infectious fevers with acute inflammation and ulceration; general invasion of the body, including the blood stream, but marked local changes in the small intestine	Typhoid and paratyphoid fever (enteric fever)
Dysentery bacilli	Specific acute inflammation with ulceration of the intestinal tract; exotoxin produced	Acute bacillary dysentery
Salmonella bacilli	Acute inflammation of the intestinal tract	Food poisoning
Influenza bacilli	Acute inflammation with pus	Influenzal meningitis
Abortus and melitensis bacilli	Specific inflammation of a subacute type mainly involving the glands and spleen	Undulant fever (brucellosis)
Tetanus bacilli	Powerful toxin produced with a selective effect on nerve cells	Tetanus

which was isolated in 1983. The virus attacks the lymphocytes which are required in the defence against infection. High-risk groups include homosexuals, injecting drug users and haemophiliacs. There is no cure for AIDS and treatment is aimed at temporary suppression of the HIV virus and present symptomatic alleviation of infections caused by bacteria due to the lowered immunity in these patients.

The diagnosis of most viral illnesses is evident from the typical signs and symptoms. In bacterial infections, the white cells in the blood are greatly increased (leucocytosis); however, this does not occur with most viral infections. Confirmation of the diagnosis of a virus infection is much more difficult and takes much longer than with bacterial infections.

Special techniques are required to culture viruses present in infected material. Viral antibodies can be demonstrated in the blood but usually this takes several weeks.

Table 3.3 The spirochaetes

Name	Pathological effects	Diseases
Treponema pallidum	Chronic inflammation with fibrosis and ulceration; widespread lesions, with the heart, arteries and nervous system particularly affected	Syphilis
Leptospira icterohaemorrhagiae	Toxin which particularly affects the liver to cause hepatitis and jaundice	Weil's disease (spirochaetal jaundice)
Borrelia vincentii	Acute inflammation and ulceration of the throat and gums	Vincent's angina

Specimens for a bacteriological examination

The primary object of practical bacteriological methods is to isolate the organism causing a particular disease. In order to do this it is essential to obtain the organism; if a disease is suspected of being caused by bacteria, certain methods are adopted to obtain the relevant biological fluid or specimen. A knowledge of the pathogenesis of the disease (i.e. the organ systems affected by the pathogen) usually points to the possible tissues which can be examined for the presence of the organism.

In general, the common specimens examined for the presence of bacteria are as follows.

Throat swabs

A swab is a piece of sterile cotton-wool wrapped round the end of a stick. The sterile wool is rubbed over the surface or area from which the specimen is to be taken. Fresh swabs should be delivered to the laboratory as soon as possible.

Diseases in which throat swabs are normally taken are:

(a) acute tonsillitis or any 'sore throat'
(b) diphtheria
(c) scarlet fever
(d) rheumatic fever.

Nasal swabs

These are less important than throat swabs but are taken in suspected nasal diphtheria.

Sputum

In diseases in which sputum is being coughed up this specimen should be provided for bacteriological examination. It is particularly important in:

(a) pulmonary tuberculosis
(b) pneumonia.

Sputum examination for the presence of tubercle bacilli, the bacteria which cause pulmonary tuberculosis, is of considerable importance. First, it aids in establishing the diagnosis as one of active pulmonary tuberculosis; secondly, it suggests that the case is infectious and should be treated with adequate isolation measures. In pneumonia, examination of the sputum for bacteria is often carried out to determine the causative organism.

Faeces

Many bacteria cause lesions in the intestinal tract and the organisms in these cases can often be found in the faeces. Diseases in which examination of faeces is important are:

(a) all cases of acute diarrhoea
(b) dysentery and other chronic diarrhoeas
(c) food poisoning
(d) typhoid and paratyphoid fevers
(e) tuberculosis of the intestinal tract.

Urine

The urine is frequently examined for the presence of bacteria and must be obtained using aseptic precautions. A specimen is obtained after washing the genitalia with soap and water and discarding the first urine passed (i.e. collecting a *midstream* specimen). Urine examination for bacteria is of importance in the following diseases:

(a) acute pyelonephritis and cystitis
(b) acute urethritis
(c) tuberculosis of the renal tract.

Blood

In cases where it is suspected that the bacteria may be actually growing in the blood stream, a condition known as *septicaemia*, a small quantity of blood, usually 2–3 ml, is put into a special bottle known as a *blood culture* bottle. This bottle contains a special medium, usually glucose broth or cooked meat, which allows bacteria to grow. The blood should be collected under strict aseptic conditions, as otherwise contaminating organisms may confound the results of the test. A fresh sterile syringe must be used in each case. Blood cultures are usually taken in the following diseases:

(a) all cases of suspected septicaemia
(b) bacterial endocarditis
(c) typhoid and paratyphoid fevers
(d) all cases of prolonged undiagnosed fever.

Pleural and cerebrospinal fluid

When fluid is present in the pleural cavity of the chest a sample is frequently aspirated through the chest wall in order to isolate the causative organism that may be present. Such organisms include pneumococci, streptococci, staphylococci and tubercle bacilli. All these organisms commonly cause disease of the lungs and pleura causing exudation of fluid into the pleural cavity.

Cerebrospinal fluid is withdrawn by carrying out a lumbar puncture. It is examined for bacteria in all cases of meningitis (inflammatory disease of the meninges). The bacteria often found include meningococci, pneumococci, and tubercle bacilli.

Swabs from the genital regions

With discharge from the vagina or urethra a swab is taken for examination of the presence of organisms, particularly the gonococcus. If there is a sore on the genital organs, a scraping from the sore is taken for examination for the presence of spirochaetes (syphilis).

Eye swabs

In many cases of inflammation of the eyes, and also before any operation on the eyes, swabs are obtained. Before operations are performed on the eye it is essential that no pathogenic organisms are present in the conjunctivae.

Methods of identification of organisms

Having obtained the material for bacteriological examination the specimen is then treated in the laboratory by different methods in an effort to identify the organism.

Staining of smears

In some cases the material obtained is smeared onto a slide and various stains or dyes are applied to colour and show up the organisms. By means of these stains one can differentiate certain organisms, depending on the dye they take up. For example, an important and commonly used stain is known as Gram's stain. Based on their staining properties most of the common organisms can be divided into two groups:

1. Gram-positive organisms, which turn blue on application of the stain
2. Gram-negative organisms, which turn red.

The cocci (except for the meningococci and gonococci) are usually Gram-positive, while many of the more important bacilli (but not the tubercle bacilli or *Corynebacterium diphtheriae*) are Gram-negative.

Again, by washing out the stain with acid most organisms are distinguished from the tubercle bacillus which resists the action of acid and is thus called an *acid–fast bacillus*.

Cultures

Most specimens taken are put on a special plate containing suitable material, such as blood, embedded in firm agar gel which allows the organism to grow in an uncontaminated state. The plate is placed in a special box, known as an incubator, kept at 37°C (most organisms grow well at body temperature). After 24 to 48 hours the plate is examined for growth of the organism. This method of identifying the organism is called isolation by culture. Smears or films are then taken from the culture plate and stained for examination under the microscope as outlined above. The culture plate yields useful information regarding the identity of the organisms depending on their characteristic growth patterns. For instance, the haemolytic streptococcus, an important organism causing several diseases, causes haemolysis on a blood culture plate distinguishing it from the non-haemolytic streptococcus which does not.

Agglutination reactions

An agglutination reaction can be explained by the Widal reaction, which is a typical agglutination reaction used in the diagnosis of typhoid fever. A patient suffering from typhoid fever, develops antibodies against the typhoid bacilli as part of the body's protective mechanism to fight the disease. If serum from the patient is mixed with known typhoid bacilli in a test-tube the bacilli become clumped or agglutinated owing to the action of the antibodies on the bacilli. No agglutination would occur, however, if serum and organisms other than typhoid bacilli were mixed together. The agglutination reaction can therefore be used for diagnosing several infections and is of particular value when it is difficult to isolate the actual organisms and is extensively used in cases of the enteric fevers.

Agglutination reactions become positive after the illness has lasted approximately a week, as it takes about 7–10 days for the antibodies to develop in the patient's blood.

How bacteria enter the body (mode of spread)

Organisms must enter the body to cause disease, and the different ways in which they do so are often referred to as the modes of spread.

Droplet infection. If organisms are present in the upper air passages they are expelled into the air while speaking, sneezing or coughing, and can then be readily inhaled by others. Infection can thus easily spread through close proximity to the infected person. In some cases the infected droplets can contaminate dust, and inhalation of the dust can cause infection. Fortunately most organisms die outside the body, but an important exception is the tubercle bacillus which can remain alive in dust for many months. The majority of the acute infectious diseases, such as measles, whooping cough, diphtheria, etc., are contracted by droplet infection via the respiratory tract.

Infection may spread through handling articles (*fomites*) which have become infected with the organism, e.g. clothes, bedlinen, toys, pencils, etc. Neglect in washing the hands thoroughly is very likely to spread infection.

The infecting organism may be present in the *nasal secretions*, *faeces* and *urine*. Lack of hygiene following visits to the toilet may lead to contaminated *food* or water. Contamination of *water* supplies from leaking drains is a potential cause of epidemics. *Flies* which feed on excreta are another common means by which food can become contaminated.

The diseases which are spread through contamination of food, milk or water are intestinal infections such as food poisoning, dysentery and typhoid fever.

Certain organisms, especially gonococci and the spirochaete which causes syphilis, require actual *direct contact* between the infected person and the one to be infected.

Infecting organisms may be conveyed by means of a blood-sucking *insect*, e.g. by mosquitoes carrying the malarial parasites and lice carrying the typhus organisms.

Finally, infection may spread to man from contact with *animals*, e.g. rabies from dogs and anthrax from sheep.

How bacteria cause disease (pathogenesis)

Although bacteria exist all around us they do not necessarily cause disease. This is because in order to cause disease following entry into the body, certain criteria must be met:

1. The bacteria must be present in sufficient numbers.
2. The bacteria must be virulent, that is, of a sufficient degree of activity.
3. The organisms must have entered the body via the appropriate pathway, encouraging its virulent activity and providing an optimum environment for growth; for example, gonococci when swallowed are destroyed and do not cause disease, while dysentery organisms are virulent only if swallowed.
4. The person infected must be susceptible to the organism, that is, must not be resistant (immune). This subject is discussed further under immunity.

Given the above suitable conditions, the organisms entering the body will multiply and produce toxins, which are substances that react on specific target tissues and cells (e.g. diphtheria toxin on

Droplet infection

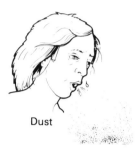

Dust

Unsterile injections

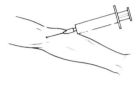

Infected skin breaks

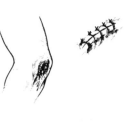

Low standards of hygiene

Inadequate sanitation

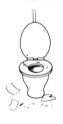

Unwashed hands

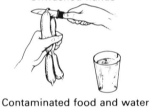

Contaminated food and water

Insufficient cooking

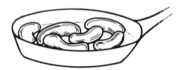

Animals

Domestic

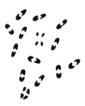

Louse

Mosquito

Fly

Sexual intercourse

Gonorrhoea

Syphilis

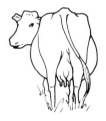

Viruses

Fig. 3.2 Some common modes of infection.

the nerves and heart). The nature of these reactions varies with different bacteria, some toxins causing inflammation, either acute or chronic, while others cause degeneration of cells.

How the body resists and overcomes infection (immunity)

We have so far considered the isolation and identity of the bacteria causing disease, the mode of entry of the organisms and the conditions necessary for these bacteria and their toxins to cause disease.

One of the conditions required before bacteria can cause disease is that the person infected must be sensitive or susceptible to the organisms. In many cases the infected person is not susceptible and does not suffer from the disease even though he is harbouring the organism. In these circumstances the person is said to be immune to the disease.

Immunity to a particular disease may be acquired naturally, or it may be acquired deliberately by artificial immunization.

THE DEFENCE AGAINST INFECTION

The body defends itself against infection by bacteria and viruses both locally and constitutionally. The local response to an infection is by the process of inflammation and the constitutional reaction is through the immune system.

Inflammation

This is the reaction of local tissues in response to an infection.

Acute inflammation is characterized by redness, swelling and increased temperature of the area involved. There is often considerable pain and impairment or loss of function. These features are caused by dilatation of the small blood vessels which exude fluid.

Chronic inflammation Early white blood cells in the area are activated by the tissue damage and begin to release lymphokines which activate more white cells and make them sticky with surface adhesion factors. The white blood cells

(polymorphonuclear leucocytes) attracted to the area of inflammation (chemotaxis) engulf the foreign material or bacteria; an excess of dead polymorphs and tissue cells leads to the formation of an abscess. Lymphocytes produce antibodies which neutralize the toxins present and prevent the bacteria from spreading. Fibrous tissue cells form strands of dense connective tissue which wall off the infected area and lead to scar formation. If this is extensive, distortion and deformity of the area results.

The nature and degree of the inflammation depend mainly on the type of agent or bacteria responsible. Some diseases, such as tuberculosis, cause gradual and chronic inflammation, while others, such as staphylococcal infections, can cause acute and severe inflammation. Sometimes an inflamed area can give rise to a discharge or exudate which may be:

1. *Serous.* When the pleura or peritoneum is inflamed, there is an effusion of clear yellow fluid.

2. *Purulent.* The exudate contains infective organisms, masses of polymorphs and debris of dead cells.

3. *Haemorrhagic.* A bloodstained exudate sometimes occurs with bacterial infections, but it is particularly common in malignant growths (carcinoma).

Repair If the inflammation is mild, then the protective mechanisms of the body can overcome the disease and healing can occur with very little permanent change in the affected area. If it is more severe, permanent changes, principally fibrosis or scarring, may occur. If this scarring is extensive, owing to severe inflammation, it can interfere with the proper functioning of the part. This may lead to a serious disability, perhaps with fatal results, if a vital organ is affected. For example, disease causing chronic inflammation of the valves of the heart can give rise to scarring and deformity, with a resultant malfunctioning heart which may over a long period lead to chronic heart failure.

Immunity

Most organisms, though not all, on entering the

body stimulate the lymphocytes to produce substances which react with these toxic invading organisms and destroy them. These substances are called antibodies and antitoxins. The organisms are said to act as *antigens* to stimulate the production of *antibodies* (and produce *humoral immunity*). They can also arm cells for direct attack (*cellular immunity*).

The antibodies and antitoxins produced, e.g. against the diphtheria organism, have a specific effect against the organism or toxin respectively. Although antibodies do not persist indefinitely some are produced by the white cells for many years, while others are produced for only a few weeks or months.

Antibodies are a type of protein known as gamma globulin and the types of white cell which produce them are lymphocytes and plasma cells. Different groups of cells are capable of producing different antibodies to deal with different kinds of antigens that enter the blood stream. The thymus gland plays an important part in the development of these cells in the fetus, and the lymph nodes, spleen and the gastrointestinal tract are a factory for the activation of these lymphocytes in the adult.

Naturally acquired immunity Skin acts as an important natural barrier and serves as the first line of defence against invading bacteria. Natural immunity to a particular disease may be acquired in several ways:

1. The individual has an actual attack of the disease. When the body is invaded by an infection, protective antibodies are produced by the lymphocytes to counteract and neutralize the invader. Antibodies will only protect against the particular organism to which they can bind, i.e. to which the lymphocytes were exposed previously. If there is considerable antibody stimulation, the patient will probably be immune from subsequent attacks by the same organism. However, not all infections give rise to long-lasting immunity, and further attacks of the same disease may occur.

2. The individual is exposed to repeated infection in small doses, so that an actual attack of the disease does not occur. By repeated stimulation of the body's immune systems by trivial infections, too short-lived to cause overt disease (subclinical infection), a complete development of antibodies can occur over a period of time. These can then resist a subsequent full dose of infection, which would normally cause pathological disease. This method of developing immunity to a particular disease explains why some people are immune or resistant to a disease without ever having suffered from an actual attack.

3. Resistance to a disease may be inherited. For example, an infant may be immune for a short period owing to the passage of the mother's protective antibodies into its circulation via the placenta or through the mother's milk.

4. In addition to the above, certain animals possess natural immunity to diseases such as syphilis and gonorrhoea, while others are highly susceptible. For example, sheep and cattle are very susceptible to anthrax while dogs and rats are practically immune.

Artificially acquired immunity (active and passive) Artificial immunity is the result of a deliberate and successful attempt by the body to develop antibodies against infectious organisms. The history of the discovery of this process is of great interest and helps in understanding immunity.

In 1798 Jenner observed that people who suffered from the mild disease known as cowpox, contracted from cattle, rarely suffered from the much more serious and often fatal disease known as smallpox. If they did contract smallpox the attack was usually mild. From this he inferred that the cowpox attack in some way conferred a resistance or immunity to smallpox in the person concerned. He also believed that probably the organism causing cowpox was almost identical to that causing smallpox, but of a milder nature. Jenner then proceeded to inoculate a boy with cowpox, and after the boy had overcome the mild infection, demonstrated that he could not be infected with smallpox. This experiment led to the development of vaccines.

Another major advance in artificially acquired immunity was Pasteur's discovery in 1885 that certain bacteria could be altered and rendered harmless by several means, so that they could be

Naturally acquired

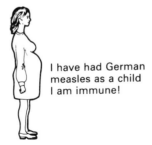

I have had German
measles as a child
I am immune!

Passive immunity

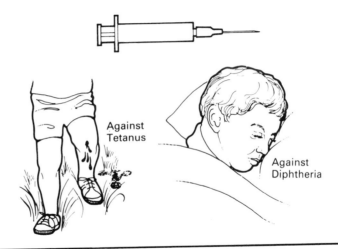

Against
Tetanus

Against
Diphtheria

Active immunity

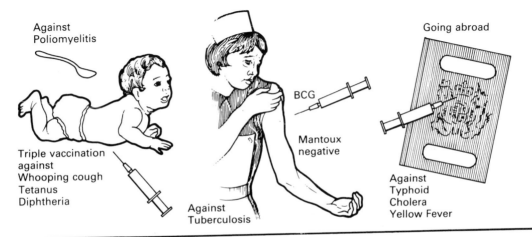

Against
Poliomyelitis

Going abroad

BCG

Mantoux
negative

Triple vaccination
against
Whooping cough
Tetanus
Diphtheria

Against
Tuberculosis

Against
Typhoid
Cholera
Yellow Fever

Fig. 3.3   Some types of immunity.

injected into human subjects safely. Although these bacteria could no longer cause disease, they retained their capacity to stimulate the formation of antibodies. Thus, infecting a person with this modified type of organism led to an immunity or resistance in the individual without causing overt disease. Pasteur adopted to modify the virulence of an organism by heating the organism, adding an antiseptic, or infecting an animal prior to its entry into a human being. Infection of an animal modifies the infecting organism so that it is no longer capable of causing active disease in man but can still result in immunity.

The term *vaccine* is given to a suspension of modified avirulent organisms, and the procedure of inoculating is termed *vaccination* or *immunization*.

Toxins produced by organisms can themselves be suitably modified to render them inactive and may be used to produce immunity instead of the altered avirulent organisms. Modified toxin as used in immunization procedures is known as *toxoid*.

In addition to the type of artificial immunity referred to above, which is called active immunity, there is another form known as passive immunity which will be discussed later (see p. 50).

Clinical use of vaccination (immunization) and serum treatment Vaccination is the method frequently used to produce immunity to certain infectious diseases which can become widespread and serious. To protect against typhoid fever, dead typhoid bacilli are used to prepare a vaccine; when inoculated with the vaccine the body forms antibodies which afford protection against typhoid fever for over a year. In areas where typhoid fever is rampant inoculation must be repeated at intervals to renew antibody formation. This type of immunity is known as active immunity since it depends on the activity of the host's lymphocytes to produce the appropriate antibody.

Diseases in which vaccination (active immunity) is of value include:

diphtheria
cholera
tuberculosis
typhoid

Table 3.4 Immunization schedule

Age	Visits	Vaccine	Intervals
2–12 months	3	Three administrations of DTP + OPV + *Haemophilus* b	6–8 weeks and 4–6 months
12–24 months	1	MMR vaccination	
First year at school	1	Booster DT + OPV	
10–13 years	1	BCG for the tuberculin negative	
Girls: 11–13 years	1	Rubella vaccination	
15–19 years or on leaving school	1	TT + OPV	

DTP = diphtheria, tetanus, pertussis (triple vaccine);
DT = diphtheria, tetanus vaccine; MMR = measles, mumps, rubella; OPV = oral poliomyelitis vaccine; TT = tetanus toxoid.

tetanus
whooping cough
poliomyelitis
rubella.

An individual who has recovered from an infection will have specific antibodies circulating in his blood (e.g. a child recovering from measles has abundant antibodies against the organism causing measles circulating in his blood). This blood can be withdrawn from the infected child and the serum containing the antibodies (*convalescent serum*) can be inoculated to prevent the development of measles in another child who has been exposed to this infection. This is known as *passive immunity* since the antibodies are not actively produced by the child who receives the serum.

Diseases in which antitoxin serum (passive immunity) can be used are:

diphtheria
tetanus.

Convalescent serum is no longer used to prevent measles for fear of transmitting other infections. Instead, the protein which contains the antibodies (gamma globulin) is isolated from the serum, purified and stored for future use.

In diphtheria, the horse is used as a source of antitoxin serum. After being repeatedly inoculated with inactivated diphtheria bacilli to let sufficient antitoxin form the horse is bled, the serum sterilized and stored for emergency use in severe diphtheria (p. 54). Human normal immunoglobulin is used for measles and virus A hepatitis, while human specific immunoglobulin can be used for chicken pox, virus B hepatitis, tetanus and rabies.

Organ transplantation

As discussed earlier, the introduction of bacteria or other foreign material (known as the antigen) leads to the production of antibodies, chiefly by the lymphocytes. These antibodies block the effect of the antigen. Any material introduced into the body acts as an antigen unless it is a natural part of the body, or sufficiently similar to the natural product as to be indistinguishable from it. For example, transfusion of blood into an individual from another person will produce serious antibody reactions unless the blood is of a similar group. This specific property of the body to recognize foreign protein and destroy it by means of antibodies makes organ transplantation difficult. For example, transplantation of a kidney from a road accident case into a patient suffering from terminal kidney failure is technically easy but unless the kidney is from an identical twin, antibodies are formed by the recipient which react with the transplanted kidney and lead to an antigen–antibody reaction resulting in *rejection* of the transplanted kidney. Several approaches are being tried to overcome rejection:

1. Steroids, such as prednisone, help to suppress the antigen–antibody reaction but have to be given in large doses. Cyclosporin has a similar action.

2. Certain cytotoxic drugs, especially azathioprine, prevent the production of antibodies (this is termed *immunosuppression*). They have toxic effects and have to be administered cautiously.

3. Antilymphocytic serum may be given to suppress the lymphocytes which produce the antibodies. Human lymphocytes injected into a horse lead to the production of antibodies to these lymphocytes in the horse's serum. This becomes the source of antilymphocytic serum. In order to prevent the rejection of a transplanted organ, antilymphocytic serum is injected and treatment begun with prednisone and azathioprine.

With these precautions, transplanted organs may function well for a period of time (i.e. show *tolerance*) and temporary success has been recorded with transplants of organs such as the kidney, liver, pancreas, lung and heart. Many problems remain to be overcome before this operation can become a routine procedure. At present, the organ to be transplanted must be removed soon after the donor's death as no method is available for preserving it for more than a few hours without reducing its viability.

Anaphylaxis, serum sickness, hypersensitivity and allergy

All the above conditions are in some way related to each other and the terms are often interchangeable. This is particularly so with the term *allergy*. To explain the above conditions, which are rather difficult to understand, it is best to describe how they are encountered in clinical practice.

Anaphylaxis

In some individuals given a serum injection, a subsequent injection administered 10 to 14 days later may manifest a very severe and often fatal reaction known as *anaphylaxis*. The essential features of the reaction are a spasm of smooth muscle and a dilatation of small capillaries leading to difficulty in breathing and circulatory collapse and convulsions, and, in some cases, death.

These effects are due to the presence of a foreign protein in the serum which produces an excess of sensitive antibodies following the first injection, which, when injected again, causes a severe antigen–antibody response leading to the violent reaction. However, if the second injection is given before 10 days have elapsed, the anaphylactic reaction does not develop. This may be because the protein has not produced an adequate initial sensitization.

Anaphylaxis is very rare, the immediate injection of adrenalin (0.5 to 1 ml of 1:1000 dilution) is of great value in the treatment. When injecting serum of any kind, adrenalin should always be readily available.

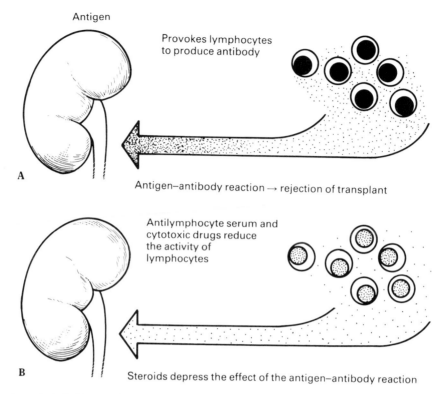

Fig. 3.4 Organ transplant. **A.** Causes of rejection. **B.** Prevention of rejection.

Serum sickness

About 7 to 14 days after an injection of large amounts of serum the person may develop an urticarial reaction involving the skin, joint pains, fever and enlarged glands. These symptoms follow the first injection. As in anaphylaxis, they are due to a sensitization of the body against a foreign protein in the serum. Serum sickness, however, unlike anaphylaxis, is never fatal.

The antihistamine drugs (Phenergan, Benadryl, etc.) often relieve symptoms, and adrenalin is useful by injection. Should these measures fail, cortisone or related drugs are usually prescribed.

Hypersensitivity

Anaphylaxis and serum sickness, just discussed, are of the nature of hypersensitive reactions, but these terms are usually reserved only for sensitiveness following serum injections. Many individuals, however, are sensitive to a great many different foreign proteins present in foods, dust,

flowers, drugs, etc. When they come in contact with these offending substances by eating, inhaling or touching them, they develop certain characteristic reactions such as:

(a) laboured breathing (asthma)
(b) wheals (urticaria)
(c) vomiting and diarrhoea
(d) severe running from the nose and eyes
(e) fever.

These individuals are said to have an idiosyncrasy to the offending substance or to be 'allergic'. Certain diseases such as asthma, urticaria, hay fever and eczema are often due to a sensitivity to a plant, drug, foodstuff etc., and are therefore called allergic diseases. The protein causing the allergy is termed the 'allergen'.

CHEMOTHERAPY

Chemotherapy is the treatment of infections by

substances which destroy or suppress bacteria.

The sulphonamides were the first group of chemical drugs to be used successfully in the treatment of common infections. They exert their effect by inhibiting the growth of invading bacteria, thus allowing the defence mechanism of the body to overcome susceptible organisms. Unfortunately the sulphonamides are ineffective against many dangerous bacteria.

The discovery of penicillin represented a major accomplishment in the fight against bacteria, and greatly increases the range of bacteria which can be overcome. Penicillin is not a chemical drug but is the product of a living mould. It is called an *antibiotic* and acts by preventing bacterial cell wall synthesis or by suppressing particular aspects of bacterial cell function such as inhibition and transpeptidase. A considerable number of potent antibiotics are now available. Streptomycin was the first agent to be found effective against the tubercle bacillus, while chloramphenicol suppresses the typhoid group of bacteria. The tetracycline antibiotics have further extended the scope of chemotherapy. One of the problems following the use of antibiotics is that in some cases bacteria that are initially susceptible to a particular antibiotic become resistant to it following repeated exposure. For example, nowadays staphylococci grown from hospital dust are nearly always resistant to penicillin.

The sulphonamides

The original sulphonamide drugs were often toxic, but they have been gradually replaced by much safer preparations. There are now many sulphonamides available, all with slightly different properties; some act best in the kidneys and some in the bowel, some are less powerful and therefore can be given safely for long periods.

Sulphonamides are less expensive than antibiotics and are usually given orally in tablet form or liquid suspensions.

Sulphadimidine and sulphadiazine

These sulphonamides are used for acute systemic infections, such as pneumonia, meningococcal septicaemia, streptococcal tonsillitis, and pyelitis. A large initial dose of 2 to 3 g is followed by a smaller dose varying from 1 to 1.5 g 4- to 8-hourly. In successful cases the temperature falls very quickly with obvious improvements in the patient's condition. Treatment should be sustained for several days but should not be normally continued for more than a week, especially if there is no effect, in view of the possibility of toxic effects. Sulphadiazine is well absorbed into the cerebrospinal fluid and so is particularly useful in the treatment of meningococcal meningitis.

Sulphafurazole and sulphamethizole

These preparations are rapidly concentrated in the kidneys and are therefore valuable for treating renal infections. Prolonged treatment at low doses may be necessary.

Sulphaguanidine and phthalysulphathiazole

These are poorly absorbed from the intestinal tract and so exert their effect locally in the bowel. For this reason they can be given in high doses (e.g. 2 g 4- to 6-hourly) in infections of the intestinal tract such as dysentery or enteritis. Usually the temperature falls and the diarrhoea ceases within a few days of treatment.

Co-trimoxazole (septrin)

This is a combination of trimethoprim with a sulphonamide sulphamethoxazole. Trimethoprim enhances the antibacterial action of sulphonamides and the combination is effective against a wide range of Gram-positive and Gram-negative bacteria. It is particularly useful as the treatment of choice in bronchopneumonia in the elderly and is widely used for chest and renal infections. It is normally prescribed in tablet form to be taken twice a day but is also available as an intravenous infusion for very ill patients. When given intravenously it has to be diluted and given by drip transfusion.

Toxic effects of sulphonamides In some patients

sulphonamides may cause nausea or even vomiting, and skin rashes may develop. Particularly following high dosage or prolonged treatment, agranulocytosis may occur wherein the number of white cells diminish disposing the patient to other infections; however this is rare.

Antibiotics

Penicillin was first used in the treatment of infections in 1943 and since then an increasing number of antibiotics have become available. Some forms of bacteria are resistant to the action of penicillin from the start, while others become insensitive to its action after prolonged treatment. Hence there is a need for more effective antibiotics in these situations.

The first step in the treatment of an infection is to isolate and to identify the causative organism. It can then be cultured and its sensitivity tested to various antibiotics. The appropriate bacteriological specimen (sputum, urine, throat swab, pus, blood culture, cerebrospinal fluid, etc.) is sent to the laboratory and the organism is cultured by incubation in a suitable medium. Small discs of filter paper impregnated with the various antibiotics or sulphonamide are placed on the culture plate; if the organism is sensitive to an antibiotic or sulphonamide preparation, it fails to grow in the immediate vicinity of the disc impregnated with that antibiotic or sulphonamide preparation. On the other hand, if the organism is resistant to an antibiotic, growth of the organism will not be affected. Unfortunately, these sensitivity tests take a few days to perform and if the patient is ill, it may not be wise to wait for the results to come through. Consequently, the physician has to choose a chemotherapeutic agent on his estimate of the likely bacterial cause of the infection and on the severity of the illness. If it is evident that the patient is not responding to this initial treatment, the antibiotic can be changed in the light of the sensitivity tests.

Antibiotics may be divided into two types according to their action on bacteria. *Bacteriostatic* antibiotics inhibit the growth and multiplication of bacteria, while *bactericidal* antibiotics destroy bacteria in the process of multiplication. Thus tetracycline is bacteriostatic and penicillin is bactericidal. They should not be given together since the action of tetracycline in inhibiting multiplication of bacteria actually protects them from the effect of penicillin.

Some antibiotics (e.g. penicillin) are effective mainly against Gram-positive bacteria, and others (e.g. streptomycin) against Gram-negative bacilli. In seriously ill patients, therefore, where the infective organisms are not known, both antibiotics may be given together. A knowledge of the action of the antibiotic and of the type of bacterial infection will enable the physician to decide the treatment to be prescribed. In making his choice of antibiotic he will also be influenced by the cost of the drug (some antibiotics are very expensive), by its possible toxic effects and by knowledge of whether the patient is known to be sensitive to any particular preparation. For example, if a patient is known to be sensitive to penicillin and has had a reaction to it in the past, some alternative antibiotic must be chosen.

Penicillin

Penicillin acts by preventing the organisms from growing and also by actually destroying the organisms. Its action varies with different bacteria, being highly effective against some while having little or no effect against others.

Uses of penicillin Table 3.5 gives the main diseases and their causative organisms for which penicillin is prescribed.

Penicillin has little or no effect on organisms such as:

1. the enteric fever, dysentery or food poisoning group
2. the *E. coli* group, which are frequently responsible for urinary tract infections (pyelitis, cystitis) and also some cases of septic peritonitis
3. the tubercle bacillus
4. the whooping-cough bacillus
5. any of the viruses which are the causative organisms of many acute infectious fevers (measles, poliomyelitis, chickenpox, smallpox etc.).

Doses and administration of penicillin There are

Table 3.5 Main diseases (and their causative organisms) for which penicillin is prescribed

Diseases	Causative organisms
Septic infections (wounds, abscesses); osteomyelitis; septicaemia	Streptococci and staphylococci
Acute tonsillitis; bacterial endocarditis; eye infections (conjunctivitis)	Streptococci
Pneumonia	Pneumococci, streptococci, staphylococci
Syphilis	*Treponema pallidum*
Gonorrhoea	Gonococci

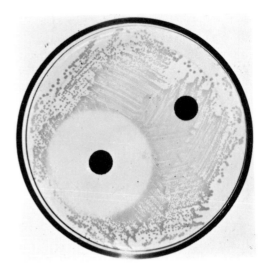

Fig. 3.6 Staphylococci resistant to penicillin, but sensitive to erythromycin. The paper disc on the right was impregnated with penicillin which failed to inhibit growth of the organisms, but around the erythromycin-impregnated disc on the left is a clear area where the organisms have failed to grow.

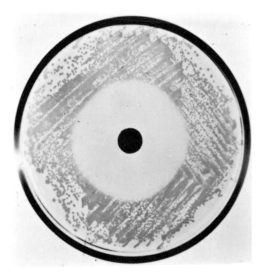

Fig. 3.5 Penicillin-sensitive staphylococci seen as an irregular growth on the surface of a nutrient gel plate. The bacteria have failed to grow near the penicillin-impregnated central black disc.

several preparations of penicillin in use, the following being most widely preferred.

1. *Crystalline benzylpenicillin.* This is the ordinary soluble sodium (or potassium) salt which is usually referred to as 'penicillin'. This form is very rapidly absorbed into the blood stream but is also quickly excreted by the kidneys. The larger the dose of penicillin given, the longer the therapeutic effect lasts, up to a limit. It is probable that even the largest doses are all excreted within

8 hours. The dose of penicillin given depends both on the severity of the infection and the frequency of the infections. The tendency nowadays is to give large doses of penicillin, at longer intervals.

For moderately severe systemic infections, 500 000 units of penicillin are normally given 12–hourly; however, in more serious infections, and particularly where the causative organism is not highly sensitive to penicillin, higher doses can be employed.

In addition to the above, crystalline penicillin is injected into the pleural cavity in cases of empyema (pus in the pleural cavity).

2. *Procaine benzylpenicillin.* (This preparation is commonly referred to as *procaine penicillin.*) Combining procaine with crystalline soluble penicillin delays its absorption so that an effective blood concentration can be maintained for a longer time. This allows fewer injections to be given, usually at 12- or 24-hourly intervals. Owing to its slow absorption, however, a higher concentration of penicillin is not usually achieved with procaine penicillin and therefore severe systemic infections are usually treated with soluble crystalline penicillin.

Procaine penicillin is thus mainly used for

treating localized infections or the less severe general systemic infections. The usual dose is 300 000 to 600 000 units at 12- or 24-hourly intervals. For an immediate effect soluble crystalline penicillin (100 000 units) is often combined with procaine penicillin.

Benzathine penicillin is another long-acting penicillin with a duration of action of 3–4 weeks. It can be used for the prophylaxis of rheumatic fever in patients who cannot be relied upon to take oral penicillin.

3. *Phenoxymethylpenicillin (penicillin V).* This preparation is fully effective when given by mouth, unlike most other forms of penicillin, which are largely destroyed by the acid gastric juice. Except for severe general infections, oral therapy with penicillin V is usually sufficient and obviates the need to give frequent intramuscular injections. This is of particular value when treating children.

Phenoxymethylpenicillin is given in 60 to 125 mg doses 4-hourly to 6-hourly. The last daily dose may be doubled to avoid waking the patient at night.

The actual structure of the penicillin molecule was worked out several years ago and therefore new forms of penicillin are common. Many of these preparations are effective in the treatment of bacterial infections resistant to the action of penicillin itself.

Ampicillin

This is effective in overcoming a wide range of bacterial infections when given orally. It is available in 250 mg capsules and can be given every 6 hours, the dose depending on the type and severity of infection. As its absorption from the bowel into the blood is variable, it should be given before meals. In severe infections, it can be given by intramuscular injection or by intravenous drip infusion. As with penicillin, it is liable to give rise to urticarial reactions.

Amoxycillin is similar to ampicillin but is better absorbed and is effective in typhoid fever.

Cloxacillin

Some bacteria produce an enzyme called penicil-

linase which can inactivate the action of penicillin. Cloxacillin is not affected by penicillinase and is effective against organisms producing this enzyme. It has to be given by intramuscular injection in doses of 250 mg every 6 hours.

Flucloxacillin is very similar to cloxacillin but can be given by mouth. One 250 mg capsule should be taken four times daily about an hour before taking meals.

Tetracyclines

This group includes tetracycline, oxytetracycline and doxycycline. These antibiotics have a very wide range of activity – they are often referred to as 'broad-spectrum antibiotics' – being effective in streptococcal, staphylococcal, pneumococcal, meningococcal, gonococcal and *E. coli* infections. In addition they are effective in rickettsial and certain viral infections.

Tetracycline and oxytetracycline are usually given orally in 250 mg doses 6-hourly. Demethylchlortetracycline is more long-acting so that 300 mg twice daily is usually sufficient. In those very severe infections where the patient cannot take oral therapy, tetracycline, erythromycin and oxytetracycline may be given by intravenous or intramuscular injection. Since local irritation and pain are likely to follow parenteral therapy, oral therapy should be started as early as possible.

The tetracycline antibiotics are also used for local application as a 1% ointment for bacterial skin diseases such as impetigo and sycosis.

Toxic effects of the tetracyclines Nausea, vomiting and diarrhoea are not infrequently seen, particularly following intensive and prolonged therapy. Tetracyclines cause the least gastrointestinal upset. With prolonged therapy, excessive growth of organisms such as fungi and staphylococci, may occur in the bowel with resultant infection of the gastrointestinal tract. This infection may cause acute inflammation of the bowel (ileocolitis) with severe fatal diarrhoea and fever.

Another adverse effect very likely to arise with prolonged therapy or with heavy dosage is vitamin deficiency, particularly vitamins B and K. This is due to the alteration of the normal intestinal bacterial flora. When the tetracyclines are given for more than a few days, vitamin B complex should be given. Tetracyclines form complexes with calcium and are deposited in developing bone and teeth and therefore should not be prescribed to children and in pregnancy.

Chloramphenicol (chloromycetin)

Chloramphenicol is similar in its action to the tetracyclines but in addition it is a very effective antibiotic in the treatment of typhoid fever. Chloramphenicol is given in oral doses of 500 mg 6-hourly.

Chloramphenicol eye drops and eye ointment are useful in the treatment of purulent conjunctivitis.

The toxic effects of chloramphenicol are similar to those of the tetracyclines, while, in addition, chloramphenicol may give rise to the more serious danger of severe aplastic anaemia. Aplastic anaemia, which is often fatal, has most often occurred in children on prolonged and heavy dosage. The use of chloramphenicol is best restricted to the treatment of typhoid fever and to infections not responding to penicillin or the tetracyclines.

Erythromycin

Erythromycin is an antibiotic effective against staphylococci, streptococci and pneumococci. Its action is in many ways similar to that of penicillin. The chief use of erythromycin is in the treatment of staphylococcal infections resistant to penicillin and the other antibiotics.

Erythromycin is given by mouth in tablets, in 200–300 mg doses 6-hourly. No serious side-effects have so far been noted and erythromycin does not materially alter the normal intestinal flora, with the result that it rarely causes diarrhoea or vitamin deficiency. Unfortunately it does cause vomiting and crampy abdominal pain due to a direct action on gut muscle but new preparations will avoid this.

Neomycin

Neomycin is an antibiotic with a very wide range of activity. It is never given by injection as it is too toxic, causing severe kidney damage and deafness.

Uses of neomycin Neomycin has the following uses:

1. Neomycin is mainly used for local application in bacterial skin infections such as impetigo, sycosis and infected eczema. Unlike penicillin, bacterial resistance to neomycin rarely develops.

2. In bacterial infections of the eye, neomycin in ointment form is very effective.

3. Neomycin is not readily absorbed when given by mouth, and toxic effects are not likely to develop when it is given orally and it can therefore be used in the treatment of gastroenteritis in infants.

4. Oral neomycin is also given before operations on the intestinal tract.

5. In severe cirrhosis of the liver, with manifest central nervous system changes, neomycin is given to sterilize the bowel and reduce toxic absorption.

Lincomycin

Lincomycin is particularly effective against *pyogenic* (pus-forming) Gram-positive pathogens which are resistant to the action of penicillin. It is valuable in the treatment of bone infections (osteomyelitis) and can be given by mouth (500 mg every 8 hours) for mild infections or intramuscularly (600 mg twice daily) for severe cases.

Clindamycin is a similar preparation and can be given by mouth (300 mg every 6 hours) in the treatment of chronic wound infections not responding to penicillin.

Cephalosporins

This group of broad-spectrum antibiotics have a structure similar to that of penicillins; they include cephaloridine and cephaloxin. Cephaloxin is active against Gram-negative organisms such as E. coli and is used in the treatment of resistant urinary tract infections and bronchitis. It can be given by mouth (250 mg every 6 hours).

Gentamicin

Gentamicin is a powerful antibiotic against many

Gram-negative organisms, including those resistant to other antibiotics. It has to be given by injection but is liable to give rise to deafness and vertigo if the dose is too high or too prolonged. This is particularly prone to occur where kidney function is impaired. It is advisable to monitor the dose given by measuring the level of gentamicin in the blood and discontinuing this treatment if the blood levels are likely to be toxic to the auditory nerve.

Streptomycin

Streptomycin was the first antibiotic to be successful in the treatment of tuberculosis and is still used extensively. However, many other alternative and effective drugs are now available (see p. 134).

Streptomycin has to be given by intramuscular injection and is effective against many Gram-negative bacilli. As with gentamicin, it has a toxic effect on the auditory nerve and can cause vertigo, tinnitus (noises in the ear) and deafness.

Other antituberculous drugs are described in the treatment of pulmonary tuberculosis.

Quinolones

The most frequently used of this group of broad-spectrum antibiotics is ciprofloxacin. Although expensive these antibiotics are effective against both Gram-positive and Gram-negative organisms and they have few side-effects.

Other chemotherapeutic agents

Urinary tract antiseptics

Nitrofurantoin and *nalidixic acid* are two chemotherapeutic drugs excreted in the urine in an active form and of value in the treatment of persistent urinary tract infections.

Antifungal agents

One of the disadvantages of antibiotic treatment of bacterial infections is that they allow infection by various fungi to flourish. Strangely enough, many antibiotics, themselves derived from fungi,

are effective in the treatment of fungal infections.

Imidazoles and tiazoles This group includes clotrimazole, econazole, isoconazole, retoconazole and several others. These are used locally for vaginal candidiasis (thrush) and dermatophyte (skin fungal) infections, such as athletes foot. Flucanzole is active by mouth and used to treat systemic fungal infections.

Nystatin *Candida albicans* is a fungus which can affect the mouth (thrush), the bowel (candidiasis) and the vagina (*Candida* vaginitis). Nystatin is available for appropriate treatment in the form of an oral liquid suspension, tablets for intestinal infection and pessaries for vaginal infection. Nystatin is effective treatment and can be given prophylactically to prevent fungal infection in patients on long-term antibiotic therapy.

Amphotericin B This can be used for rare systemic fungal infections and has to be given by intravenous drip infusion.

Griseofulvin This oral antibiotic is effective in ringworm and other fungal infections of the skin, nails and hair. It has to be taken four times a day (250 mg) and, to be effective, treatment must be continued for many months.

Drugs acting on protozoa

Malaria Effective drugs are available both for protection against and treatment of malaria (see p. 64).

Amoebic dysentery Drugs such as *emetine* and *metronidazole* (see p. 65) are effectively used in overcoming intestinal amoebiasis.

Anthelmintics

These are drugs used in the treatment of various worm infestations (see p. 175–177).

Anti-viral drugs

There is no effective systemic treatment for most viral infections. *Acyclovir* and *idoxuridine* can be applied locally for herpes zoster (shingles) and herpes simplex (cold sore) to relieve the discomfort and, if applied early, may shorten the duration of the symptoms; they are also active against varicella zoster virus infection. *Ganciclovir* is helpful for cytomegalovirus.

Amantadine has been used in epidemics to prevent influenza infections.

Zidovudine, formerly known as *azidothymidine* (AZT) is used in the treatment of AIDS.

4

Infectious illnesses (acute infectious fevers; tropical diseases; skin diseases; sexually transmitted diseases)

ACUTE INFECTIOUS FEVERS

The term *acute infectious fever* might be used to describe any viral or bacterial infection; in practice however, it refers to a group of particular diseases easily spread from person to person, often occurring in epidemics and particularly common in babies and children. In the developed part of the world, these ailments no longer lead to the high death rate in children as a result of:

1. Improved standards of nutrition: children receive better nutrition today and therefore are better able to resist infection.

2. Improved private and public hygiene, including a clean water supply; high standards of cleanliness in the sale and provision of food; proper sanitation in homes, public places and places of work; and an efficient sewage system and methods of disposal of refuse. All these are important factors which contribute to reduce the spread of infection.

3. Protection of children by an organized programme of immunization against common infections. Ailments such as diphtheria, smallpox and poliomyelitis, causes of a high mortality in infants and children in the past, have now almost been eradicated owing to immunization.

4. The introduction of chemotherapy for the treatment of various complications following these infections.

The term *acute infectious fever* is usually reserved for those infections which tend to display the following characteristics:

1. The onset is acute and is associated with a rise in temperature.

2. The disease is caused by a specific bacterium or virus.

3. It tends to run a definite course and often occurs in epidemic form.

4. It is very infectious (i.e. it can easily spread from person to person).

5. In many cases a single attack confers immunity from subsequent ones, although exceptions do occur.

Certain terms are frequently used while discussing infectious fevers and are best explained at the outset.

Epidemic. When a large number of cases occur at the same time, to be followed by a period in which few or no cases occur.

Endemic. Area where the disease is found at regular intervals.

Sporadic. When scattered cases of the disease are observed.

Pandemic. When there is a worldwide distribution of the disease.

Isolation and period of isolation. Most cases of infectious disease are isolated to prevent the disease spreading to other people. The period of isolation required varies with different diseases, but generally lasts until the patient no longer harbours the infecting organisms. With some people, however, the organisms may persist indefinitely, even after having fully recovered from the illness. Such people are called *carriers*, because they carry virulent organisms capable of spreading disease to others. These people can also carry virulent organisms without ever having had the active disease because they have a natural resistance or immunity to the disease.

Incubation period. The incubation period is the length of time which elapses between the individual becoming infected and the appearance of the first symptom. The incubation period varies with different diseases.

Quarantine. Quarantine is the restriction of the activities of people who have been in contact with a case of infectious disease until such time as it is known whether or not they have acquired the disease. The period of quarantine is just longer than the incubation period. In practice, strict quarantine of contacts is not usually en- forced except in cases of serious infectious diseases such as smallpox or typhus. Known contacts of most other infectious diseases are nowadays kept under medical observation so that they can be isolated as soon as any symptoms develop. In most cases, close observation with prompt isolation if necessary, is just as effective in controlling the incidence of infectious diseases.

Notifiable diseases. Certain diseases, usually the infectious diseases, need to be notified to the public health authorities. This is to enable the authorities to take precautionary measures to prevent spread of the disease. Some diseases are notifiable only at certain times, e.g. when they are prevalent or there is a large epidemic of the disease.

General features of acute infectious fevers

Infectious fevers start with a rise in temperature, general malaise, headache, loss of appetite or vomiting, a dry mouth, a hot dry skin and a diminished output of urine. In rubella, a rash appears on the first day; in measles, the rash is not apparent until the fourth day of the illness. In adults with severe infection the onset may be a rigor (see p. 4) while in small babies, a convulsion or fit may occur.

General principles of treatment

In nursing patients with infectious illnesses, precautions must be taken to avoid spread of infection to others. The patient is best isolated in a separate room (barrier nursed), particularly for enteric fevers. Disposable eating utensils and bedpans should be employed, but if these are not available care should be taken to ensure that the patient's utensils are marked and adequately sterilised after use. All people attending the patient should wear gloves and gowns and wash their hands before leaving the room.

Most fevers occurring in children can be treated at home but admission to hospital becomes necessary if the infection is severe or home conditions are unsuitable.

Measles (Plate 1)

Cause

Virus infection.

Spread and incidence

Spread is by direct contact through droplet infection from sneezing or coughing. It is very contagious, especially in the catarrhal stage before the rash appears. The maximum incidence of the disease is between the ages of 8 months and 5 years. Attacks are common in winter and spring when widespread epidemics may occur.

Incubation period

10–14 days.

Symptoms and signs

1. The onset is usually abrupt with the following predominant catarrhal symptoms:
    a. coryza (common cold)
    b. conjunctivitis
    c. photophobia
    d. bronchitis.
With these symptoms the child presents a picture of running eyes and nose, coughing and sneezing. In some cases a laryngitis with hoarseness is present.

2. Before the rash appears, many cases manifest the typical Koplik's spots which are distinct features of measles. These are small white spots on the mucous membrane of the mouth beside the molar teeth. They often disappear when the rash appears.

3. The temperature rises on the first day, often to 100–103°F (37.8–39.4°C). It usually falls slightly on the third day, to rise again on the fourth day with the onset of the rash.

4. The rash appears around the fourth day of the illness and is seen first on the forehead and behind the ears and soon spreads all over the face and body. The rash is a dusky red macular eruption which gives a bloated, swollen appearance to the face.

5. The rash gradually fades and disappears in a week while the temperature comes down more gradually. The infection varies in severity from mild to seriously ill cases.

Complications

1. Bronchopneumonia, particularly frequent in young children, is an important complication of measles.
2. Acute gastroenteritis is particularly liable to occur in infants and children under 2 years of age.
3. Conjunctivitis, blepharitis and corneal ulceration.
4. Otitis media and mastoiditis.
5. Stomatitis.
6. Inflammation of the brain and spinal cord (encephalomyelitis) is a rare complication of measles, as it is of many of the other infectious fevers.
7. In the undernourished state, measles may precipitate a condition called kwashiorkor (protein-energy malnutrition).

Treatment

The patient is nursed in strict isolation in a well-ventilated room. The usual nursing care as outlined in the general treatment of a fever case with regard to diet, bowels, sleep etc. is necessary.

In view of the risk of conjunctivitis, corneal ulceration and stomatitis, particular attention should be paid to the eyes and mouth. Discharging eyes should be bathed in warm water and direct sunlight on the eyes should be avoided.

A careful watch must be kept on the breathing as quickening of the respiratory rate often suggests the onset of bronchopneumonia. Penicillin or other antibiotics should be given if there is a suspicion of pneumonia or other bacterial complication.

Pain in the ear, discharge from the ear or swelling behind the ear strongly suggests otitis media or mastoiditis, and one of the antibiotic drugs will be given to clear up the inflammation. In those cases which do not rapidly clear up, lancing the ear drum (*myringotomy*) to provide proper drainage may be necessary.

The patient is kept in bed until the temperature

has been normal for several days and until all signs in the chest have subsided. This may take several weeks in moderately severe cases.

All clothes, linen, utensils, etc. are disinfected at the end of the illness as with any infectious case.

Preventive treatment – immunization

Active immunization A live attenuated measles vaccine is now available and offers effective protection. A vial contains the dried powder for a single dose and this is dissolved in water for injection. It may give rise to a slight elevation in temperature and should not be used in babies under 1 year.

Passive immunization A passive immunity to measles can be acquired by intramuscular injection of human normal gamma globulin. Gamma globulin is that part of the serum protein which contains the antibodies, and is prepared from the serum of healthy adults who have had measles.

If gamma globulin is given to contacts within 5 days of exposure to infection, an attack of measles can be completely prevented. However, if the gamma globulin is given between 6 and 9 days after exposure, a modified mild attack of measles develops. In practice, full protection is usually given to infants under 2 years, when the risk of developing bronchopneumonia and gastroenteritis is high. Full immunization is not usually carried out over the age of 2 years unless the child has contracted another disease.

Rubella (German measles)

Cause

Virus infection (*Togavirus*).

Spread and incidence

By direct contact and droplet infection on coughing, sneezing, etc. Adults and children are affected. The disease is most prevalent in spring and early summer.

Incubation period

14–19 days.

Symptoms and signs

1. The onset is less acute than in measles. There are general symptoms of a mild infection, such as malaise, headache, nasal catarrh and a slight temperature.

2. The rash appears on the first day of the illness. It begins on the face and spreads to the trunk and limbs. It is a discrete, pink, papular eruption, not usually as confluent and widespread as in measles. Koplik's spots do not occur.

3. The occipital and cervical lymph glands are characteristically enlarged.

Course and complications

The illness is usually mild and complications are rare. However, if rubella occurs in the first 3 months of pregnancy it causes congenital deformities (particularly congenital heart disease) in some cases. In view of this risk, it is desirable for girls to have had rubella while they were young and therefore to have developed immunity before conception. A vaccine against rubella is available for girls between their 10th and 13th birthdays. Immunity is also checked in early pregnancy.

Treatment

Isolation for 5–6 days is usually sufficient along with the routine treatment for a mild fever case.

Whooping cough

Cause

The pertussis bacillus (*Bordetella pertussis*).

Spread and incidence

Usually by droplet infection after coughing; less commonly the disease is spread by contact with infected clothes or other articles (fomites). The disease is most prevalent in spring and autumn. Children under the age of 5 are the usual sufferers, but adults may also be affected. Since the decline in the severity of scarlet fever and the reduction in the number of diphtheria cases through active immunization, whooping cough is nowadays one of the causes of serious acute specific fever in children.

Incubation period

7–14 days.

Symptoms and signs

Catarrhal or preparoxysmal stage This stage usually lasts a week, when the child appears to be afflicted with a bad cold. Fever is often present, while the cough tends to be very persistent and may be associated with vomiting.

Paroxysmal stage This stage is characteristic and there is little doubt about the nature of the illness. Paroxysmal attacks of severe coughing occur, the child going blue in the face and holding his breath. When it appears that the child might suffocate, a long deep inspiration with a loud 'whoop' is observed. Vomiting frequently occurs at the end of the paroxysm and thick sticky mucus is expectorated. There may be as many as 20 or more of these bouts (frequent at night) in a severe attack leaving the child utterly exhausted.

Course

The paroxysmal stage usually lasts 3 or more weeks, the bouts gradually becoming less severe. The younger the child the more severe the disease, most of the deaths occurring in children under 1 year.

Diagnosis

This is obvious in the paroxysmal stage. Prior to this stage, whooping cough should be suspected in any child with a severe cold and cough associated with vomiting. A swab suitably curved for insertion into the postnasal region is obtained and cultured in a special medium in the laboratory.

Complications

1. *Bronchopneumonia* is the outstanding complication of whooping cough and is responsible for many deaths among infants.

2. *Bronchiectasis.* Collapse of part of the lung may occur in the acute stage owing to the thick mucus obstructing a bronchus. If the lung fails to re-inflate, the permanent collapse may lead to bronchiectasis.

3. *Gastroenteritis.* In children under 2 years, whooping cough often leads to gastroenteritis, particularly in the summer months when enteritis is prevalent.

4. *Convulsions.* Repeated convulsions are serious and may prove fatal.

Treatment

In mild cases, where the paroxysms are few and the child's general health is good, the patient should be exposed to fresh air. In severe cases with frequent paroxysms and fever, the child is put to bed. A well-ventilated room is particularly important in the treatment of whooping cough.

Diet is of particular importance because of the frequent vomiting. The child is best fed with small, frequent, light meals immediately after each bout of coughing. Skilled attention is needed to encourage the child to take sufficient nutrition, particularly with infants. Routine bottle feeds may need to be abandoned and the infant fed whenever it is responsive.

To reduce the paroxysms of coughing, various drugs have been tried. Phenobarbitone given 30 mg twice a day (15 mg for infants), may be effective. Convulsions are adequately treated with oxygen and by giving phenobarbitone (60 mg) immediately, followed by smaller doses. Sedatives should not be given in quantities as to make the child too drowsy, as the resultant depressed cough reflex results in retention of the thick bronchial mucus.

Penicillin is given at the first suspicion of pneumonia. The tetracycline antibiotics are sometimes given in severe attacks as it is believed by some that these drugs reduce the number and severity of the paroxysms.

Preventive treatment

An effective vaccine is available for active immunization. The vaccine is usually combined with those against diphtheria and tetanus (triple vaccine) and three injections are recommended for complete protection given at monthly intervals from 8 weeks. Very rarely, inoculation has been followed by encephalitis (brain damage), but the benefits of inoculation in preventing fatalities from whooping cough and long-term lung complications are factors in favour of vaccination.

Scarlet fever

Cause

A streptococcal strain that causes destruction of red blood cells (*Streptococcus haemolyticus*).

Spread and incidence

Mainly by droplet infection. Less often, fomites (infected articles such as toys, books, etc.) may be responsible. Milk infected by a carrier may cause a widespread outbreak of the disease. The organism generally enters the body through the throat and a streptococcal sore throat is an initial symptom of the disease. In puerperal women the infection may occur via the genital tract – puerperal scarlet fever. Primarily in children, especially during the winter.

Incubation period

2–4 days.

Symptoms and signs

1. The onset is nearly always sudden, with fever, severe headache, vomiting and sore throat.
2. The pulse rate is rapid and out of proportion to the degree of fever.
3. The throat is inflamed, and exudate is usually present on both tonsils, often giving the appearance of a membrane.
4. The tongue is heavily furred, and the red papillae seen through the fur gives the appearance referred to as the strawberry tongue. After a few days the tongue peels, becoming red and raw – *red strawberry tongue*.
5. The rash appears on the second day and

has the following characteristics:

a. The face is spared of the rash but is flushed, except around the mouth (circumoral pallor).
b. It appears first around the neck and chest and soon spreads rapidly all over the body.
c. It is a bright red erythema which blanches on pressure.
d. It fades in about a week, to be followed by the typical desquamation; here the skin peels off, either in large scales or in a small form which produces 'pin holes' in the skin.

Types of scarlet fever

Simple This is the ordinary, relatively mild type with symptoms and signs described above.
Toxic Severe toxaemia is present in these cases and many patients die. This form is rare in Great Britain but is still common in Eastern Europe.
Septic In this type the septic complications are a predominant feature.

Diagnosis

The diagnosis is usually clinically evident by the sore throat accompanied by the erythematous rash. If the rash is missed, the occurrence of desquamation later on in the illness is suggestive of scarlet fever.
Dick test This is similar to the Schick test used in diphtheria. Scarlatinal toxin is injected into the skin, and if the person is susceptible to scarlet fever a bright erythema develops in 12 hours and disappears by 24 hours. The test can be employed up to the third day after onset of the disease provided the toxin can be injected into an area of skin devoid of rash.

Complications

Scarlet fever may be accompanied by septic infections or followed by toxic or allergic disorders.

1. Septic. The septic complications are caused by the infection spreading to the surrounding

tissues. They usually develop in the early stage of the disease, unlike the toxic complications which tend to appear in the second and third weeks. The primary septic complications are:

a. Septic cervical adenitis
b. Otitis media, which may spread to cause mastoiditis
c. Quinsy (peritonsillar abscess).
2. Toxic and allergic. The main complications in this group are:

a. Acute myocarditis and endocarditis. The heart involvement in scarlet fever is closely related to that in acute rheumatic fever and is treated in the same way.
b. Acute nephritis. This is identical to the ordinary form of acute nephritis described in Chapter 11.
c. Arthritis.

Treatment

The patient is nursed in bed with isolation procedures and nursing care usual in a fever case. In view of the mild form of scarlet fever encountered these days, patients are not usually nursed in hospital where there is a significant risk of cross-infection from other strains of haemolytic streptococci. Penicillin is most valuable in the treatment of scarlet fever and reduces the risk of complications considerably. Isolation for 2 weeks is usually sufficient except when septic discharges contain the organisms, which requires longer periods.

Erysipelas

Cause

Haemolytic streptococcus.

Spread and incidence

By direct contact, entry into the body usually through a skin abrasion or wound. Erysipelas was formerly a very common infection in hospitals, especially in surgical wards where infected wounds and abscesses spread the disease. Nowadays, however, with proper aseptic techniques, and particularly with the introduction of the sulphonamides and antibiotics, the disease is less common and can be quickly controlled.

Symptoms and signs

1. Erysipelas is most frequently observed in middle-aged and elderly people, and the presence of some debilitating disease or chronic alcoholism is particularly likely to give rise to the infection.
2. The onset is usually sudden, with fever, general constitutional upset and rigors.
3. The characteristic lesion is a bright red erythema of the skin which is swollen and tense with a well-defined border. The face is a frequent site of this local lesion and often spreads over the nose and cheeks (butterfly distribution). Another common site is around the margin of a surgical wound.

Treatment

Penicillin usually clears up the infection in a few days and reduces the risk of spread. The general treatment consists of bed rest and the routine care for an acute fever case.

Diphtheria

Cause

Infection with the diphtheria bacillus (*Corynebacterium diphtheriae*) of which there are several strains, the *gravis* strain producing the most severe infection.

Spread and incidence

Mainly by droplet infection. Indirect spread (e.g. from sucking infected pencils) can also occur. Children are chiefly affected, although diphtheria may also be seen in adults, especially during epidemics. Winter is the most usual season for diphtheria.

Incubation period

2–4 days.

Pathology

The illness takes the form of a typical local lesion with a severe general toxaemia. The local lesion is a membranous exudate (diphtheritic membrane) which usually occurs in the throat causing faucial diphtheria. Less often it is situated either in the nose (nasal diphtheria) or in the larynx (laryngeal diphtheria). Combined lesions may occur, and rarely skin diphtheria may develop.

Although the organisms remain in the membrane, they produce a very powerful toxin which causes a general toxaemia. The toxin particularly attacks the heart muscle (myocardium), causing an acute myocarditis (showing characteristic ECG changes), and the nervous system, causing various forms of paralysis.

Symptoms and signs

1. The onset may be insidious without associated fever, but the pulse is rapid and there may be marked exhaustion, restlessness, irritation and general malaise.

2. Examination of the throat reveals the tonsils covered by a greyish-white membrane. This membrane may extend over the soft palate and cannot be wiped off with a swab. The breath has a musty smell.

3. The tonsillar glands in the neck are enlarged, giving the neck a swollen appearance.

4. In nasal diphtheria, the membrane is confined to the nose, causing a blood-stained nasal discharge.

5. When the membrane involves the larynx, breathing becomes obstructed and the trachea may need to be opened surgically (tracheostomy) to allow the patient to breathe.

6. Myocarditis may be caused by the toxins produced by the diphtheria bacilli in the first week. The pulse is thready and rapid, blood pressure falls and death can follow.

7. Paralysis of the nerves and muscles, due to the toxins, may lead to difficulty in breathing and swallowing.

Diagnosis

The clinical diagnosis is confirmed by a throat swab which reveals the characteristic growth pattern of the bacillus on culture.

Treatment

Once the diagnosis of diphtheria is suspected it is important to start treatment immediately without waiting for the result of the throat swab to avoid the deleterious effects of the toxin which can spread rapidly. Diphtheria antitoxin (usually a dose of 24 000 units) is injected intramuscularly while in more severe cases a bigger dose may be given intravenously. In addition, penicillin should be administered to overcome the spread of the bacilli and prevent secondary infection. Intensive nursing is essential and the patient must be isolated to avoid spread of infection.

Prevention

Although epidemics of diphtheria used to be a feature many years ago enforcement and practice of a strict immunization programme has lead to a very low incidence of the disease today. Inoculation against diphtheria is combined with vaccines against whooping cough and tetanus (triple vaccine) and administered to babies at monthly intervals from 8 weeks of age. Booster doses may be given at 5, 11 and at 18 years.

Rabies

Cause

Virus infection (*Rhabdovirus*).

Spread and incidence

The virus infection is transmitted to man by the bite of an infected dog or cat. Dogs in turn are infected from exposure to foxes which constitute the reservoir in Europe. The disease is not seen in the UK because of the strict quarantine enforced on dogs brought into the country.

Incubation period

20–60 days (may range up to 1 year).

Symptoms and signs

Initial symptoms are non-specific with headache, malaise and insomnia. After 2–4 days the patient becomes agitated, confused and lucid in turn. This is followed by typical 'hydrophobia' (fear of water) characterized by involuntary spasms of the main and accessory muscles of respiration brought on by attempts to drink water or even the sight or sound of water. Paralysis and bizarre patterns of breathing follow ending in death due to respiratory failure within 10–14 days.

Diagnosis

Virus particles can be grown from saliva, and viral antigen can be identified in skin biopsies by direct fluorescent antibody techniques. Increasing titres of antibodies to the virus in blood also confirms the diagnosis.

Prevention and treatment

Management at the time of biting is important and prevents rabies. First aid involves thorough washing of the wound with soap and water for 5 minutes followed by washing with clean water and the application of 40–70% alcohol or 0.01% povidone iodine. The wound should not be sutured to avoid inoculation of the organism to skeletal muscle. Tetanus prophylaxis should be started. In cases where attack was unprovoked or exposure was due to licks or minor bites a vaccine (killed virus grown in human diploid cells (HDCV)) is given and the animal observed for 5–10 days. If the animal remains healthy or brain examination by direct immunofluorescence microscopy is negative for *negri bodies* the vaccine is discontinued.

Major bites or attacks by wild animals should be followed by administration of vaccine and antirabies immunoglobulin (preferably obtained from a human source).

Tetanus

Cause

The tetanus bacillus (*Clostridium tetani*).

Spread and incidence

The bacteria, which are present as commensals in the gut and which are also found in the soil, enter the body through trivial wounds caused by a splinter, nail in the boot or a garden fork and can also follow septic infection. Tetanus is rare in the UK and is observed mostly in farmers and gardeners.

Incubation period

2 days to a few weeks.

Symptoms and signs

1. Severe muscle spasms usually starting in the jaw muscles causing difficulty in opening the mouth – hence called 'lockjaw' (trismus).

2. The spasms spread to involve other muscles of the face, neck and trunk leading to a board-like rigidity of the abdominal wall.

3. Violent spasms may be brought on by moving the patient or even making a noise resulting in severe, sometimes fatal exhaustion of the patient.

Pathology

Following entry through the wound the bacilli may remain localized, leading to local stiffness, but have an affinity for nerve cells and migrate to motor nerve endings and nerve cells. The involvement of the anterior horn cells in the spinal cord results in rigidity and convulsions.

Diagnosis

Usually made on clinical grounds following a history of an old injury.

Treatment

1. After the diagnosis is suspected a single intravenous injection of immune serum containing 1000–3000 i.u. of antitoxin is given.

2. The wound is thoroughly cleaned.

3. Metronidazole or benzylpenicillin is given to prevent secondary infection.

4. Spasms are controlled by placing the patient in a quiet room with subdued lighting. All manipulations should be carried out gently with due warning to the patient preferably in an intensive care unit involving expert nursing care.

5. Serious cases of spasms may require diazepam or curare.

6. Nutrition and fluids are maintained. If the laryngeal muscles are involved a tracheostomy may be needed to ensure a clear airway.

Prevention

Preventive inoculation of babies in the first year with tetanus toxoid (with vaccines against diphtheria and whooping cough) has reduced the incidence. Where there is a possibility of tetanus in any wound, injured children and adults should receive 1 ml tetanus toxoid if they have been adequately immunized within the previous 10 years. Otherwise they should be given ATS (antitetanus serum), followed after 6 weeks by a course of three injections of toxoid to avoid the need for future injections of ATS. Repeated injections of ATS lose their effect and frequently give rise to serum sickness. Adults should receive a booster dose every 10 years.

Chickenpox (Plate 2)

Cause

Virus infection (*Varicella zoster*).

Spread and incidence

By droplet infection or contact through the hands and clothing of attendants. The disease is very common, attacking all age groups, but especially children under 10 and is most prevalent in autumn and winter.

Incubation period

12–21 days, usually around 14.

Symptoms and signs

The onset is usually mild, the patient merely feeling 'unwell' with a mild pyrexia. In children, quite often the first sign of the disease is the appearance of the rash which has the following characteristics:

1. It appears first on the trunk, particularly the back, and then spreads to the face and limbs. The eruption is particularly dense on the trunk and the upper parts of the limbs.

2. Red papules appear first, which rapidly change to vesicles and pustules. Within a few days the pustules dry up and form scabs which quickly fall off.

3. The rash appears in crops so that all types of lesion – papules, vesicles, pustules and crusts – are observed together.

Complications

Chickenpox is nearly always a mild disease, severe toxicity being rare. The most frequent complication is infection of the rash due to scratching. Chickenpox pneumonia may develop in patients with a compromised immune status.

Diagnosis

The most important aspect in diagnosis is to distinguish a severe case of chickenpox from a mild case of smallpox. The differentiation can usually be made on observing the order of appearance, the distribution and, in smallpox, the protracted development of the rash.

Electron microscopy can be used to establish the presence of the virus in the vesicle fluid, tissue culture incubation being used for identification of the virus.

Chickenpox may also be mistaken for various skin diseases such as impetigo, urticaria and scabies.

Treatment

Treatment of chickenpox mainly concerns prevention of secondary infection of the lesions. Patients are advised not to scratch the lesions, and in children, finger nails should be cut short and, if itching is severe, gloves or splints should be applied. The itching may be alleviated by using a soothing lotion such as calamine with 1% phenol. If the lesions are profuse, penicillin may be required to prevent secondary infection. Acyclovir can be used in severe cases with pneumonia.

Isolation is necessary till all the crusts have separated.

Smallpox (Plate 3)

Cause

Virus infection (*Vaccinia*).

Spread and incidence

By direct contact and droplet infection through the respiratory tract. Smallpox was the most infectious disease and was a major cause of death for many years. However, a vigorous programme of vaccination by the World Health Organization in countries where smallpox was endemic and also an international agreement that all travellers to and from such countries had to be vaccinated has eradicated the disease.

Symptoms and signs

The rash of smallpox is similar in appearance to that of chickenpox but there are distinct differences. The vesicles are more dense on the face and the limbs than on the trunk. The vesicles are larger and deeper and become purulent, leaving scars when they heal (pockmarks). The initial rash develops sequentially into papules, vesicles and pustules followed by scabs unlike chickenpox which manifests all lesions at the same time. There are serious constitutional manifestations with high fever, headache and prostration.

Successful eradication of smallpox (vaccination)

It was the study of smallpox by Jenner which led to the initial instances of the prevention of disease by vaccination. In vaccination against smallpox the vaccine used was a suspension of a virus which caused cowpox in cattle. The virus of cowpox (vaccinia) appears to be similar to the virus of smallpox except that its effect on human beings is much less virulent. Inoculating a person with a vaccine containing the virus of cowpox caused an attack of vaccinia and led to the formation of antibodies. As a result the person became immune when exposed to the much more serious disease, smallpox, thereby preventing its spread.

A similar virus causes monkeypox in primates in Central Africa. The virus of smallpox is now maintained in specific laboratories in order to differentiate such disorders as monkeypox from smallpox.

Mumps (Plate 4)

Cause

Virus infection.

Spread and incidence

By droplet infection through the respiratory tract. Mumps is predominantly seen in children between the ages of 5 and 15 years and also in young adults. Epidemics occur mainly in schools and institutions.

Incubation period

12–28 days.

Symptoms and signs

1. In some cases the first sign of the disease may be the swollen face. Usually, however, the initial symptoms of pyrexia, headache and sore throat occur a few days before the characteristic swelling of the parotid glands.

2. The enlarged parotid glands produce a swelling below the angle of the jaw and the skin over the glands becomes tense and shiny. One gland is usually enlarged for a short time before the other. There is often a complaint of pain while eating and it may be difficult to open the mouth.

3. The enlargement of the glands usually subsides within 7–10 days. The temperature falls when the glands begin to subside generally within a few days.

Complications

Orchitis, or inflammation of the testis, is a well-recognized complication frequently seen in older children and adults. With the onset of orchitis, fever returns along with pain and swelling of the testis. Rare complications include mastitis (inflammation of the breast), oophoritis (inflammation of the ovary), pancreatitis and encephalitis.

Treatment

There is no specific treatment for mumps. Oral hygiene is important to prevent secondary infection. Children are nursed in bed till the temperature has subsided and are kept away from school until all the swelling has subsided. Adults, however, in view of the likelihood of complications, are usually kept in bed for a longer period until the parotid swelling has completely subsided. Aspirin or codeine may be needed to relieve pain. If chewing is difficult, a soft diet is given and fluid can be sucked through a straw.

If orchitis develops, testicular support and cortisone or related steroids often bring about rapid relief of the swelling and pain.

Prevention

A live vaccine given in combination with measles and rubella in the second year of life is useful,

Influenza

Cause

Infection by a virus, of which there are several different strains.

Spread and incidence

By droplet infection. Influenza is a highly infectious disease. It occurs throughout the world in widespread epidemics, which vary considerably both in their clinical picture and fatality rates. Pandemics (world-wide epidemics), with a very high mortality rate, also occur occasionally; the last one occurred in 1918, when large numbers died. In localized outbreaks influenza is fairly mild.

Incubation period

1–3 days.

Symptoms and signs

1. The onset is usually sudden, with symptoms similar to those of the common cold or an acute bronchitis. The symptoms tend to vary, however, with different epidemics.
2. The general constitutional upset is more severe than one would expect with an ordinary cold. Headache, chills and lethargy are common.
3. A cough, sneezing, running eyes and nose, and laryngitis are usual symptoms.
4. Nausea, vomiting and abdominal pains are a feature of some outbreaks.

Complications

Bronchopneumonia is the most important complication and is responsible for many mortalities. The pneumonia is usually caused by secondary infection with such organisms as the influenza bacilli, streptococci and staphylococci. Elderly people are more prone to develop pneumonia.

Treatment

All patients are best nursed in bed with the usual nursing care for a fever case. Isolation is often not possible owing to the rapidity of development of the disease and the difficulty of early diagnosis.

There is no specific treatment for influenza. Aspirin or codeine is useful for the headache. Penicillin or other antibiotics are usually given for the treatment of secondary infections. As the immunity to influenza lasts for a short period recurrent attacks are not unusual.

Prevention

Vaccines are available against some strains of influenza. They offer partial immunity for some months and are of limited value when there is an epidemic.

Glandular fever (infectious mononucleosis)

Cause

Virus infection (Epstein–Barr virus).

Spread and incidence

By droplet infection and direct contact. Predominantly seen in children and adolescents of either sex. It occurs both sporadically and in epidemics.

Incubation period

5–10 days.

Symptoms and signs

1. The onset is usually gradual with general malaise, tiredness, loss of appetite and rise of temperature.

2. In some cases there is a sore throat, which may be covered with exudate. A measles type of rash may develop.

3. The lymph glands become enlarged, usually after a few weeks. The cervical glands are particularly enlarged but axillary and inguinal glands are also affected. The spleen enlarges.

4. Blood examination reveals an increased number of white cells (leucocytosis), and especially the monocytes hence the name *mononucleosis*. There are also unusual forms of lymphocytes which the pathologist can recognize as typical of this virus infection.

5. The diagnosis can be confirmed by an agglutination test called the *Paul-Bunnell test*, though this is not always positive.

Course and treatment

Patients should be kept in bed while the temperature is raised. Unfortunately many patients continue to feel unwell and tired for several weeks or even months, with occasional fever. There is no specific remedy and simple analgesic remedy is used to relieve discomfort in the upper respiratory tract.

Typhoid fever

Cause

Salmonella typhi.

Spread and incidence

Typhoid fever is spread mainly through the contamination of water, milk, or food with sewage. Human carriers excrete the organisms in the faeces or urine, and if proper hygiene and sanitation are lacking, contamination of water or food results. For this reason typhoid fever is particularly likely to arise in armies during times of war and also in areas where there is inadequate sanitation.

Incubation period

Usually 10–14 days.

Pathology

The bacilli enter the blood stream from the bowel and cause septicaemia with fever. They settle mainly in the small intestine where they cause inflammation leading to ulcers. Bacteria may also invade the gall bladder (which is a source of chronic excretion of bacilli), and the bones, sometimes forming abscesses. The heart may be affected by bacterial toxins.

Symptoms and signs

1. The onset is gradual with headaches, slowly rising fever and marked malaise. The pulse may be slow in relation to the temperature.

2. The abdomen may be distended and tender. Constipation is often present in the early stage.

3. Usually after a week, diarrhoea supervenes with frequent watery motions ('pea soup' stools) sometimes streaked with blood. The patient at this stage has a high temperature and is dehydrated and exhausted. He may lapse into a comatose confused state.

4. A rash usually appears on the abdomen, consisting of small round red areas ('rose spots').

5. Complications are common in the untreated case. Haemorrhage from the bowel, intestinal perforation, bronchopneumonia and heart failure can lead to a fatal termination.

Diagnosis

1. *Blood culture.* The bacilli circulate in the blood stream during the first week. In suspected cases, several blood specimens should be sent to

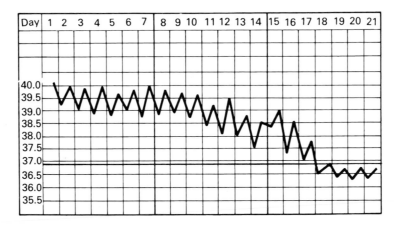

Fig. 4.1 Temperature chart from a case of uncomplicated typhoid fever, not treated with chloramphenicol. The temperature became normal on the 18th day.

the laboratory for culture and identification of the typhoid bacilli if present.

2. *Widal test.* Antibodies to typhoid bacilli develop in the blood and are present in appreciable amounts after the first week of the infection. These antibodies can be measured by the Widal reaction and confirm the diagnosis if they have increased over the first week. There is a difficulty. Antibodies are induced in any person who has been vaccinated against typhoid and this fact has to be borne in mind in interpreting the result.

3. *Stool examination.* Specimens sent in the third and fourth weeks usually show a positive growth on culture.

4. *Blood count.* A decrease in the number of neutrophils is observed (*neutropenia*).

Treatment

Typhoid cases must be nursed in isolation with strict barrier nursing and disposable eating utensils, urinals and bedpans are advisable. Suitable disinfectants should be added to excreta, and the nurse should wear gloves and a gown when attending to the patient.

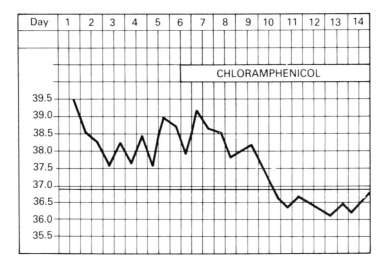

Fig. 4.2 Temperature chart from a case of typhoid fever showing the response to chloramphenicol.

Chloramphenicol is a very effective antibiotic in the treatment of typhoid fever and is given by mouth in capsule form 0.5 g every 6 hours for a week or more. Prolonged treatment with chloramphenicol may give rise to agranulocytosis (absence of white cells), so other drugs have been tried such as ampicillin and co-trimoxazole (see pp. 12 and 39).

Carriers

Some people harbour typhoid bacilli in the bowel or in the gall-bladder without any detriment to their own health. However, they may be a great danger to others and, particularly if they are employed in handling food, can cause an outbreak of typhoid fever. Treatment with an antibiotic if often effective in clearing the infection, but sometimes a cholecystectomy (removal of gallbladder) is necessary. Carriers should be warned of the danger they can bring to others if strict personal hygiene is not observed; indeed, carriers are forbidden by law from handling food on sale to the public.

Prevention

An active immunity to typhoid fever can be created by means of the highly effective vaccine available. It is necessary, however, to revaccinate once a year if an effective immunity is to be maintained. Vaccination against typhoid is usually practiced in any circumstances wherein the sanitation and hygiene are such that they cannot be relied upon to prevent the disease arising. For troops during war and for people who, because of travel, may be exposed to contaminated food or water, typhoid vaccination is essential.

Paratyphoid fevers

Paratyphoid fevers are caused by infection with the paratyphoid bacilli, referred to as *Salmonella paratyphi* A, B and C. These bacilli are very similar to the typhoid bacillus in their action. Paratyphoid fevers and typhoid fever are often grouped together under enteric fever. Typhoid fever, which was formerly the common type of enteric fever seen in Great Britain, is now less frequent; on the other hand, paratyphoid B infection is now more prevalent.

Paratyphoid infection tends to be much less severe and toxic than typhoid, but the general symptoms and treatment are similar. The exact diagnosis of the specific organism causing the enteric fever can be made on bacteriological examination.

Bacillary dysentery

Cause

Shigella bacillus, of which there are several types, including *Shigella sonnei*, *Shigella flexneri* and *Shigella shiga*.

Spread and incidence

The method of spread of the disease is similar to that of enteric fever. The bacilli are excreted in the faeces, and through defective sanitation and bad hygiene, food and water can then become contaminated. Flies, too, frequently cause contamination of food and are a prevalent mode of spread of the disease.

Although dysentery is common in tropical countries it is becoming more frequent in the UK, especially in camps, nurseries and large institutions subject to overcrowding. *Sonnei* infections in children are commonly seen in this country, while *flexneri* dysentery, which usually occurs in adults, is less common but more severe. The most virulent infections are caused by the *shiga* bacilli, but these are rarely seen outside the tropics.

Pathology

There is an acute inflammation of the large intestine with ulceration in severe cases.

Symptoms and signs

In *sonnei* dysentery in children the disease is usually mild, with few constitutional symptoms and slight fever. The predominant feature is diarrhoea, with the passage of blood and mucus

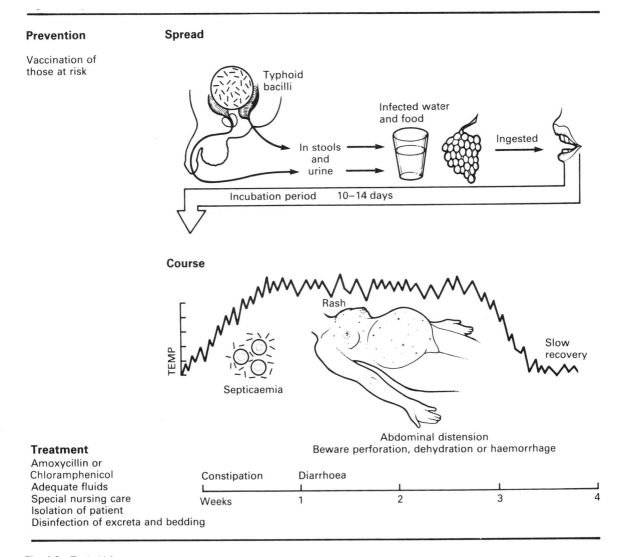

Prevention

Vaccination of
those at risk

Spread

Typhoid
bacilli

Infected water
and food

In stools
and
urine

Ingested

Incubation period   10–14 days

Course

TEMP

Rash

Septicaemia

Slow
recovery

Abdominal distension
Beware perforation, dehydration or haemorrhage

Treatment
Amoxycillin or
Chloramphenicol
Adequate fluids
Special nursing care
Isolation of patient
Disinfection of excreta and bedding

Constipation   Diarrhoea

Weeks   1   2   3   4

Fig. 4.3 Typhoid fever.

in the stools. The number of stools passed in the day rarely exceeds five or six. Slight abdominal colic is usually present.

In *flexneri* infections, toxaemia is more marked, associated with headache, loss of appetite, thirst and lassitude all present. Severe abdominal colic with the rapid onset of urgent diarrhoea are the main symptoms. As many as 15 to 20 stools a day may be passed. The typical stool is small and consists entirely of blood and mucus or muco-pus, without faecal matter. In severe cases shreds of mucous membrane are present. *Shiga* infec-

tions are usually accompanied by profound prostration and dehydration.

Diagnosis

Laboratory examination of the stools or of a rectal swab is carried out in all cases and usually reveals the causative organism.

Treatment

The usual nursing care and isolation precautions outlined under typhoid fever are necessary. The

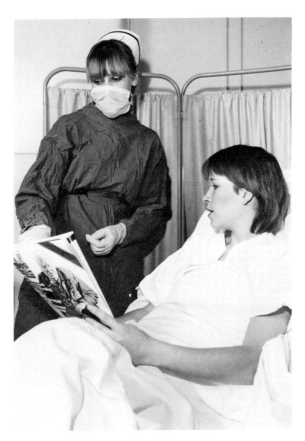

Fig. 4.4 Barrier nursing.

form of dysentery usually seen in the UK (i.e. due to *sonnei*) is highly infectious, and when dealing with the disease in children it is most important that different nurses should attend to the feeding and to changing of clothes etc. Disposable napkins should be used.

In the acute stage a fluid diet is given, but as soon as the stools become more solid, additions to the diet are quickly made in the form of soft, bland, low-residue foods. For severe cases, where dehydration is present, intravenous fluids may be necessary.

Ampicillin usually leads to a rapid improvement but occasionally resistant bacteria need an alternative antibiotic.

The patient is considered infectious until successive bacteriological examination of the stools are negative.

Food poisoning

Cause

Food poisoning is caused by the contamination of food with bacteria, or with the toxins of bacteria. The most common causes of food poisoning are the *Salmonella* group of bacilli and the toxins produced by *Staphylococcus*. The rare form of food poisoning known as botulism is caused by the botulinus toxin and is usually caused by the improper canning of foods.

Incubation period

Usually 24–36 hours.

Spread and incidence

Food poisoning may arise through contamination of food due to lack of proper hygiene in carriers. Animals such as rats and mice may also infect food. Foods such as reheated pies, cooked meats and duck eggs are particularly liable to contamination by *Salmonella* organisms, while cakes, custards and ham are most frequently infected by staphylococcal toxin.

Symptoms and signs

Food poisoning due to staphylococcal toxin causes a severe acute gastroenteritis with vomiting, abdominal colic and diarrhoea. These symptoms usually start within a few hours of the eating of the offending food. Usually all the people who eat the food are similarly affected.

Food poisoning caused by the *Salmonella* bacilli produces a picture similar to acute gastroenteritis. The onset, however, is not as rapid as in staphylococcal poisoning, since it takes 6–24 hours to develop, and the symptoms may persist for a longer period over several days.

In botulism the symptoms usually develop about 24 hours after the poisoned canned food was eaten. The predominating symptoms are various forms of paralysis; in most cases the outcome is fatal.

Diagnosis

The diagnosis of food poisoning can be made

when vomiting, abdominal pain and diarrhoea occur in several people after they have consumed food from the same source. Dysentery, which also causes abdominal colic and diarrhoea, is differentiated from food poisoning by the absence of vomiting and the presence of blood in the stools, which is rarely observed in food poisoning.

Treatment

Most patients with food poisoning recover fairly rapidly following rest in bed and a fluid diet.

In staphylococcal cases which do not respond to treatment rapidly, erythromycin or terramycin, may be used with some effect. In *Salmonella* food poisoning there is no specific therapy, but chloramphenicol or the tetracycline antibiotics may be of value in some cases.

Preventive treatment is important and entails the proper handling and storage of all foods. Adequate hygienic measures must be employed in all kitchens, and food should be stored out of reach of flies, rats and mice. In addition, people handling food must be free from any infection.

TROPICAL DISEASES

With the widespread use of international air travel, diseases previously found commonly in tropical or subtropical areas are now appearing in the UK as well.

Malaria

Malaria is one of the commonest diseases in tropical countries and is responsible for much ill health and many deaths each year.

Cause

It is caused by a parasite, *Plasmodium*, of which there are several species – *vivax, ovale, malariae* and *falciparum.*

Spread and incidence

The disease is spread by the bite of the female *Anopheles* mosquito which acts as a vector. It can also spread transplacentally or via transfusions. Malaria occurs throughout the tropical areas and can be imported into temperate regions by tourists, business travellers or immigrants.

Incubation period

12–28 days, depending on the species causing the disease.

Life cycle of the parasite

All species undergo a complex life cycle, with division and cyst formation. Part of this life cycle takes place in the blood cells and liver of a human (asexual cycle), and part in the stomach and salivary glands of the *Anopheles* mosquito (sexual cycle). When the infected anopheles mosquito bites a human, the parasite is introduced into the blood stream and causes malaria. At the same time, when the mosquito sucks infected blood from a man with malaria the parasite completes the other part of the cycle in the mosquito.

Symptoms and signs

Of the four different species of plasmodia, the two common types give rise to benign and malignant varieties of the disease. Tertian malaria is characterized by recurrent bouts of high fever occurring every third day. This fever is accompanied by severe rigors, profuse sweating, prostrating headaches, and vomiting. The attack then subsides and the temperature becomes normal for a few days until the next attack.

In malignant tertian malaria, the parasite can invade the brain, leading to convulsions, coma and death.

Treatment

In areas where malaria is rife, suppressive therapy to protect against an attack of malaria should be given. From the 17th century until modern times Cinchona bark or quinine has been the traditional remedy, but this has now been largely replaced by more effective drugs. Chloroquine is currently the drug of choice in an acute attack and can be combined with Primaquine to treat *vivax* and *ovale* malariae. In cases of chloroquine resistance, drugs with a quinine base along with Fansidar is useful.

For those entering an area where malaria may be present, it is important to take preventive tablet treatment (Proguanil (Paludrine) 100 mg daily) during the stay and for 4 weeks after returning home.

Prevention

1. Measures must be taken to prevent the breeding of *Anopheles* mosquitoes by drainage of stagnant water or larviciding pools that do not drain.
2. Protective measures must be observed by people against mosquito bites such as sleeping under nets and wearing protective clothing.
3. Insistence that visitors to malarial areas take preventive tablets before, during and after their visit.

Amoebiasis

Cause

Amoebiasis is caused by a parasite (*Entamoeba histolytica*).

Spread and incidence

The disease spreads from the consumption of contaminated vegetables and water. The motile parasite is found in the stool of the infected patient but the cyst is the infective form. The disease is seen worldwide, particularly in places with low standards of sanitation.

Incubation period

14–28 days.

Pathology

The parasite invades the colonic mucosa and causes multiple flaskshaped ulcers. The disease can spread to the liver causing an abscess or can result in an amoeboma which consists of granulation tissue with a few amoebae.

Symptoms and signs

Characterized by abdominal discomfort and frequent loose stools containing blood and mucus. The condition can become severe with dehydration, anaemia and septicaemia. Sigmoidoscopy reveals the typical scattered ulcers surrounded by mucosal erythema. Chronic cases are characterised by loss of weight, malaise and intermittent episodes of diarrhoea.

In amoebic liver abscess pain is a significant feature with fever, sweats, lethargy and anorexia. The liver becomes enlarged and tender.

Complications

Extension of the abscess to the brain can occur and the skin around the perianal region may be involved with resultant local ulceration. The liver abscess can rupture into the chest cavity.

Diagnosis

A fresh stool specimen is examined under the microscope and the diagnosis can be made by identifying the entamoeba.

In cases of amoeboma cysts may be found in the stools. In amoebic liver abscess liver function tests are altered (example, high bilirubin and alkaline phosphatase levels and low plasma albumin levels). Imaging techniques such as ultrasound and computerised tomography can be used to localise the abscess or cyst from which the fluid can be aspirated to study the resolution following treatment.

Treatment

Metronidazole or tinidazole is effective treatment for amoebic dysentery and should be given by mouth. It is also effective for amoebic hepatitis but when abscess formation has occurred, surgical drainage may be necessary.

Prevention

1. Untreated water should be boiled and filtered before consumption.
2. Safe disposal of sanitary waste should be practiced.

3. Cyst passers should be treated with Dilox-anide furoate and metronidazole.

Cholera

Cholera can be an extremely severe and some-times fatal disease seen in the tropics.

Cause

A bacillus (*Vibrio cholerae* or *Vibrio el tor*).

Spread and incidence

Infection is spread through contamination of water in particular, and food. The disease still occurs in endemic form in tropical countries.

Incubation period

1–2 days.

Pathogenesis

The cholera bacillus secretes an exotoxin which binds to the surface of the intestinal cells. The intestine becomes a site of net secretion of isotonic fluid containing sodium, chloride, bicar-bonate and water. Up to one litre can be secreted in an hour in severe cases. The effect of the toxin lasts for 3–4 days (i.e. lifespan of the intestinal epithelial cell) and the cycle recurs. The *el tor* biotype causes a milder form of the illness.

Symptoms and signs

1. Vomiting starts in the first 24 hours, fol-lowed by sudden diarrhoea.
2. The typical 'rice-water' stools free of faecal matter are characteristic of cholera. The *el tor* biotype causes a less severe diarrhoea.
3. As dehydration progresses features of iso-tonic fluid depletion supervene such as increased thirst, sunken eyes, loss of skin turgor, dry mucosae, muscle cramps, a rapid thready pulse and reduced urine output.

Diagnosis

In severe cases a clinical diagnosis is possible based on rapid progression to dehydration in endemic areas. In milder forms stool examination by culture or dark ground microscopy to demon-strate the typical motility of *V. cholerae* is re-quired.

Treatment

Moderate dehydration can be managed with oral rehydration solutions. Severe cases need intrave-nous infusions such as Ringer's lactate to restore the lost blood volume. Tetracycline reduces the duration of diarrhoea and decreases the faecal excretion of the bacilli.

Prevention and control

A clean water supply and the safe disposal of faecal waste are essential prerequisites for ade-quate control of the disease in an endemic area. Education of the population relating infective diarrhoeal diseases to personal and general sani-tation practices is useful to prevent recurrence.

A vaccine can be used for those at risk. Booster doses are required every 6 months for people in endemic areas and travellers.

Typhus fever

Cause

Included in the term *typhus fever* are many different forms, all of which are caused by a group of organisms called Rickettsiae.

Spread and incidence

These organisms are found in rats and other rodents, and are conveyed to man through the bites of lice, fleas, ticks and mites. The forms of typhus which are spread by lice and rat fleas are especially prone to occur in overcrowded camps and institutions where there is a lack of proper hygiene. Different forms of typhus are seen in different parts of the world under the names of tropical scrub typhus, Rocky Mountain spotted fever (America, Canada), Q fever (Australia, America), Scrub typhus (Asia) and Trench fever (Africa and Central America).

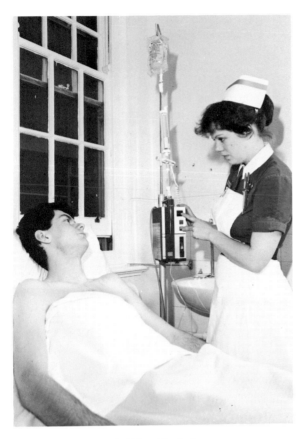

Fig. 4.5 Intravenous fluid for dehydration.

Incubation period

10–14 days.

Symptoms and signs

The severity of the different forms varies in different outbreaks from a mild to a fatal disease. The characteristics of most forms consist of a sudden abrupt high fever (40°C), severe toxaemia and a purpuric rash which spreads initially on the axillary folds and the trunk and then spreads to the limbs. The fever usually runs a course of 2–3 weeks. Haemorrhagic manifestations and hypotension lead to renal involvement with a reduced urine output.

Diagnosis

The clinical features are diagnostic and can be confirmed by serological tests using group-specific rickettsial antigens.

Treatment

The specific treatment of typhus consists of the administration of one of the tetracycline antibiotics or chloramphenicol, which have a rapid effect in most cases.

Prevention and control

General nursing care is very important in order to maintain the patient's resistance. Strict measures are necessary to prevent the nurse and other patients being bitten by lice or fleas. Thorough delousing of all patients is necessary.

Thorough and regular washing of clothes in hot water with detergent kills lice and their eggs.

Plague

Cause

A bacillus found in rats (*Yersinia pestis*).

Spread and incidence

Plague is a highly infectious and often fatal disease seen in tropical areas. It often occurs in widespread epidemics. The infection can be conveyed to man by the bite of the rat flea (*Xenopsylla cheopis*).

Incubation period

2–8 days.

Symptoms and signs

The *bubonic* form of the disease starts with a systemic upset fever, chills and headache. Within 24 hours the patient finds a 'bubo' (swelling of the lymph glands), usually in the groin, which is very tender. Severe cases manifest with hypotension and shock.

The *pneumonic* variety results from spread of the organisms to the lungs. Cough, chest pain and blood in the sputum (haemoptysis) are usual features. A severe bronchopneumonia may result.

Diagnosis

The organism can be isolated from material aspirated from a bubo and stained or cultured in standard media to confirm the diagnosis.

Treatment

Streptomycin is effective, and tetracycline and chloramphenicol are alternative choices along with the routine nursing care of a severe infectious fever case.

Prevention and control

In preventing the spread of infection the suppression of rats and their eradication is important. Vector (flea) control using insecticides helps in minimizing the transmission in towns and cities.

Leprosy

Cause

A bacillus (*Mycobacterium leprae*).

Spread and incidence

Droplet infection from upper respiratory tract. It is a disease found in tropical and subtropical areas with high ambient temperature and has almost completely disappeared from Europe.

Incubation period

60 days to 2 years.

Pathogenesis

The mycobacterium affects cutaneous nerves over the face and the upper and lower limbs in areas where the nerves are close to the skin and therefore cooler (i.e. posterior aspect of the elbow and the knee). The infection leads to indeterminate leprosy which then progresses depending on the hypersensitivity reaction to one of three types – tuberculoid, borderline or lepromatous leprosy.

Symptoms and signs

Tuberculoid leprosy is characterized by a hypopigmented hairless anaesthetic lesions. Single lesions are usual and are observed over the extensor regions of the arm, elbow and knee. It is a chronic disease mainly affecting the skin and nerves. The face especially becomes thickened and nodular. Affection of the nerves causes loss of sensation leading to trophic ulcers. Acute reactions characterized by inflammation and oedema of the skin lesions with increased tenderness of the nerves are a feature of the lepromatous variety.

In advanced cases destruction of the bones of the nose and face develops and blindness may result.

Diagnosis

The clinical features are diagnostic in advanced cases. In cases with early skin lesions a skin smear taken from the edge of the lesions or from the ear lobe may show the presence of the bacillus.

Treatment

Multidrug therapy is the rule and medication needs to be supervized to ensure compliance. Tuberculoid leprosy is treated with rifampicin and dapsone for 6 months. The lepromatous type needs longer treatment (2 years) with rifampicin, dapsone and clofazamine. Acute reactions may need to be controlled by steroids.

Prevention and control

Education regarding the importance of continuous treatment is essential for full resolution of the disease. BCG vaccination has been shown to reduce the incidence of leprosy.

Brucellosis

Brucellosis, formerly known as undulant fever, is primarily an animal disease which is caused by infection with the Brucella organism (*Brucella abortus*), of which there are several types. The organisms are present in infected cows, pigs and goats, and the infection is carried to man through handling or ingestion of contaminated milk, cheese, meat, or pork. Farm workers and packing house employees are frequently affected.

The chief symptoms are a prolonged fever, often with few constitutional signs. Severe sweating and joint pains are a feature in many cases. The spleen is usually enlarged. The diagnosis is confirmed by finding the organisms in the blood (by means of a blood culture) or, more often, by an agglutination reaction similar to the Widal reaction of typhoid.

The specific treatment is the administration of one of the tetracycline antibiotics. Relapses are, however, commonly seen.

Yellow fever

Cause

A mosquito-borne RNA virus (Flaviviridae).

Spread and incidence

The disease is transmitted by a mosquito which acts as a vector. The fever is predominantly seen in West Africa and South America. The *Aedes* mosquito acts as the chief carrier.

Incubation period

3–6 days.

Pathogenesis

Following entry into the body by the mosquito bite the virus replicates in lymph nodes and large organs such as the liver and the kidney. The virus replicates rapidly and destroys the normal structure with resultant malfunction of the organs involved.

Symptoms and signs

It may start as a non-specific febrile illness with chills, headache, muscle ache (myalgia) and nausea which continues for several days. A brief remission is followed by relapse with increasing toxicity, vomiting, abdominal pain, dehydration and jaundice.

In severe cases shock, coma and convulsions precede death.

Diagnosis

Liver function tests are abnormal. The virus can be detected in the serum during the first few days by enzyme-linked immunosorbent assay (ELISA). Viral culture confirms the diagnosis.

Treatment

Supportive treatment is important and severe cases may require intensive fluid and electrolyte therapy.

Prevention

A live attenuated vaccine (a single 0.5 ml subcutaneous injection) called yellow fever 17D is useful and provides life-long immunity.

Japanese B encephalitis

Cause

A flavivirus (*Japanese B encephalitis virus*).

Spread and incidence

The infection is introduced by an infected mosquito (Culicine species). The disease occurs in epidemic and endemic forms throughout Asia.

Incubation period

7–14 days.

Pathogenesis

Following entry into the body the virus replicates at a high rate and enters the blood stream (*viraemia*) and localizes in the endothelial cells of the brain capillaries particularly the cerebral cortex, thalamus, basal ganglia and the brain stem.

Symptoms and signs

Non-specific flu-like symptoms like fever, headache, malaise and nausea last a few days. The neurological symptoms have a sudden onset with increasing headache and confusion. Seizures, neck stiffness and rigidity supervene.

In severe cases the patient is comatose with loss of sensation of the limbs (quadriparesis) or one half of the body (hemiparesis).

There is considerable mortality due to respiratory failure and uncontrolled convulsions. Some patients develop intellectual impairment, personality changes or epilepsy.

Diagnosis

A history of travel to endemic areas is significant. Cerebrospinal fluid examination for anti-Japanese encephalitis antibody can confirm the diagnosis.

Treatment

No specific antiviral therapy is available. Patients are managed by intensive respiratory care, control of convulsions and careful monitoring of fluid balance. Cases with high temperature may require prolonged use of antipyretics.

Prevention

Children and non-immune adults who are entering an endemic area should receive vaccination. Two doses of an inactivated mouse-brain preparation vaccine given subcutaneously one week apart, one month before travel provides adequate safety for 8–12 weeks.

SKIN AND SEXUALLY TRANSMITTED DISEASES

Ringworm infection

Cause

A dermatophyte infection (*Tinea*).

Spread and incidence

The dermatophytes (so called because they can digest keratin) belong to three genera. Man is host to some while others are incidental pathogens to man. The infection spreads in places where bathing facilities are shared.

Symptoms and signs

The characteristic annular lesion is usually present and associated clinical manifestations depend on the part of the body affected.

Tinea pedis This is an infection of the feet, common in males. A unilateral itchy, inflamed, fissured and moist toe space is usually the presenting feature although a vesicular pattern involving the instep or the sides of the toes may also occur.

Tinea cruris infects the groin and adjacent areas and is more common in males. Itching is usual and inflammation with a well-defined margin with a central clear area may be observed.

Tinea corporis is of animal origin and the lesions are multiple and present all over the body, though not always ring-shaped.

Tinea capitis may be secondary to any of the species and involves the scalp and hair. Affected hairs break off just above the scalp, producing a short stubble. There may be a marked degree of inflammation resulting in a lesion-like a boil, called *kerion*. Tinea can also affect the hands and nails.

Diagnosis

The typical lesions can be modified by the use of steroids and may be difficult to diagnose based only on clinical features. Microscopic examination of the scrapings. The fungi can be grown in Subaroud's medium.

Treatment

Topical anti-fungal agents such as Whitfield's ointment and the imidazoles are useful in localised infections. Oral griseofulvin is the treatment of choice for hair, nail, widespread skin and chronic infections. A weak topical steroid is indicated in cases with inflammation.

Candidiasis

Cause

The infection is caused by a yeast (*Candida albicans*).

Spread

The yeast is a commensal (normally present without causing disease) in the intestine, mouth and the vagina. It may become pathogenic when topical steroids are used for long periods or in cases of use of immunosuppressives, oral contraceptives, systemic steroids, broad-spectrum antibiotics and in the extremes of age.

Symptoms and signs

Candidiasis can present in several ways depending on the area of infection. White patches present on the oral mucosa can be scraped off to reveal inflamed mucous membrane (*thrush*). Soreness and fissuring at the angles of the mouth results in angular stomatitis. Sore, red marginated skin with pustules is termed intertrigo. Anogenital areas can become itchy and sore with a curd-like discharge (*vulvovaginitis*) or show tiny red papules and pustules on the glans and prepuce of the penis (*balanitis*). Involvement of the nail leads to a painful swollen nail bed (*paronychia*).

Diagnosis

This is usually based on clinical findings and a history of the predisposing factors.

Treatment

Any remediable predisposing factors must be dealt with to avoid recurrence. Locally active agents include nystatin, amphotericin B and the imidazoles. In cases of vaginal thrush treatment of sexual partners is important.

Pityriasis versicolor

Cause

A commensal yeast (*Pityrosporum orbiculare*).

Spread and incidence

An altered immune status changing the pathogenicity of the surface commensal seen in the tropics and subtropics.

Symptoms and signs

Usually seen in young adults as distinctive hypo- and hyperpigmentation over the upper trunk, arms and neck. Lesions are sharply demarcated and scaly.

Diagnosis

Scrapings show clustered spherical yeasts under the microscope.

Treatment

2.5% Selenium sulphide usually clears the condition.

Syphilis

Cause

A spirochaete (*Treponema pallidum*).

Spread and incidence

It occurs in all parts of the world and is transmitted during sexual intercourse with an infected person. It can also be transmitted to the foetus via the placenta from an infected mother.

Incubation period

7–90 days.

Symptoms and signs

These can be described in four stages:

1. In the primary stage a firm, painless ulcer, called a *chancre*, appears on the penis in the male or the labia in the female. The chancre may bleed easily and gives rise to painful enlargement of the inguinal lymph glands. Occasionally this primary sore appears on the lips, the breasts or the fingers. It usually occurs about a month after the intercourse and takes a few weeks to heal. Unless treated it is followed by:

2. The secondary stage, usually a few weeks after the appearance of the chancre. There may be generalized enlargement of the lymph glands, general malaise, mild fever and a skin rash. The

rash usually appears on the trunk, it is ham-coloured and does not itch.

3. The late tertiary stage is characterized by the gumma which is a punched-out lesion. Involvement of the bones and joints lead to fractures and joint destruction.

4. The quaternary stage. Some years after the original infection, serious constitutional effects may occur, including involvement of the aorta which may lead to aortic aneurysm and aortic regurgitation (see p. 102), and involvement of the spinal cord leading to tabes dorsalis of the central nervous system (p. 206).

Congenital syphilis

Syphilis may be transmitted to the fetus by an infected mother. If the baby is born alive, it may develop disorders of growth, of the eyes or of the nervous system.

Diagnosis

In the primary stage, dark ground microscopy of a scraping from the chancre may reveal the presence of the spirochaete.

Reliable blood tests are available to establish the diagnosis. The older tests (Wasserman and Kahn) are not specific for syphilis and although positive in syphilis, usually give rise to false positives (i.e. positive in other diseases).

More specific tests such as the TPI (*Treponema pallidum* immobilization test) should be performed if the WR (Wasserman reaction) is positive. Late stages require serological testing such as the VDRL test and the *Treponema pallidum* haemagglutination assay (TPHA) or the fluorescent treponema antibody absorption (FTA-abs) test.

Cerebrospinal fluid examination is required if neurosyphilis is suspected.

Treatment

Procaine penicillin given daily for 14–21 days by intramuscular injection is successful treatment both to cure the disease in the primary and secondary stages and to arrest the damage and promote healing in the tertiary stage. Oxytetra-cycline can be given to patients sensitive to penicillin.

Careful supervision and follow-up is necessary until the blood tests show that the infection has been safely overcome.

It is important to examine the sexual partner when possible to avoid re-infection.

Non-specific urethritis

This is common in young men and is due to a non-gonococcal infection of the urethra, perhaps in some cases to an unidentified virus. The symptoms are those of frequency of micturition, burning discomfort on passing water and a mucopurulent urethral discharge. These features are sometimes associated with conjunctivitis and acute arthritis, and this condition is termed *Reiter's syndrome*.

Although the symptoms subside after a few weeks, they frequently recur and the joints can become chronically inflamed.

Tetracycline is often prescribed but the response is not consistent and alternative antibiotics may be needed. Female partners should also be treated due to the risk of pelvic inflammatory disease.

Gonorrhoea

Cause

A gonococcus (*Neisseria gonorrhoeae*).

Spread and incidence

Gonorrhoeal infection in the adult results from sexual intercourse with an infected person resulting in acute and chronic disorders.

Incubation period

7–10 days.

Symptoms and signs

Acute gonorrhoea The main lesions in acute gonorrhoea are as follows:

1. Acute inflammation of the urethra (acute urethritis) in the male and of the cervix of the uterus in the female. This inflammation causes a thick, purulent, yellow discharge often combined with painful micturition, and is the predominating sign of gonorrhoea.

2. The inflammation often spreads to neighbouring organs, causing prostatitis and epididymoorchitis in the male, and salpingitis and oophoritis in the female. The latter leads to pelvic peritonitis. Blood-stream infection develops in some cases, resulting in:

  a. Septicaemia, with the organisms growing in the blood. This may lead to infective bacterial endocarditis and meningitis.
  b. Acute septic arthritis ('gonococcal rheumatism').
  c. Inflammation of the eyes – iritis and conjunctivitis are common.

Chronic gonorrhoea In the late stages the common results of gonorrhoea are a urethral stricture and chronic prostatitis with prostatic abscess in the male, and chronic salpingitis with sterility in the female.

Gonococcal ophthalmia of infants (ophthalmia neonatorum) An acute inflammation of the eyes may result in an infant due to contamination during birth in cases where the mother suffers from acute gonorrhoea.

Complications

Severe conjunctivitis, iritis and corneal ulceration can result and lead to blindness. The presenting sign is a discharge from the eyes in a newborn infant. This may, however, be caused by other organisms, but in all cases swabs obtained from the eyes are necessary to establish the causative organism.

Diagnosis

Microscopic examination of smears (for example from the endocervix in infected females) shows pus cells and intra- and extracellular Gram-negative diplococci.

Treatment

Prophylactic treatment Antenatal care, by de-

tecting cases of active gonorrhoea, is an important practice in the prevention of gonococcal ophthalmia of infants.

Curative treatment Most cases of acute gonorrhoea respond to one or two injections of procaine penicillin with probenescid. In the chronic stages, penicillin in larger doses given for a longer period is also very effective. In cases of penicillin resistance kanamycin is useful.

In the chronic stage, a urethral stricture may require dilatation with bougies.

For infants with ophthalmia, penicillin is effective. If only one eye is affected the good eye must be protected by a shield (*Buller's shield*) and the infant is made to lie on the affected side.

Proper isolation of all cases of active acute gonorrhoea is important. Care must be taken in handling dressings and soiled linen since most discharges contain the infective organisms.

All cases of discharge from the eyes in newborn infants must be treated with strict isolation measures as infection can spread rapidly to other infants. It should be borne in mind that eye discharges can also occur in infants due to infection by other organisms such as the streptococci or staphylococci. These cases are also extremely infectious and must be treated with strict isolation techniques to prevent spread of infection.

AIDS (acquired immune deficiency syndrome)

Cause

A virus (human immunodeficiency virus; HIV).

Spread and incidence

The condition is transmitted through the blood of an infected person. It is spread from a homosexual to another from blood in the anal region during intercourse as well as in heterosexuals. It occurs in drug addicts who use a non-sterile needle infected by the virus from a previous user. It can also occur in haemophiliacs who need repeated blood transfusions and receive infected blood. Cases have been reported in which the virus appears to have spread from cuts or sores in people living in crowded and insanitary conditions.

The disease can be distinguished as progressing in distinct stages with characteristic manifestations:

Primary HIV infection

The period between infection and development of detectable levels of antibody to HIV is variable – 2 to 6 months. A small percentage may remain negative for a longer period. Clinical manifestations appear with a positive antibody test in 50% of cases.

Approximately 50% develop an acute illness distinguished by frequent oral and oesophageal ulceration; a maculo-papular rash, which may become generalized, on the trunk and generalized enlargement of the lymph glands.

Conventional HIV antibody tests become positive 2–6 weeks after the onset of the illness. Biopsy of the enlarged lymph glands show preserved architecture with infiltration of CD8+ lymphocytes.

Early HIV disease

Once the individual recovers from the early illness described above they enter a so-called 'asymptomatic phase' characterized by mild symptoms. Generalized lymph node enlargement is associated with unpredictable and irregular fever. Hypersensitive reactions may develop with worsening of previous eczema or folliculitis.

The HIV virus may be detectable in the plasma. There is an increase in the levels of immunoglobulins (IgG and IgA) and the numbers of CD8+ cells increases.

Intermediate stage (AIDS-related complex)

The patient is more susceptible to pathogens and the patient may manifest infections secondary to pneumococcus, *Shigella*, *Salmonella* or *Haemophilus*. Vaginal thrush and pelvic inflammatory disease are common. Childhood exanthemas are more serious and Kaposi's sarcoma may occur at this stage.

The HIV virus is easier to isolate from the plasma, and the delayed-type hypersensitivity reactions to common antigens such as mumps virus, diphtheria and tuberculin are lost.

Late phase of HIV infection

Opportunistic infections The late phase is a stage of severe immune deficiency and infected individuals become easily susceptible to infections – *opportunistic infections*. Depending on the level of CD4+ lymphocytes, a hierarchy of opportunistic infections can occur.

At cell levels of less than $300/\mu l$ tuberculosis and syphilis may be reactivated; at levels below $200/\mu l$ pneumonia due to *Pneumocystis carinii*, and fungal infections are common. At low levels of immunity – 50 cell/μl gastrointestinal disease and cytomegalovirus infection may supervene.

Infection of the CNS A dementing illness may manifest, and spinal cord involvement may result in muscle weakness.

Kaposi's sarcoma This infection is more common and aggressive in this late stage. It produces purplish tumours that may affect any organ, typically the skin. This is more common in homosexuals with multiple partners.

Prognosis

The conventional measure of prognosis is the time from infection to development of an AIDS-defining condition such as an opportunistic infection. The prognosis is also dependent on geographical location, life-style, cultural practices, housing and health-care facilities.

Five years following exposure, 15% will have progressed and half as many may have died. Ten years after exposure 50% will have progressed to advanced stages and 80% of them would have succumbed.

A number of predictors of progression have been defined. For example, a consistent predictor of the risk of progression is the level of CD4+ lymphocytes. The lower the counts the greater the chance of progressing to an advanced stage. Oral thrush is a strong predictor and approximately doubles the chances of progression.

Medical intervention

This can be divided into three categories:

1. anti-retroviral therapy (especially the use of zidovudine)
2. prophylactic therapy against *Pneumocystis carinii* infection
3. ancillary care, including earlier diagnosis and better symptomatic treatment of opportunistic infections.

Zidovudine may prolong survival by, on average, over 2 years. The advantage of survival is greater if the therapy is started before AIDS has developed.

Disease in the returned traveller

Fever

Many individuals feel warm and feverish after return from a tropical country. Individuals with a definite raised body temperature need to be investigated further.

Malaria

Falciparum malaria is an important infection which can present within 1 month or invariably within 2 months after returning from the tropics. Paroxysmal fever associated with rigors is usual in vivax malaria and can occur up to 2 years after leaving an endemic area.

Typhoid fever

Symptoms due to typhoid fever begin within 3 weeks of return. Initial symptoms may be non-specific, such as cough, headache and mild malaise. Blood cultures are essential to establish the diagnosis.

Amoebiasis

Fever is invariably present, and if the cause is not easily detectable, serological testing for antibodies to *Entamoeba histolytica* is advisable in individuals who have visited the tropics or subtropics in the preceding year. There may be pain in the right upper abdomen.

Jaundice

Travellers who develop jaundice within 2 months of leaving various parts of the world with low standards of hygiene are presumed to have hepatitis A. Other causes are falciparum malaria, non-A non-B hepatitis, leptospirosis and secondary syphilis. The latter causes are usually associated with significant fever compared to that observed in hepatitis A.

Lassa fever

Symptoms begin within about 3 weeks after leaving the savannah region of West Africa. History of travel associated with fever without a definite cause should be referred to a specialist tropical disease hospital for further investigation.

Table 4.1 Recommended immunization and prophylaxis for travellers

	Essential	Recommended
Southern Europe		#
Central and South America	+ ○	* #
Middle East		* #
India and Pakistan	1	* #
South East Asia	+	* #
China		* #
North Africa		* #
West Africa	+ ○	* #
East and Central Africa	2	* #

1 = malaria prophylaxis: chloroquine only; 2 = malaria prophylaxis: mefloquine 250 mg/week; + = malaria prophylaxis: chloroquine 300 mg/week and proguanil 200 mg/day; # = polio; * = typhoid; ○ = yellow fever.

Table 4.2 Precautions against diseases while abroad

Disease	Vectors	Precautions
Hepatitis B, HIV	Blood	Injection with unused needle
Dysentery Enteric fever Hepatitis A Traveller's diarrhoea	Contaminated water and food	Consume pure water (boiling/iodination); peel fruits and wash salads in pure water
Malaria	Mosquitoes	Use insect repellants; wear protective clothing; use mosquito nets
Rabies	Domestic dogs	Avoid contact with animals
Sexually transmitted diseases (Hepatitis A, HIV)	Human	Avoid new sexual contacts and prostitutes

5

Diseases of the circulatory system

ANATOMY AND PHYSIOLOGY

The heart is a muscular pump which propels the blood throughout the body, and the arteries are the pipelines by means of which fresh blood is carried to all organs and tissues. Used blood is returned to the heart in the veins. The blood in the arteries has been oxygenated in the lungs and supplies the tissues with oxygen necessary for metabolism. Arterial blood is bright red because of its oxygen content. The blood in the veins contains carbon dioxide, the waste product of metabolism, and venous blood is darker in colour than arterial blood because of the lack of oxygen in it. The exchange of oxygen for carbon dioxide takes place while the blood is in a fine network of vessels, called capillaries, which connect arteries with veins.

THE CIRCULATION

The right ventricle drives venous blood through the lungs to be oxygenated. The left ventricle propels fresh oxygenated blood through the body. This continuous process is known as the circulation.

   1. The left ventricle drives fresh oxygenated blood through the aortic valve, into the aorta and thence in the arteries to all parts of the body.
   2. Arterial blood supplies oxygen to the tissues in exchange for carbon dioxide and is then returned by the veins to the right atrium.
   3. Venous blood from the right atrium passes through the tricuspid valve into the right ventricle.
   4. The right ventricle drives the venous blood

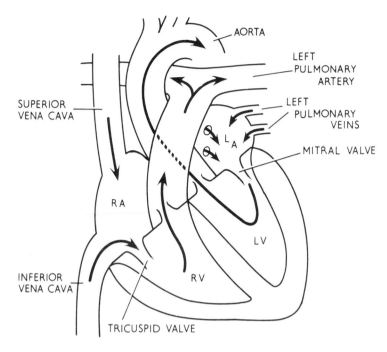

Fig. 5.1 Diagram of the circulation. (RA = right atrium; LA = left atrium; RV = right ventricle; LV = left ventricle)

through the pulmonary valve into the pulmonary arteries and so through the lungs.

5. Blood having been oxygenated by the lungs is carried by the pulmonary veins to the left atrium.

6. Oxygenated blood from the left atrium passes through the mitral valve to the left ventricle.

The heart cycle is divided into two periods – systole and diastole. The systolic period is when the heart is contracting to propel the blood out into the arterial circulation. The right and left ventricles contract at the same time. The pulmonary and aortic valves are open during systole to allow the blood to pass through. The atrioventricular valves (mitral and tricuspid), however, are closed. This is to prevent blood being forced back into the atria when the ventricles are contracting. When the ventricles cease to contract the period of rest or diastole begins. At this stage the pulmonary and aortic valves close to prevent regurgitation of blood back into the ventricles. On the other hand, the atrioventricular valves, which were closed during systole, now open to refill the empty ventricles in time for the next

systole of the heart. The function of the valves is, therefore, to prevent a backward flow of blood.

CONDUCTION SYSTEM

The heart normally beats at a regular rate, usually between 70 and 80 times a minute. There is a specialized mechanism in the heart which is responsible for the proper initiation and conduction of the electrical impulse which activates muscle contraction. The electrical impulse normally starts in the upper part of the right atrium, in what is called the sino-atrial (SA) node, or pacemaker of the heart. The normal rhythm is called sinus rhythm. The impulse quickly spreads out over both atria causing them to contract. The impulse then passes to a second area of specialized tissue known as the atrio-ventricular (AV) node, which lies close to the septum between the atria. From here the impulse passes to the ventricles by a special pathway in the ventricular septum called the 'bundle of His'. Other than this pathway, the atria are electrically insulated from the ventricles. The bundle of His divides up into two branches, right and left, to carry the impulse to both ventricles. The contraction of the ventricles is, therefore, normally controlled by an impulse which arises in the atria, thus causing the atria and ventricles to beat at the same rate and in regular sequence. When the conducting pathway is diseased, so that the passage of the impulse is interfered with, the atria and ventricles may cease to beat at the same rate. In extreme cases, where disease in the conducting pathway may completely block the passage of all impulses from the atria to the ventricles (complete heart block), the latter start to beat of their own accord and at their own rate. If this occurs, the ventricular rate is not around the usual 70 to 80 beats a minute, but is approximately 40 beats a minute.

The pacemaker of the heart (the sino-atrial node) is under the influence of two nerves, the vagus, which slows, and the sympathetic, which quickens the heart rate.

Electrocardiogram (ECG)

The spread of the electrical impulse, first from the sino-atrial node to the atrio-ventricular node and then through the bundle of His to the ventricles, is associated with changes in electrical voltage, which may be recorded.

The electrocardiogram is an instrument which records the electrical changes produced during the contraction and relaxation of the heart muscle as it beats. Electrodes are attached to the limbs and chest of the patient, and the electrical changes are amplified and recorded on a moving paper to yield a permanent tracing. The normal tracing shows characteristic waves, given letters to identify them. The first wave is called the 'P' wave and is associated with atrial contraction. This is followed by the 'QRS' complex associated with contraction of the ventricles. Finally, the 'T' wave is formed as the ventricle relaxes. Important information as to the heart's action can be gleaned from study of the electrocardiogram pattern, especially in disease.

SPECIAL CARDIAC INVESTIGATIONS

There are now many tests available, apart from

the ECG, which give detailed information of the heart's function and structure. Some of these require special instruments and techniques involving a specialist cardiac team. Invasive investigations may carry a very small risk and it is important that the benefits of the procedure outweigh the risks.

Phonocardiography

This means a method of recording visually heart sounds and added sounds such as murmurs so that the physician can analyse and interpret them in detail. Microphones are applied to the chest and the sounds are reproduced on a recorder. An electrocardiogram is taken at the same time so that the relation of the murmur to systole and diastole can be determined.

Echocardiograph

The heart contractions and the movement of the valves can be determined by photographing reflected sound waves. Using an ultrasound beam, the operator can take a recording of the pericardium, the walls of the ventricles and the valves. This technique can be used in the diagnosis of pericardial effusion, abnormalities of the ventricles or of mitral or aortic valve disease, as well as other conditions.

Cardiac catheterization

The cardiac catheter is introduced into a vein in the arm or leg to investigate the right ventricle; or into an artery for investigation of the left ventricle. The catheter is manipulated into position under an X-ray monitor and provides information as to the pressure in the atria, the ventricle and the main vessels. This information is vital to the surgeon before making a decision whether or not to operate in congenital heart disease or on the valves.

Angiocardiograph

A special catheter is introduced into the heart, either through a vein or an artery and a fluid is introduced which shows up on X-ray. This is

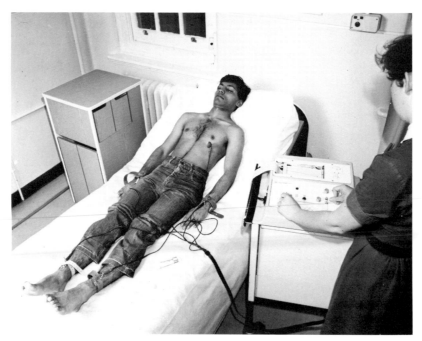

Fig. 5.2 Taking an electrocardiogram.

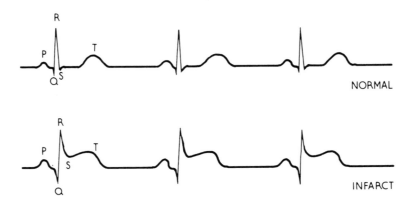

Fig. 5.3 Electrocardiogram tracings in the normal heart and after a myocardial infarct.

recorded either on a cine film or on multiple X-ray plates and enables a precise diagnosis to be made of many structural abnormalities, whether congenital or acquired.

Coronary arteriography

In this procedure the tip of the catheter is placed in the origins of the right and left coronary arteries and a fluid injected which shows up on X-ray. It enables the surgeon to see if the coronary arteries are obstructed and suitable for surgery.

Holter monitoring

Two sets of ECG leads are connected to a miniature portable ECG machine with a cassette tape. This can be worn by patients strapped to a belt similar to a Walkman personal stereo. The cassette records the patients ECG for 24 hours while he or she carries out normal activities. The tape can be played back in the hospital to look for any abnormal rhythms that may have occurred during the day or night. The patient is usually told to make a note of whenever they have any symptoms such as palpitations to see what heart rhythm was responsible.

IRREGULAR HEART ACTION

The following are the more common forms of irregular heart action:

1. sinus arrhythmia
2. extrasystoles
3. atrial fibrillation
4. atrial flutter
5. heart block
6. paroxysmal tachycardia
7. ventricular fibrillation.

Sinus arrhythmia

Sinus arrhythmia is a very common phenomenon wherein there is an increase in the rate of the heart on inspiration, with a corresponding slowing of the heart rate on expiration. It is most frequently seen in normal young children and needs no treatment.

Extrasystoles

Extrasystoles (extra beats) are one or more or premature beats which occur before the next normal beat is due. After the premature beat there is usually a long pause in the heart action. This premature or extra beat may be so weak that the impulse does not travel to the pulse at the wrist so that there is a 'missed' beat. If the extra (ectopic) beats are very numerous the patient may complain of palpitations due to the irregular heart action.

The causes of extrasystoles may be conveniently divided into two groups, important and unimportant, as follows.

Important causes of extrasystoles

Here the extrasystoles are of significance and there is usually heart disease present.

1. In acute myocardial infarction and after cardiac surgery, the onset of ectopic beats may predate more dangerous and prolonged irregularities, particularly ventricular fibrillation. Hence the presence of these extrasystoles may require appropriate treatment.

2. Thyrotoxicosis, by its effect on the heart, commonly causes numerous extrasystoles as well as atrial fibrillation.

3. Digitalis poisoning. Overdosage with digoxin often produces an extrasystole after every other heart beat so that a characteristic coupling of the pulse rhythm occurs – *pulsus bigeminus*. The presence of this irregularity calls for a reduction in the dose of the drug.

Unimportant causes of extrasystoles

Extrasystoles are often present without any evidence of heart damage and no significance need then be attached to them. Extrasystoles may occur in those who smoke.

Atrial fibrillation

Atrial fibrillation is an important and common type of irregular heart rhythm and is usually associated with heart disease.

Instead of the normal contraction of the atria which follows when the pacemaker impulse starts in the sino-atrial node, the atria undergo a very rapid twitching called fibrillation. There is no proper contraction of the atria. The ventricles are continuously stimulated by these rapid twitchings but respond only to the stronger impulses. The result is that the ventricles contract in a most irregular fashion both in rate and in force.

Causes of atrial fibrillation

1. Rheumatic heart disease, especially associated with mitral stenosis, is a common cause before the age of 50.

2. Thyrotoxicosis, when the atrial fibrillation may recur in paroxysmal attacks or may be permanent.

3. Coronary arteriosclerosis and hypertension in later life.

Ectopic ventricular beats

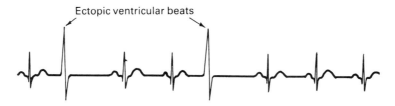

Fig. 5.4 Ectopic ventricular beats.

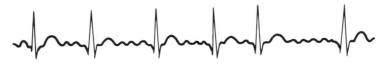

Fig. 5.5 Atrial fibrillation. Note absence of regular P waves.

Atrial fibrillation may be caused by any form of heart disease, but the above are the most frequent causes.

Symptoms and signs

The diagnostic clinical sign is the complete irregularity of the heart's action in both the rate and the force. The rate in untreated cases is often 120 to 160 beats a minute. There is, in most cases, a difference between the rate as counted by the pulse at the wrist and that counted directly over the heart with a stethoscope (apex beat), which is known as a 'pulse deficit'. The pulse deficit may be as much as 20 beats a minute. The pulse deficit is caused by some heart beats being too weak to be transmitted to the pulse at the wrist. It is thus better to monitor such cases with the apex beat.

As most cases of atrial fibrillation are associated with heart disease, signs of the latter are usually present. Very often the onset of atrial fibrillation precipitates congestive heart failure.

Treatment

Digoxin Unless due to thyrotoxicosis, the specific drug for the treatment of atrial fibrillation is digitalis. The most commonly used preparation of digitalis is digoxin and this is available in three strengths; 0.25 mg or 0.125 mg tablets are usually prescribed for adults and a weaker 0.0625 mg tablet is available for children or the elderly.

Ampoules of 0.5 mg digoxin are also available for intravenous use. These must be diluted in saline or dextrose and given by slow intravenous infusion.

Digoxin delays conduction from the atrium to the ventricle, thus reducing the number of impulses reaching the ventricle. Slowing of the heart rate results and the action of the ventricles becomes stronger and more efficient. In patients not already taking digoxin and where the heart rate is very rapid, the initial dose of digoxin may be given as a slow intravenous infusion, usually 0.5 mg over an hour. In less urgent cases, digoxin is given as tablets by mouth, often at an initial dose of 0.5 mg and then 0.25 mg 6-hourly until the heart rate has slowed.

Once the heart rate is controlled at a suitable rate, digoxin may be given at a daily dose of 0.25 mg or less each day. To establish a safe and efficient dose, the level of digoxin can be measured in the blood. If the dose of digoxin is too high, toxic effects may follow. Particularly in patients who have been taking digoxin regularly for some years, it is easy to forget the potential poisonous effects of digoxin and to ascribe the symptoms to some other cause. The results of digoxin overdose include:

1. loss of appetite, nausea and vomiting
2. marked slowing of the heart rate with a pulse rate of less than 50
3. numerous ectopic ventricular beats sometimes with pulsus bigeminus in which every normal beat is followed by an ectopic beat.

Electrical cardioversion The cardioverter is an apparatus which passes an electric current through the heart and may successfully restore sinus rhythm in the majority of cases of acute atrial fibrillation. In patients where the fibrillation has been present for a long time, the rhythm usually relapses into fibrillation again after treatment. This being so, the treatment is usually reserved for patients where the atrial fibrillation is of recent origin. Cardioversion is performed under short term anaesthesia so that the patient is not aware of the procedure. When sinus rhythm has been restored, drugs such as quinidine, amiodarone or disopyramide may be prescribed daily to prevent relapse.

Anticoagulation When the heart is enlarged and the atrium is not contracting properly because it is fibrillating, blood clots may form on the wall of the atrium (*mural thrombi*). Slowing the heart either by digoxin or by cardioversion can occasionally lead to dislodgement of the clot, forming an embolus which may reach and obstruct the cerebral circulation, causing a stroke. To avoid the possibility of this disaster, anticoagulant therapy with warfarin or heparin is sometimes used.

Thyrotoxicosis When atrial fibrillation is due to thyrotoxicosis, treatment of the thyroid disorder leads to restoration of sinus rhythm. If it does not, quinidine may be administered or cardioversion can be applied.

Atrial flutter

Atrial flutter is due to the same causes as atrial fibrillation and has a similar type of action except that the heart is often regular instead of irregular. The treatment is the same as for atrial fibrillation.

Heart block

Disease affecting the conducting mechanism of the heart may interfere with the proper conduction of the cardiac impulse, so that blocking of the beats may occur. There are very many different types of heart block but only the main types will be covered here. In incomplete heart block, isolated impulses fail to reach the ventricles from the atria; consequently, the ventricles

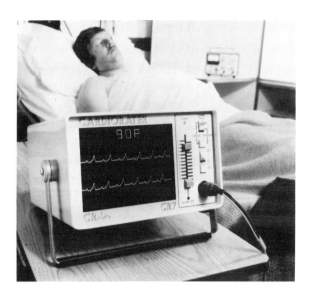

Fig. 5.6 Monitoring the heart rhythm by continuous electrocardiogram.

fail to contract, with the result that a beat is missed or dropped. The rhythm of the heart rate in incomplete heart block is usually irregular. In complete heart block no impulses reach the ventricles from the atria and the ventricles beat at their own independent rate, usually about 40 beats a minute. The rhythm of the heart in complete block is regular.

Stokes–Adams syndrome

In Stokes–Adams syndrome the ventricles fail to contract for a period as the result of a severe degree of heart block. In most of these patients coronary arteriosclerosis is the cause of the heart block. In severe cases the patient falls unconscious and a convulsion or fit may occur, usually with cyanosis. If the heart fails to beat within minutes the patient dies; less severe attacks usually cause a feeling of faintness and giddiness with a transient 'black-out'. The diagnosis may be made with a holter monitor.

Treatment

An artificial pacemaker is used. This is a small electrical device, placed in the heart and powered by a battery. The pacemaker provides rhythmic stimulation directly to the heart when its natural pacemaker fails, and so prevents dangerous failures of contraction. A temporary pacemaker wire may be inserted into the patient in an emergency.

Paroxysmal tachycardia

Paroxysmal tachycardia is a common irregularity of the heart but is not often seen by the nurse, as most of these patients do not require in-patient hospital treatment. Paroxysmal tachycardia may not be associated with any other evidence of heart disease.

Symptoms and signs

1. Sudden onset of extreme tachycardia (fast heart rate) so that the heart beats about 180 to 200 times a minute.
2. Rhythm of the heart is absolutely regular.
3. The attack may last from several minutes to several hours, or even in severe cases for days. During the attack the patient may complain of palpitations and/or dyspnoea.
4. The attack passes off as suddenly as it occurs.

Treatment

Stimulation of the vagus nerve in an effort to slow the heart rate may occasionally stop an attack. This may be induced reflexly by firm pressure over the carotid artery in the upper part of the neck or by painful pressure over the eyeballs.

If the rapid heart rate can be shown to start in the atrium, intravenous verapamil is usually successful in slowing the heart to its normal rate. If the tachycardia originates in the ventricle (as shown on the electrocardiogram), drugs such as lignocaine may be given intravenously. If all these measures fail to restore rhythm, cardioversion may be necessary. The patient is given a short anaesthetic and a direct electric current shock is applied to the chest. This is usually effective in restoring the heart rhythm.

HYPERTENSION (High blood pressure)

The blood pressure, measured with a sphygmo-manometer, depends on two main factors:

1. The strength and rate of the contraction of the heart, known as the cardiac output.
2. The peripheral resistance to the blood flow, which is determined by the calibre of the smaller arteries (arterioles).

The more constricted the arterioles, the greater the peripheral resistance. The blood pressure rises when the cardiac output increases or when there is vasoconstriction of the peripheral arterioles, i.e. increased resistance. It is conventional to write a systolic pressure of 120 mmHg and a diastolic pressure of 80 mmHg as 120/80.

As we get older, the arteries become thicker and less elastic, a condition known as arteriosclerosis. This leads to an increase in blood pressure and explains why the blood pressure tends to be higher in older people. Thus a blood pressure of 170/90 might be regarded as 'normal' for a man of 70 but would certainly be abnormal for someone aged 20. Consequently, in defining what is meant by the term hypertension, the age of the patient is an important factor. As a number of factors, including anxiety, elevate blood pressure, the reading must be consistent after rest and reassurance. Below the age of 50, the diastolic pressure is normally less than 90 mmHg.

Causes of hypertension

In the majority of patients with high blood pressure, no obvious cause can be found. This type of hypertension is known as essential hypertension. Some forms of kidney disease lead to high blood pressure, particularly chronic nephritis or pyelonephritis. Consequently, particularly in young people, the presence of hypertension will lead to investigation of the kidneys and their function. Hypertension itself can cause damage to the kidneys so that sometimes it is difficult to know which came first, the high blood pressure or the kidney ailment. Certain endocrine disorders can cause hypertension. Phaeochromocytoma is a tumour of the adrenal medulla which produces large amounts of adrenaline, and a rise in blood pressure which may be episodic. In Cushing's syndrome, excess cortisone causes re-

Commonest cause

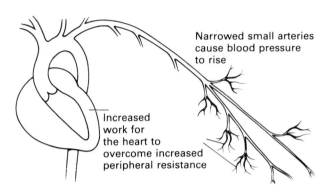

Narrowed small arteries
cause blood pressure
to rise

Increased
work for
the heart to
overcome increased
peripheral resistance

Complications

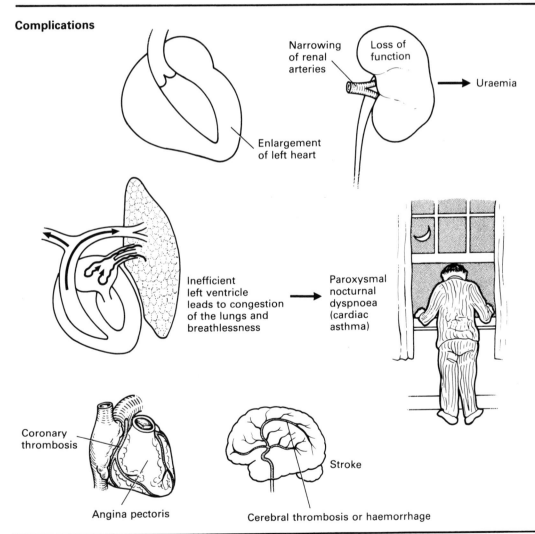

Narrowing
of renal
arteries

Loss of
function

Uraemia

Enlargement
of left heart

Inefficient
left ventricle
leads to congestion
of the lungs and
breathlessness

Paroxysmal
nocturnal
dyspnoea
(cardiac
asthma)

Coronary
thrombosis

Angina pectoris

Stroke

Cerebral thrombosis or haemorrhage

Fig. 5.7 Hypertension.

tention of salt and fluid, leading to hypertension. Hence, although in most cases of hypertension no other abnormalities can be found, sometimes investigation is indicated to exclude possible causes.

Pathology

The effects of the increased pressure in the arteries are numerous and in most cases serious.

1. The left ventricle of the heart hypertrophies (thickens) and dilates to counteract the extra pressure in the arteries. Eventually, if the strain becomes too severe the heart cannot cope and heart failure sets in.

2. The renal arteries, due to increased pressure, become thickened and narrowed, which leads to a diminished blood supply to the kidneys. This causes, in turn, a loss of function and may lead to chronic renal failure (*uraemia*).

3. The raised pressure commonly causes rupture of certain arteries, especially the cerebral arteries. This results in cerebral haemorrhage (stroke).

4. The continuous raised pressure often aggravates or predisposes to sclerotic changes in the arteries with the result that angina pectoris, coronary thrombosis and cerebral thrombosis are all frequently seen in association with hypertension.

Symptoms

Hypertension is often present for many years – perhaps 10 to 15 – during which time it may cause few symptoms. Headache, giddiness, ringing in the ears and epistaxis (nose bleeds) are symptoms which usually occur only when the blood pressure is very high. Eventually, however, due to the persistently increased pressure against which the heart has to work, heart failure develops. Even mild exertion leads to breathlessness, and attacks of 'cardiac asthma' may supervene. In addition, the patients may complain of cardiac pain (angina) resulting from coronary arteriosclerosis, since hypertension predisposes to the occurrence of coronary arteriosclerosis. For the

same reason, coronary thrombosis is common in hypertensive people, whilst another frequent result of hypertension is stroke caused by a cerebral haemorrhage.

In severe cases of hypertension, attacks known as *hypertensive encephalopathy* may arise. Severe headaches, vomiting, convulsions, paralysis and papilloedema are usually present. These attacks also occur in the form of hypertension called malignant hypertension. Here, in contrast to the prolonged course of the more usual type of essential hypertension (often called *benign essential hypertension* to contrast it with the malignant form), the whole tempo of the disease is much more rapid, and death takes place within a few years of the onset. The kidneys are especially affected in malignant hypertension and renal failure is a frequent feature. Malignant hypertension also tends to affect much younger people than the benign form.

Treatment

Effective drug treatment is now available for lowering the blood pressure, and must be instituted in view of the hazards of hypertension. However, this forms only a part of the measures that may be taken. The patient should reduce weight if he is obese, he should give up cigarette smoking and try to lead a less stressful life.

Many drugs are now available for the treatment of hypertension but there is a good deal of variation in individual response. Quite often a combination of drugs is more effective than a single one. The hypotensive drugs most frequently used at present include:

1. Beta-blockers (e.g. atenolol). This is one of many drugs which block the constricting effect of adrenaline on blood vessels and slow the heart rate. They are effective not only in reducing the blood pressure but also in relieving angina.

2. Oral diuretics (e.g. chlorothiazide). These may be given in addition to beta-blockers, and may require potassium supplements.

3. Calcium antagonists (e.g. nifedipine). These work by relaxing the muscles in the blood vessel walls, hence reducing peripheral resistance.

4. Angiotensin converting enzyme (ACE) in-

hibitors (e.g. captopril). Angiotensin II is a potent constrictor of peripheral arterioles. These drugs work by blocking its production. They are also useful in the treatment of heart failure.

5. Other drugs. These may be given for more severe hypertension.

During the initial period of stabilization on hypotensive drugs, care must be taken to increase the dose only gradually, since the blood pressure may fall suddenly. If the patient is in hospital, the blood pressure must be recorded regularly.

CORONARY ARTERY DISEASE

Coronary artery disease has become the major cause of death in middle and old age in the Western world. The coronary arteries are the first arteries to come off the ascending aorta and they carry fresh oxygenated blood to supply the entire myocardium. The left coronary artery divides into two branches, the anterior descending and the circumflex. These branches supply the left ventricle. The right coronary artery supplies blood to the right ventricle. In coronary artery disease, thickening and narrowing of the coronary vessels

occurs so that the blood supply to the heart muscle is diminished. This process, known as arteriosclerosis, begins in early middle age and usually shows gradual progression with the years. Most men and women over the age of 50 show some arteriosclerosis of the coronary arteries, though there are great individual variations. When the coronaries become very narrowed, the blood flow in them may become sluggish and a thrombosis or clot may form in one branch. This coronary thrombosis may deprive part of the heart muscle of its blood supply: the myocardium involved cannot survive and this is known as a myocardial infarction.

Factors disposing to coronary artery disease

The increasing frequency of coronary thrombosis as a cause of death in the developed countries has led to an intensive search into all the factors which could explain this increase.

1. Diet. One of the features of arteriosclerosis is the deposition of fatty plaques on the inner lining (intima) of the coronary arteries. These

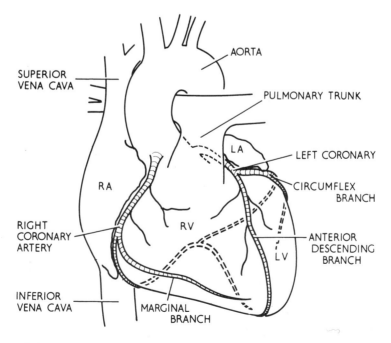

Fig. 5.8 The coronary arteries.

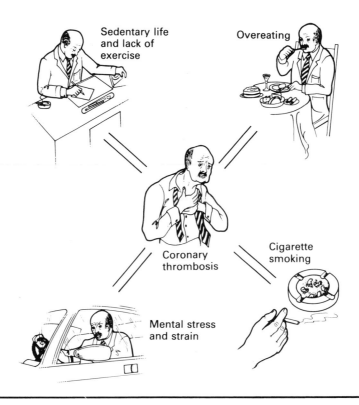

Sedentary life and lack of exercise

Overeating

Coronary thrombosis

Cigarette smoking

Mental stress and strain

Other factors   High serum cholesterol   Familial tendency   Hypertension

Fig. 5.9 Factors disposing to coronary thrombosis.

deposits are formed from the products of fat in the blood and, in particular, cholesterol. Cholesterol is partly derived from the animal fats in our food, particularly meat, fat, butter, eggs, milk and cream. Some people have a familial tendency to form high levels of blood cholesterol even though their diet is not to blame. It is thought that excess blood cholesterol may be deposited in the lining of the coronary arteries.

2. Cigarette smoking predisposes to coronary thrombosis, and the risk for smokers of dying from coronary disease is about double that of non-smokers. Stopping smoking tends to reduce the risk.

3. Lack of exercise. There is a tendency today for many people to go to and from work by motor transport, to sit at a desk during the day and to sit in a chair watching television in the evenings. This sedentary existence predisposes to coronary artery disease.

4. Obesity. Fat people are more prone to heart disease than those who are thin.

5. The stress and strain of modern life predisposes to coronary thrombosis. Persons with a anxious personality are more prone to heart disease.

6. Patients with hypertension have a greater incidence of heart disease.

7. Diabetic patients are more liable to coronary artery disease.

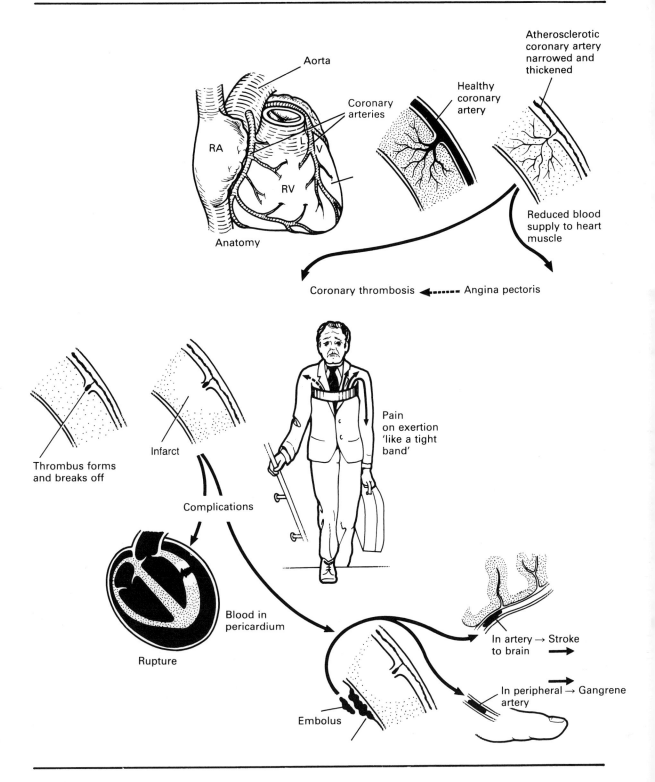

Fig. 5.10 Coronary artery disease.

ANGINA PECTORIS

This is a clinical syndrome produced by a reduction in the blood supply to the muscle of the heart. When a muscle has to work with a deficient oxygen supply, a severe cramping pain occurs. This pain, due to oxygen deficiency, is common to all muscles: an example can readily be provided by applying a blood-pressure cuff to the arm and opening and shutting the hand several times. This, after a time, brings on severe pain in the hand which is due to lack of oxygen caused by cutting off the local blood circulation by the bloodpressure cuff. In angina, the pain is characteristically felt behind the sternum (breastbone), and it most frequently radiates down the left arm. It may also radiate into the right arm, into the neck, or, more rarely, into the upper abdomen. It is of a severe gripping nature. It may occur at first only during exertion, the patient usually stating that he notices it when he goes up an incline or climbs stairs, particularly in cold weather. The pain is relieved by rest. The patient usually stops, and after a minute or so the pain passes off. In more severe cases, the pain may come on at rest. This is known as 'unstable angina'.

Causes of angina

The majority of cases are due to arteriosclerosis of the coronary arteries, which become too narrowed to provide an adequate blood supply to the heart muscle. High blood pressure is another factor in producing angina, since this leads to enlargement of the heart and greater oxygen requirements. Other less common causes of angina are aortic aneurysms (which may be associated with narrow openings of the coronary arteries), severe anaemia (the blood carries less oxygen) and aortic stenosis (the pressure falls in the coronary arteries).

Treatment of angina

Much can be done medically and surgically to relieve the pain and to prevent extra strain on the damaged heart. The patient is warned to avoid exertion which will bring on the pain, though it is important that the patient should lead as normal and active a life as possible. Regular moderate exercise is to be encouraged. In patients of an anxious temperament where emotional upsets cause angina, beta-blocking drugs such as atenolol are useful. Diet is also of importance in angina. Obesity, if present, throws an added strain on the heart, and therefore a low calorie diet is given to reduce the patient's weight to normal or slightly below normal. Individual meals must always be light, because a heavy meal increases the work of the heart to an appreciable extent; indeed, anginal pain may be noticed after a heavy meal, the patients imagining they suffer from 'indigestion'.

Cigarette smoking increases the risks of angina. Although it is not easy for habitual smokers to give up cigarettes, angina patients must be urged to do so. If the blood pressure is raised, treatment should be given to reduce it.

Several drugs are used in the treatment of angina, which act by producing a dilatation of the coronary arteries and thus improving the blood supply to the heart. Glyceryl trinitrate (trinitrin) (0.5 mg) in the form of a tablet, which can be allowed to dissolve under the tongue, may be very effective in relieving an attack of angina. When angina is more frequent and persistent, use of the beta-blocker drugs often provides relief of symptoms. There are many varieties of beta-blocker drugs. Atenolol or oxprenolol are two in common use. Beta-blockers and newer vasodilator drugs (e.g. isosorbide) may be given in long-acting forms. Sometimes angina is unrelieved by any medical treatment and becomes persistent. The patient's activities and enjoyment of life are seriously curtailed. In such cases, the possibility of surgery must be considered. The first step is to perform coronary arteriography. The operation consists of bypassing the obstructed vessel, using a length of saphenous vein taken from the leg. One end is inserted into the aorta and the other into the coronary artery beyond the obstruction. This operation relieves the symptoms in the majority of angina patients and enables them to lead a fuller life.

Patients with unstable angina require admis-

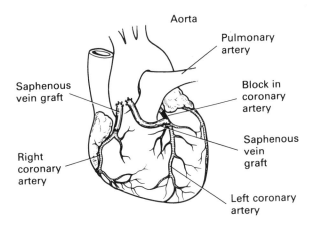

Fig. 5.11 Saphenous vein graft for coronary artery disease (by-pass operation).

sion to hospital and urgent treatment with intravenous nitrates and heparin. Without such treatment there is a high rate of progression to myocardial infarction.

CORONARY THROMBOSIS

In patients with narrowed coronary arteries there is always the danger of clot formation (coronary thrombosis) completely blocking one of the branches of the coronary tree. If a major branch is suddenly occluded, the heart will be unable to maintain its action and sudden death occurs. If only a small branch is blocked, the region of heart muscle supplied by it becomes dead: this area is known as a myocardial infarct. After a time, the dead heart muscle is replaced by a fibrous scar. If the scar is not a large one, it may interfere very little or not at all with the action of the heart. If it is a large one, however, the force of the heart beat may be seriously impaired and congestive heart failure may follow. The predisposing factors of coronary thrombosis are illustrated in Figure 5.9.

Symptoms and signs

A coronary thrombosis may occur unexpectedly in someone who has always thought himself to be in good health. Indeed, coronary thrombosis is a common cause of unexpected sudden death. In other patients, a coronary thrombosis is the culmination of months or even years of angina.

The onset of coronary thrombosis may occur at any time, while moving about or while at rest, during the day or in bed at night. The patient experiences pain in the chest which may spread into the neck or into the left arm. The pain may be no more than a dull ache, often mistaken for indigestion, or it may be of great and unbearable severity. It lasts much longer than an attack of angina and usually persists for several minutes or even hours.

In a severe case, the patient may be in severe pain, restless and sweating. There may be signs of shock with a rapid pulse of poor volume, a low blood pressure and the skin cold and clammy.

The course of the progress of a myocardial infarction can be treacherous. Although the signs and symptoms may be mild at the start, the thrombosis can spread leading to increased pain, irregularity of the heart action and collapse.

Diagnosis

1. The site of the pain, its persistence over several hours and other associated features usually make the diagnosis clear on clinical grounds.

2. Changes occur in the electrocardiogram which confirm that a myocardial infarction has occurred.

3. The infarcted myocardium releases enzymes from the breaking-down of muscle fibres and these can be detected and measured in the blood. The enzyme released first is known as *creatine kinase* (CK) and it can be elevated within a few hours of a myocardial infarction. Others are known as *transaminases* and are elevated in the blood after the first day of the infarction, remaining raised for several days.

4. The white count is increased since the polymorphs are mobilized to help absorb the damaged muscle.

Course and complications

Many patients who develop a coronary thrombosis die within a few hours of onset and before they can be taken to hospital. In others, the pain is not severe and the course is uneventful. Various complications are liable to occur, particularly in the first few days.

Arrhythmias

Irregularity of the heart rhythm is common and may vary from occasional extra beats to total irregularity of the atrial and ventricular beats. Ventricular fibrillation is the state in which the ventricles contract rapidly and irregularly and unless controlled quickly leads to a fatal outcome.

Thrombosis and emboli

Patients lying immobile with a low blood pressure are particularly liable to form a clot (thrombosis) in the deep veins in the legs or in the heart itself over the infarcted area. Part of the thrombotic clot may become detached from the vein into the blood stream and cause a pulmonary embolus in the lung. A clot from the heart travelling into the cerebral circulation may give rise to a stroke.

Heart failure

The patient goes into shock with cold extremities, a low blood pressure, rapid or irregular pulse and breathlessness. The urine output drops. The outlook is grave.

Treatment

1. Relief of pain. Where this is persistent, diamorphine (5–10 mg subcutaneously, or a smaller dose intravenously) should be given at regular intervals. Diamorphine is preferable to morphine since it is much less liable to cause nausea or vomiting. If nausea is troublesome, an antihistamine such as cyclizine can be given as well.

2. Patients should be nursed in a comfortable position. If there is evidence of breathlessness (left ventricular failure), the patient is best propped up in bed or allowed to sit up in a high arm chair. Diuretics are prescribed, sometimes intravenously, for the fluid in the lungs. Where there is evidence of shock and a low blood pressure, the patient is kept flat with the foot of the bed elevated.

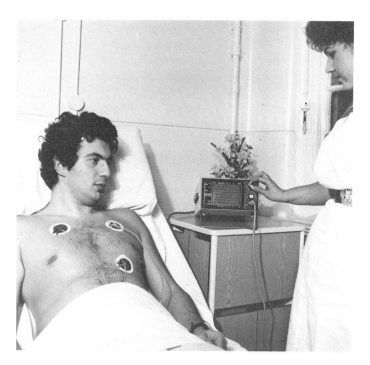

Fig. 5.12 Monitoring for arrythmias after myocardial infarction.

3. Drugs can now be used to dissolve the clot formed in the coronary arteries provided less than 24 hours have elapsed since the onset of the pain. This is known as *thrombolysis*. Aspirin 300 mg is given by mouth and streptokinase (1.5 million units) is given by intravenous infusion over one hour. These must not be given if the patient is at risk of bleeding, for example if he has a stomach ulcer that has recently bled. Intravenous or subcutaneous heparin is given for 48 hours after thrombolysis to prevent re-occlusion.

4. In severe cases, oxygen may be administered through a disposable face mask in the hope of improving the oxygen supply to the myocardium.

5. Treatment of arrhythmias. Especially over the first 48 hours, all but the mildest of cases should be monitored for the early detection of irregularity of rhythm. The patient is supervised on the oscilloscope which displays a constant electrocardiograph on a bedside screen. This takes the place of constant pulse taking but requires regular supervision just the same. When ectopic ventricular beats begin to occur, lignocaine is the treatment of choice. It is best administered in an intravenous infusion, perhaps with an initial dose of 100 mg and then at a dose level of about 2 mg every minute.

With atrial fibrillation, digoxin is administered, usually intravenously initially and then by mouth.

If ventricular fibrillation occurs electric cardioversion must be applied immediately. A strong electric current is passed through the chest and is usually successful in restoring normal rhythm though sometimes the fibrillation recurs after a time. In some cases of heart block an emergency pacemaker wire may be inserted.

6. Anticoagulants should be administered to prevent deep vein thrombosis whether or not thrombolysis is given. Heparin is given subcutaneously for the first 48 hours and then warfarin. Leg exercises are encouraged and elastic stockings are worn to help prevent deep vein thrombosis (Table 5.1).

7. Apart from cases in shock, patients should be allowed to feed themselves and to use a bedside commode, although the nurse may help with washing and shaving according to the general state of the patient.

Subsequent management

In an uncomplicated case with no pain after the onset, a regular pulse and a good blood pressure, there is no advantage in keeping the patient confined to bed after the first few days. It is good for his morale if he is told from the start that he has had a coronary thrombosis, that he will make a complete recovery, that he will be able to go home in one week (or thereabouts) and that he will be able to lead a full life.

In more severe cases, advice will have to be modified by the degree of myocardial damage. Arrhythmias such as atrial fibrillation may persist, angina pectoris may occur and there may be evidence of left ventricular failure. Patients with these disabilities may not be well enough to continue with a job demanding a good deal of physical effort.

A coronary thrombosis imposes a severe strain on the patient's confidence and morale. He may feel afraid to be active lest he precipitate another attack and well-meaning advice to take it easy can reinforce these fears. In fact there is no evidence that ordinary activity disposes to coronary thrombosis: indeed the contrary is more likely to be the case. Regular moderate exercise is to be encouraged and the patient should be advised to lead as normal a life as possible.

Cigarette smoking is known to predispose to coronary thrombosis and patients should be strongly discouraged from this habit. As far as diet is concerned, obese patients must reduce weight. As there is evidence that a diet containing a high proportion of saturated fats (dairy produce such as butter, eggs, meat, fat and cheese) increases the cholesterol in the blood and may predispose to atherosclerosis, some physicians prescribe a restricted diet in this respect.

Patients should be encouraged both to replace saturated fats with unsaturated fats and to reduce total fat consumption where possible.

Coronary care units

Some hospitals have special units of four to six

Table 5.1

	Administration	Rapidity of action	Danger	Antidote	Clinical use	Control	Average dose
Heparin	By continuous intravenous injection or every 4 to 6 hours, or intramuscularly every 8 to 12 hours	Immediate	Haemorrhage	Immediately neutralised by intravenous injection of 5 ml of protamine sulphate	Best given at onset of attack of thrombosis till other oral drugs take effect		Depends on the clotting time. Usually 5000 units every 4 to 6 hours intravenously, or 12 500 units intramuscularly
Phenindione (or warfarin)	By mouth in single or divided doses	Takes effect in 24 to 36 hours	Haemorrhage especially haematuria	Vitamin K_1, 5 to 20 mg orally or intravenously, repeated if necessary. Takes 2 to 6 hours to act. Blood transfusions essential with severe haemorrhage	Better than heparin for long-term treatment, as it can be given by mouth	Prothrombin estimations (a form of clotting time) essential	Depends on the prothrombin time. Maintenance dose about 12.5 to 50 mg daily for phenindione and 3 to 10 mg daily for warfarin

beds specially for the care of the more severe coronary cases. These are sometimes part of an Intensive Treatment Unit where other emergencies are also treated. These units allow round-the-clock supervision and apparatus is at hand to keep the airway clear, to administer oxygen, to provide resuscitation and to treat cardiac arrhythmia. Most importantly, by means of a central series of oscilloscopes, one nurse can supervise the cardiac rhythm of several patients simultaneously. However, it is neither feasible nor necessarily desirable for all patients with coronary thrombosis to be treated in special units, since adequate supervision and treatment can be undertaken in a general ward, or even sometimes at home.

Cardiac resuscitation

Occasionally, after an attack of coronary thrombosis, during an operation, after severe electric shock, or in other conditions, the heart stops beating. Providing not more than a few seconds elapse, in some cases the heart beat can be restarted. If cardiac resuscitation is to be effective, action must be prompt and efficient. The patient must be laid supine on the floor or any firm surface and external cardiac massage commenced. Two hands are placed on the sternum and strong rhythmical pressure exerted at the rate of 60 to 80 per minute. At the same time another operator performs mouth-to-mouth artificial respiration. The head of the patient is extended and the nose held. After a deep inhalation the mouth is placed on the patient's mouth and the breath is blown out forcibly into the patient's lungs. If it is available, a Brook airway should be used for this purpose, since it is less unpleasant and more effective than direct mouth-to-mouth. This airway contains a valve which allows the operator to blow into the patient's lungs, but any expired air from the patient is diverted to a side outlet. These methods are first-aid treatments and are designed to keep the patient alive until more effective remedies are made available. A cardiac resuscitation team is usually formed for such emergencies and will contain an anaesthetist as well as a physician. Special apparatus, including an oscilloscope, a defibrillator, intubators and ventilators are kept in readiness with the necessary drugs.

When the heart starts beating again in response to first-aid treatment, the rhythm is often irregular. The patient must be monitored by the

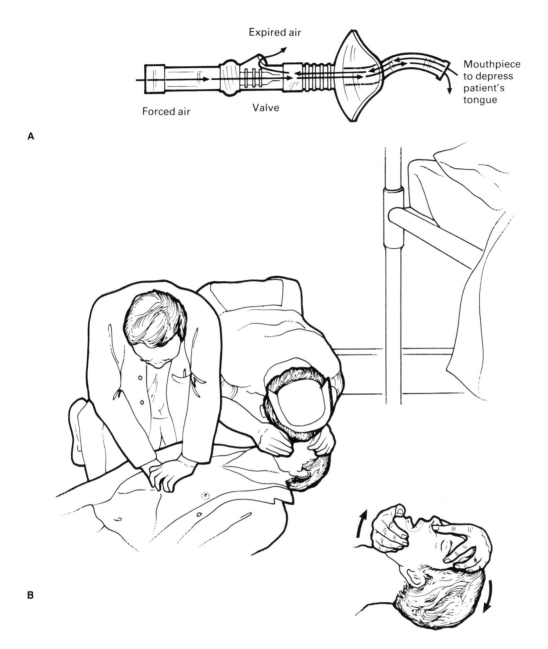

Fig. 5.13 Cardiac resuscitation: first-aid treatment. **A.** Brook Airway. **B.** Position of patient's head and nurse's hands. Shaded area to be covered by nurse's mouth if airway not available.

oscilloscope which displays a continuous electro-cardiogram on a screen. Appropriate drugs (such as adrenalin, atropine, digoxin, lignocaine and practolol) can be given intravenously to restore an effective circulation. Fibrillation of the ventri-cles is very much more serious than atrial fibril-lation and electric shocks must be administered to restore normal ventricular action through elec-trodes placed on the chest from the defibrillator.

Intubation is performed by the anaesthetist by

inserting a tube into the larynx. This makes sure the airway is kept patent and mucus can be sucked out. Ventilation can be assisted and oxygen administered by pressure from a bag attached to the tube.

Severe acidosis occurs during cardiac arrest and this may be overcome by the slow intravenous infusion of sodium bicarbonate. It can be seen that to be successful, cardiac resuscitation requires skill, time and organisation, as well as expensive apparatus. Nevertheless, many lives have been saved by these methods and by the speedy action of nurses and doctors.

Prevention of coronary thrombosis

Advice as to care of health can do much to avoid the dangers of developing this common disorder in middle age.

1. Diet. Particularly in those with a family history of coronary disease and in those known to have a high cholesterol in the blood, a diet should be recommended with a low sugar and animal fat content. Cream should be avoided entirely, butter replaced by a vegetable margarine and eggs restricted to no more than five a week. Cooking fats such as lard should be replaced by olive oil since this helps to reduce the blood cholesterol.

2. The weight must be kept down to a level appropriate to the height and age, and obesity must be avoided.

3. Regular exercise should be taken, suitable for the age and fitness of the patient.

4. Cigarette smoking should be discontinued entirely.

5. Treatment should be given for diabetes and hypertension where these are present.

PULMONARY HEART DISEASE

The right ventricle has to propel blood through the pulmonary circulation. When this circulation is impeded, a strain is imposed on the work of the heart.

Pulmonary embolism

A pulmonary embolus most commonly arises from a blood clot detached from a thrombosis of a deep vein in the leg or the pelvis (Fig. 5.20). When it lodges in the pulmonary artery, the blood flow to the lung, and oxygenation, is reduced. A massive pulmonary embolus causes sudden tightness in the chest and breathlessness: this can be followed by collapse and death. Smaller emboli may cause very little symptoms at the time but may be associated with increasing breathlessness and *haemoptysis* (coughing up blood).

The diagnosis can be confirmed by finding evidence of phlebothrombosis in the leg or pelvic veins and by the chest X-ray and lung scans which show shadows typical of pulmonary infarction. The electrocardiogram may also show characteristic changes.

It should be remembered that women taking the contraceptive pill may be slightly more prone to develop venous thrombosis in the legs and pulmonary emboli may follow. Once the diagnosis has been confirmed, anticoagulant treatment should be maintained for several months.

Cor pulmonale

This is the name given to the form of heart failure occurring in patients with lung disease, commonly chronic bronchitis and emphysema. These patients may become very cyanosed because the heart failure exacerbates the already impaired pulmonary function. Oedema and ascites usually are present and although these may respond in part to diuretics, the ultimate outlook depends on the state of the lungs.

RHEUMATIC HEART DISEASE

Rheumatic heart disease is an important cause of heart disease in young and middle-aged people. Rheumatic heart disease occurs in two main forms – acute and chronic.

Acute rheumatic heart disease

Rheumatic heart disease is usually caused by rheumatic fever, but occasionally it also occurs in chorea. Chorea is described under Diseases of the

Nervous System, and it appears to be related to rheumatic fever in that both complaints are due to streptococcal infection. New cases of these diseases are now rare in Britain.

Rheumatic fever usually follows a streptococcal sore throat after a lapse of 7 to 21 days. One attack gives no immunity; in fact there is a definite susceptibility to recurrences. Most cases occur in young children and the disease is unusual after the age of 25. The younger the patient and the more frequent the attacks, the greater the liability that permanent heart damage will result.

Pathology

Rheumatic fever is a general infection which can permanently damage the valves of the heart; the myocardium and pericardium may also be affected. The joints are swollen in the acute stage of the illness but the effect is temporary. Hence the old adage 'Rheumatic fever licks the joints but bites the heart'.

Rheumatic endocarditis

Endocarditis is an inflammation of the endocardium of the heart, affecting particularly the valves of the heart. Endocarditis, as we shall see later, has many causes, but rheumatic endocarditis is the commonest form in young and middle-aged people.

Characteristic lesions called *vegetations* occur on the valves as a result of the endocarditis. Vegetations are small clots (*thrombi*) which look like a row of beads on the valves. These vegetations are composed of fibrin, red cells and platelets, and in contrast to the vegetations which form in bacterial endocarditis, comparatively rarely break off to travel in the circulation. The valves themselves become swollen and distorted due to the inflammation. As a result, the normal heart sounds are altered when heard through the stethoscope, and a blowing murmur can be detected.

Rheumatic myocarditis and pericarditis

In the acute stage of rheumatic heart disease the heart muscle (myocardium) is affected and acute myocarditis is present. Acute myocarditis is of particular importance because death in the acute stage of rheumatic heart disease is usually due to failure of the heart muscle. The unduly rapid and occasionally irregular pulse seen in rheumatic fever is a most important sign of an underlying acute myocarditis.

Inflammation of the pericardium (*pericarditis*) occurs generally in the more severe cases of acute rheumatic fever. The pericarditis may be dry or wet (*pericardial effusion*). A large pericardial effusion may press on the heart causing severe embarrassment to an already poor circulation.

Symptoms and signs of acute rheumatic fever

1. The onset is often preceded, as mentioned earlier, by a sore throat 7 to 21 days beforehand.

2. There is a general malaise with a high temperature and heavy sweating.

3. The involvement of the joints is very characteristic and the diagnosis of acute rheumatic fever is often made on the joint lesions alone. Pains occur over the affected joints, the typical feature being their flitting nature so that different joints are affected at different times. There is swelling and tenderness of the affected joints but seldom to any severe degree. The joints never suppurate as in cases of septic arthritis.

4. The main signs of heart involvement are the very rapid pulse rate and the presence of heart murmurs. The pulse rate is faster than one would expect from the degree of fever, and the rhythm may be irregular. Any irregularity of the pulse must be carefully noted by the nurse as it may be one of the few signs of heart damage.

5. Rheumatic nodules. These are small fibrous nodules which occur around the joints and tendons, usually behind the elbows, on the back of the scalp, or ankles. They are tender and painful and their presence usually denotes a severe attack affecting the heart.

Treatment of acute rheumatic fever

Nursing

In the acute stage the patient is kept at rest in

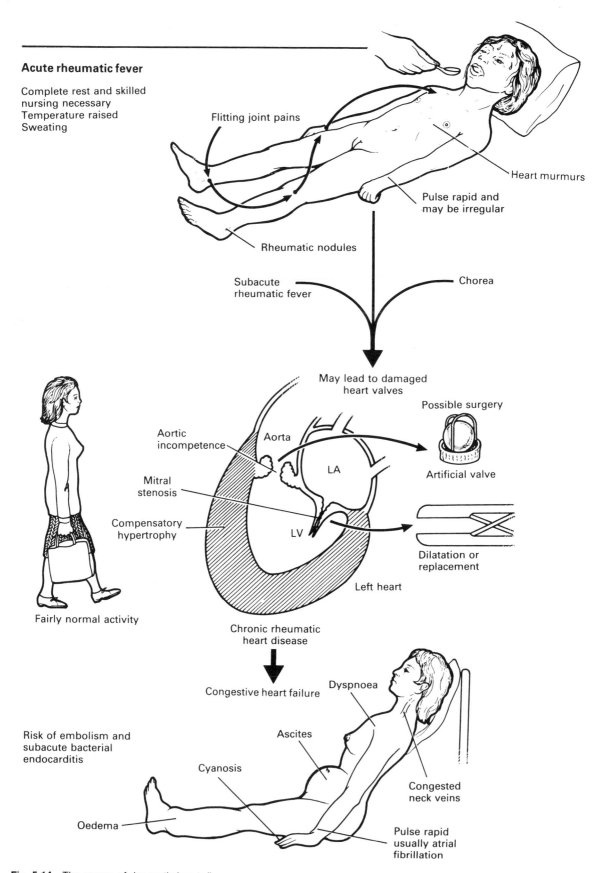

Acute rheumatic fever

Complete rest and skilled nursing necessary
Temperature raised
Sweating

Flitting joint pains

Heart murmurs

Pulse rapid and may be irregular

Rheumatic nodules

Subacute rheumatic fever

Chorea

May lead to damaged heart valves

Possible surgery

Aortic incompetence

Aorta

LA

Artificial valve

Mitral stenosis

Compensatory hypertrophy

LV

Left heart

Dilatation or replacement

Fairly normal activity

Chronic rheumatic heart disease

Congestive heart failure

Dyspnoea

Risk of embolism and subacute bacterial endocarditis

Ascites

Cyanosis

Congested neck veins

Oedema

Pulse rapid usually atrial fibrillation

Fig. 5.14   The course of rheumatic heart disease.

bed, although it requires both kindness and explanation to persuade young patients to lie quietly. Help will be needed with washing and personal hygiene but independence should be restored as soon as the medical condition allows. Children easily get bored and despondent when they have nothing to do: parents and family should be encouraged to stay or visit and the limitations of the position explained to them. If the joints are unduly swollen and painful, wrapping in warm cotton-wool is useful to relieve the pains. The affected joints should be protected from the weight of the bed-clothes by bedcradles. During the acute stage of the fever, light diet only will be needed which will be increased as the acute symptoms subside.

Drugs

There is no specific cure as yet for acute rheumatic fever, although sodium salicylate or calcium aspirin dramatically relieve the joint pains and lower the temperature. Salicylates have little or no effect on the heart lesions. Calcium aspirin is usually given in doses of 1 g every 4 hours. Toxic symptoms may occur from the large doses of salicylates used, but no real harm results as these toxic symptoms rapidly subside when the drug is reduced. Buzzing in the ears (tinnitus), deafness, nausea and vomiting are the usual toxic symptoms noticed. In severe cases of rheumatic fever accompanied by carditis, cortisone or prednisolone may be prescribed. These steroids are sometimes more effective than salicylates in suppressing pain and fever, but it is still undecided whether damage to the heart valves can be prevented.

A course of penicillin injections is often given at the start of treatment to destroy any streptococci still in the throat. It is important in children to give penicillin by mouth for up to 5 years after a severe attack of rheumatic fever to prevent further attacks and further damage to the heart.

Convalescence

Complete rest in bed is enforced until the active stage of the disease is over. This is usually revealed by the return of the pulse rate to normal and a fall in the erythrocyte sedimentation rate (ESR). When the pulse rate and the ESR have settled, the patient is allowed to sit out of bed.

Chronic rheumatic valvular disease

Chronic rheumatic valvular disease follows the acute stage, but many years may elapse before the effects are noticed. Most cases of chronic rheumatic heart disease, therefore, have a history of rheumatic fever, or chorea, in childhood. In some cases, however, there is no history of the acute stage of the disease, and in these patients it is presumed that the symptoms in the acute stage were so mild that they escaped notice.

Pathology

In chronic rheumatic heart disease it is the valves that are particularly damaged, chronic inflammation causing thickening, distortion and loss of the normal elasticity. As a result the valves cannot function properly.

Two main effects follow this chronic inflammatory change:

1. The valves may adhere together, causing a narrowing of the valve opening and obstruction to the flow of blood. This is usually known as *stenosis* of the valve.

2. Because of the loss of elasticity and distortion of the valve the latter may not close properly, so that a leakage or regurgitation of blood results. This is known as incompetence of the valve.

Chronic rheumatic valvular disease may affect all the valves of the heart but the most commonly damaged are the mitral and aortic valves. Mitral stenosis and aortic incompetence are the conditions which most commonly arise, although mitral incompetence and aortic stenosis also occur. Quite often, mitral stenosis and aortic incompetence develop in the same patient.

Symptoms, course and treatment

Until heart failure results from the added strain on the heart, chronic rheumatic valvular disease may cause few symptoms. Valvular lesions are easily diagnosed, however, if the heart is listened to with a stethoscope, whereupon the characteristic murmurs are heard. Indeed, the first indication of a valvular heart lesion may appear during the course of some routine examination, e.g. for military service or insurance purposes, the patient having previously been unaware of any disease. Enlargement of the heart may also be found, due to the compensatory muscular hypertrophy and dilatation which take place to overcome the strain on the heart. In mild cases the patient may suffer little disability and live to an advanced age, but with severe lesions heart failure develops, with death following a few years later.

During the prolonged period when there are no symptoms (the condition having perhaps been discovered only through some routine examination), the patient is advised to avoid any undue exertion which might tax the heart too much and so precipitate heart failure.

The operation of *mitral valvotomy* is often carried out in the treatment of mitral stenosis. The tightly stenosed valve is cut and dilated, thus relieving the obstruction at the valve and the engorgement in the lungs. Young patients with progressive and severe breathlessness are particularly suitable for operative treatment. This usually leads to an immediate improvement in breathing and in exercise tolerance. Valvotomy has also been performed with good immediate results in patients with aortic stenosis. Where the mitral valve has shrunken with resultant regurgitation, the whole valve can be replaced by an artificial plastic valve, usually of the ball and socket variety.

Before such surgery the patient usually undergoes investigation by cardiac catheterization, which confirms the extent of the lesion and provides information for the surgeon. Patients with artificial valves take anticoagulants regularly to prevent clot formation on them, and antibiotics before dental treatment and surgery to prevent infection.

Complications of chronic rheumatic valvular disease

Heart failure Heart failure is the eventual outcome of most cases of rheumatic valvular disease. In those cases where there is a mitral stenosis, irregular heart action in the form of artial fibrillation is usually present.

Embolism In cases of mitral stenosis, particularly if they are accompanied by atrial fibrillation, a clot (thrombus) may form in the enlarged left atrium of the heart. This clot often becomes dislodged with the result that it travels in the circulation, finally most frequently lodging in a cerebral artery, so causing cerebral embolism; the embolus also frequently lodges in a peripheral artery. Pulmonary embolism may also arise in rheumatic valvular heart disease.

Subacute bacterial endocarditis

This disease is nearly always caused by a non-haemolytic streptococcus from a group called the *viridans streptococci*. It is important to note that this organism does not attack perfectly normal valves – only those already diseased, usually from rheumatic endocarditis or some congenital lesions. The organisms settle on the valves and cause large vegetations. The vegetations are very easily dislodged into the bloodstream to cause the emboli typical of this form of endocarditis.

Viridans streptococci are commonly found in the mouth and teeth, and bacterial endocarditis frequently occurs after dental extraction or other dental treatment, which releases bacteria into the bloodstream.

Symptoms and signs

1. The illness often begins with prolonged pyrexia of unknown origin until other signs

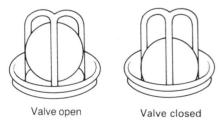

Valve open   Valve closed

Fig. 5.15 Artificial mitral valve.

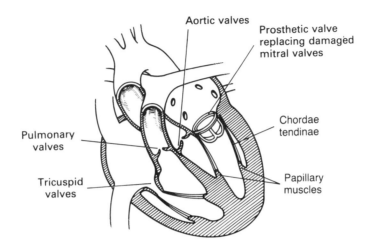

Fig. 5.16 Artificial mitral valve in situ.

appear to make the diagnosis clear. The fever is not usually high but can be accompanied by rigors and sweating. These signs are in fact those of a septicaemia, caused by the bacteria being actually present in the bloodstream.

2. The patient may complain of some generalized weakness or loss of energy.

3. At some period, signs of embolism from the dislodged vegetations appear in most cases. The exact signs depend, of course, on the organs affected by the emboli. The following are the sites most commonly involved:

   a. Brain. Paralysis in the form of hemiplegia (paralysis of one side of the body) usually occurs, the patient lapsing into coma for a temporary period.

   b. Kidneys. Emboli lodging in the kidneys cause pain in the loins with blood in the urine (haematuria).

   c. Skin. Multiple small emboli are common in the skin, producing petechial spots or larger purpuric haemorrhages. These petechial haemorrhages are especially common in the nails (splinter haemorrhages).

4. In addition to the above, there are murmurs to be heard when the heart is examined by the doctor with a stethoscope. These murmurs are due to changes in the valves.

Diagnosis

The diagnosis is often difficult in the early stages and the only sign may be continuing fever. Aids to diagnosis are:

1. A history of recent dental treatment or of previous rheumatic heart disease.
2. The presence of a heart murmur.
3. A positive blood culture. To obtain this, a small amount of blood is withdrawn from a vein under strict asepsis to prevent contamination. The blood is put into a blood culture bottle, which contains a special medium to aid the growth of bacteria. The broth is kept in a warm incubator in the laboratory and after a few days, the bacteria, if present, will multiply and form a surface scum. This bacterial growth can be identified under the microscope. Several blood cultures are often necessary before the bacteria are isolated.

Treatment of subacute bacterial endocarditis

Penicillin is usually the drug of choice. Large intravenous doses are needed, perhaps twelve million units a day in divided doses. If the temperature remains raised and the response is poor, then even greater doses may be given, perhaps with the addition of another antibiotic. Other antibiotics may have to be used if the blood culture shows a growth of bacteria not sensitive to penicillin. Whatever drug or combination of drugs is used, treatment has to be continued for a prolonged period – about 6 weeks.

Preventative measures

Patients known to have valvular disease (such as mitral stenosis or aortic regurgitation) must always have penicillin injections before any dental or other operative treatment. This will prevent bacteria entering the blood and settling on the valves. Patients who have had bacterial endocarditis should have infected teeth removed to prevent further attacks.

Summary of the course of rheumatic heart disease

The usual history is the onset in childhood of acute rheumatic fever, or chorea, which is allied to rheumatic fever. During the attack of acute rheumatic fever or chorea the heart is often damaged. The acute heart lesions may completely clear up when the acute rheumatic fever is over. In many cases, however, after the acute rheumatic fever is over the rheumatic endocarditis continues to smoulder. This chronic endocarditis gives rise to valvular heart disease (usually mitral stenosis or aortic incompetence, or both) in early adult life. At first, little disability occurs, the heart compensating for the added strain by myocardial hypertrophy. Gradually, however, signs of failure of the heart develop, causing in the early stages shortness of breath on moderate or severe exertion only. Later, however, marked dyspnoea, cyanosis and oedema occur. Whether or not heart failure will develop early, i.e. within a few years of the initial attack of rheumatic fever, depends on the severity of the damage to the heart. In milder cases, heart failure may not occur till middle age or even later still. In addition to heart failure, embolism (either arterial or pulmonary) and subacute bacterial endocarditis may complicate chronic rheumatic valvular heart disease.

SYPHILITIC HEART DISEASE

Syphilis causes a chronic inflammation of the tissues and organs which results in fibrosis or scarring. The ascending aorta is commonly affected and this produces a marked weakening of the arterial wall after many years. The high pressure in the aorta causes the weakened wall to stretch and eventually gross dilatation results. These changes in the ascending aorta may affect the heart in the following ways:

1. The marked dilatation of the aorta, which is known as aneurysm of the aorta, usually stretches the aortic valve opening and thus produces an aortic incompetence.

2. The syphilitic fibrosis commonly affects the mouths of the coronary arteries (which originate in the first part of the aorta) and so obstructs the flow of blood through these arteries. This may have a serious effect on the heart. Sudden death is a well recognized feature of syphilitic angina.

3. The aneurysm itself may rupture, leading to death.

Diagnosis

The presence of aortic incompetence in a middle-aged or elderly person with no evidence of rheumatic heart disease should be suspected as being due to syphilis. The presence of an aneurysm is detected by X-ray examination, when a dilated aorta is seen. In cases of syphilitic heart disease, the specific blood tests are positive.

Treatment

In the early stages, before the onset of heart failure, antisyphilitic treatment with penicillin is usually given. When failure occurs, this is treated in the usual way. The treatment of syphilitic heart disease is, on the whole, unsatisfactory.

THYROTOXIC HEART DISEASE

Thyrotoxicosis is due to over-activity of the thyroid gland, and is very liable to affect the heart. There is usually a persistent *tachycardia* (fast heart rate) and often atrial fibrillation. The marked increase in the general metabolism produced by the over-activity of the thyroid gland means increased work for the body, and this calls for more oxygen. To supply this the output of the heart is increased, and this is brought about by the tachycardia. If the thyrotoxicosis is allowed to go untreated, permanent damage with congestive heart failure may develop.

Diagnosis and treatment

This will be more fully discussed under Diseases of the Endocrine Glands. The patient may be given one of the antithyroid drugs such as carbimazole or an operation to remove part of the thyroid is undertaken. Radioactive iodine is also used in selected cases. Any congestive heart failure or atrial fibrillation present is treated in the usual way.

CONGENITAL HEART DISEASE

Imperfect development of the heart during fetal life leads to various deformities. The cause of such deformities is usually unknown, but sometimes when the mother contracts rubella during the first few months of pregnancy, the fetal heart is affected in this way. There are many types of abnormalities and some are so severe that they are incompatible with life, the child either being born dead or dying soon after birth. Less severe deformity of the heart may be compatible with a short period of life; in milder cases still, the normal span of life may be only slightly reduced. The common types of defect are as follows:

Septal defect. Abnormal openings in the septum separating the atria or ventricles are called atrial septal defect or ventricular septal defect respectively.

Patent ductus arteriosus. The ductus arteriosus is a normal communication present between the pulmonary artery and aorta which, during fetal life, 'shunts' the blood so that it bypasses the lungs which are not expanded. Soon after birth this opening normally closes to allow blood to go through the lungs, but in some cases it remains open, so causing signs of congenital heart disease.

Pulmonary stenosis. The pulmonary valve may be blocked so that it obstructs the blood going to the lungs from the right ventricle. This is commonly associated with other defects such as a patent septum between the ventricles, and is in these cases given the name of Fallot's tetralogy.

Coarctation of the aorta. In this form of congenital lesion there is a marked narrowing of the arch of the aorta so that the flow of blood into the lower part of the body through the normal channels is inadequate. The intercostal and other arteries become much bigger and join up with arteries in the lower part of the body so as to carry sufficient blood into the lower limbs. The dilated intercostal arteries may be seen on the chest. Coarctation of the aorta causes a severe hypertension in the upper limbs but not the lower. The pulse in the femoral artery appears later than in the radial artery, i.e. a delay.

Symptoms and signs common to many congenital heart lesions (Plate 5)

There are several symptoms and signs which lead one to suspect the presence of a congenital heart lesion:

Age of patient. In infancy or early childhood a heart lesion is probably congenital because other causes of heart disease are very rare at this age. Stunted growth and evidence of mental retardation (e.g. in Down's syndrome) are often associated with severe congenital heart disease.

Cyanosis. This is especially marked around the lips, ears and fingers, which appear bluish. Cyanosis may be due to the mixing of the arterial and venous blood as the result of an abnormal connection between the right and left sides of the heart. If the venous blood flows into the left side without passing through the lungs, there will be an abnormal amount of unoxygenated blood in the arterial system, which causes cyanosis. Cyanosis may also be caused by a poor circulation in the lungs so that there is insufficient oxygen uptake from the lungs. Cyanosis is so marked a feature of many types of congenital heart disease that the term 'blue baby' is often used to describe these patients.

Clubbing of the fingers. The ends of the fingers and even the toes are often enlarged and may look like 'drum-sticks'. The cause of this clubbing is unknown. It is also seen in some chronic respiratory and other diseases.

Diagnosis

The diagnosis of congenital heart disease is made on the presence of severe cyanosis, clubbing of the fingers, dyspnoea and the characteristic heart murmurs in an infant or young child. To diagnose the exact type of congenital lesion present is, however, except with the commoner types, more difficult. The marked advance, in recent years, of surgical treatment of congenital heart disease has, however, made such exact diagnosis of increasing importance in order to establish whether or not the lesion is of a type amenable to surgical treatment (not all types are).

To help in the diagnosis, specialized cardiac catheterization is carried out. The dye outlines the heart and its various chambers, and any abnormality may thus be visualized. The pressures in the heart chambers can be recorded and other valuable information obtained.

Complications

In many types of congenital heart disease one of the commonest complications is bacterial endocarditis. This is very common in patent ductus arteriosus, where infection occurs in the connection between the pulmonary artery and the aorta. It is also likely to complicate coarctation of the aorta.

Treatment of congenital heart disease

In the past, very little could be done for congenital heart disease, but now, due to important advances in surgery and anaesthesia, the condition can be improved and often cured. Surgery has produced the most dramatic results in cases of patent ductus arteriosus. The duct is ligatured, thus removing any abnormal strain and also preventing the development of bacterial endocarditis. Bacterial endocarditis which has already supervened on congenital heart disease is treated with penicillin or other antibiotics.

In patients with Fallot's tetralogy, an anastomosis between the pulmonary artery above the level of the stenosis and one of the main arteries, like the subclavian, is made. This allows a more adequate flow of blood into the lungs and effectively relieves the cyanosis. In severe cases of pulmonary stenosis with no septal defects a 'valvotomy' may be performed to widen the stenosed pulmonary valve and thus allow a free flow of blood into the lungs. In cases of coarctation of the aorta, successful removal of the obstructed part of the aorta has been carried out, while cases of atrial septal defect can be successfully repaired. The aims of surgery in the treatment of congenital heart disease are to relieve cyanosis and to improve the child's well-being.

CHRONIC HEART FAILURE

We have so far discussed the common causes of chronic heart disease and we have seen that many heart diseases cause symptoms only when failure of the heart develops. Before this stage the diagnosis of many forms of heart disease depends on the presence of signs which definitely indicate that the heart is not normal. Such signs include heart murmurs, irregular heart action and an enlarged heart. X-ray examination usually confirms or establishes the presence of an enlarged heart which, in nearly all cases, means that the heart is permanently damaged. Lastly, an electrocardiogram may show evidence of a diseased myocardium, particularly if it has been caused by coronary artery disease.

Chronic heart failure is usually the result of longstanding heart disease which eventually affects the heart by severe strain over a long period. The heart usually enlarges and the muscle hypertrophies to overcome the added strain. This allows the heart for a time to act more efficiently. The stage is reached, however, when the compensatory changes may fail to cope, and at this time heart failure develops.

If the strain on the heart is on the left side only, as commonly occurs in some heart diseases, then the left side of the heart may fail while the right side may continue to function normally. This stage is called 'left ventricular failure'. Ultimately, however, failure of the left side of the heart throws a burden on the right side and this in turn fails, whereupon right heart failure, or as it is more often termed, 'congestive heart failure', arises.

Left ventricular failure

Here, as noted above, the strain is on the left ventricle. This commonly occurs in:

1. coronary artery disease
2. hypertension
3. aortic valvular disease.

Symptoms and signs

These are caused by failure of the left ventricle to pump the blood from the left side of the heart into the arterial system, with the result that as the right side of the heart continues to function properly, blood accumulates in the lungs causing severe congestion. We have, then, a condition wherein the right side of the heart continues to pump blood into overloaded and congested lungs.

The cardinal symptom is breathlessness (dyspnoea), which occurs on any moderate exertion. It may also come on, however, at night, waking the patient up from sleep gasping for breath, so that he has to sit up in bed, and often goes to an open window for more air. Gradually the attack passes off. These attacks are called *paroxysmal nocturnal dyspnoea* (PND). The signs present depend on the cause of the left heart failure and may include a raised blood pressure, or signs of aortic valvular disease, such as murmurs. In addition, the pulse is usually rapid and may be irregular in rhythm. In most cases of left heart failure the left ventricle of the heart is enlarged. It should be noted that the signs of gross congestion in the venous system and the oedema, which are both so prominent in congestive (right-sided) heart failure, are absent at this stage.

Treatment

The patient must be sat up and given oxygen. Diamorphine administered intravenously is of great value. A diuretic such as frusemide helps to clear oedema from the lungs.

In the long term, diuretics such as frusemide should be taken regularly, with potassium supplements where necessary. If the blood pressure is raised, hypotensive treatment is also indicated.

Digoxin may be taken for atrial fibrillation.

Congestive heart failure

When the right ventricle fails to function properly, the right atrium becomes distended and this leads to stasis in the venous system. The pressure in the superior and inferior vena cava rises. The veins in the neck are distended, the liver becomes engorged, the legs become oedematous. This condition is known as congestive heart failure.

Causes

Any causes of the heart disease may give rise to congestive heart failure. Some of these diseases may first cause left heart failure, whilst in others the right side of the heart is affected from the start. For instance, in chronic chest diseases, especially chronic bronchitis and emphysema, congestive (right-sided) failure develops without going first through the stages of left heart failure. Figure 5.17 illustrates how mitral stenosis leads to congestive heart failure.

Symptoms and signs

1. *Dyspnoea.* Breathlessness is the cardinal symptom of congestive heart failure as it is of left heart failure. In very severe cases the patient may even be breathless lying in bed. Here the peculiar type of breathing known as *Cheyne–Stokes respiration* may be present; the respirations wax and wane so that there are periods of deep, gasping respirations followed by periods of very quiet breathing. Cheyne–Stokes breathing denotes an advanced degree of heart failure.

2. *Cyanosis.* This is due to the stagnation of the blood in the venous system, and also to the severe congestion in the lungs causing imperfect oxygenation of the blood.

3. *The pulse.* In congestive failure the pulse is usually rapid and may be regular or irregular. The commonest type of irregularity of the pulse is atrial fibrillation.

4. The veins in the neck are distended and stand out due to the venous congestion.

5. The congested lungs, in addition to produc-

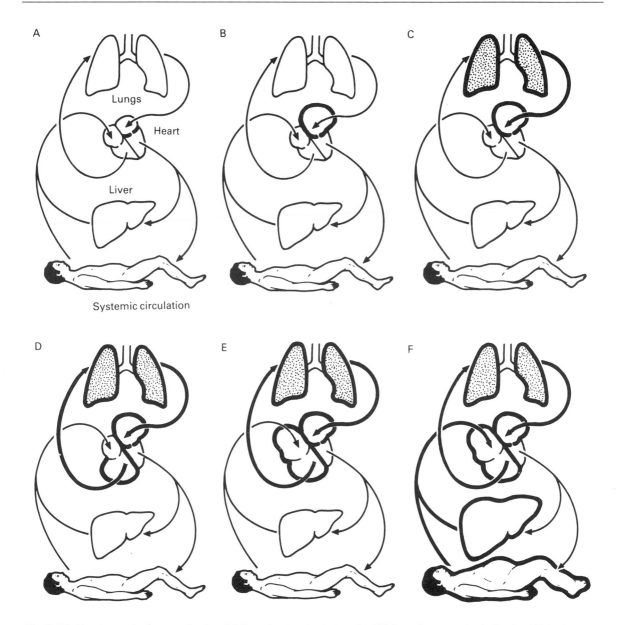

Fig. 5.17 Development of congestive heart failure due to mitral stenosis. Thickened narrowed mitral valve (**A**) leads to enlargement of left atrium (**B**). Lungs become engorged (**C**) and so the right ventricle enlarges (**D**) to meet the extra work. When the right ventricle tires, the right atrium cannot empty fully and becomes distended (**E**). The whole venous system is now engorged, leading to an enlarged liver and generalized oedema (**F**).

ing the cardinal symptoms of dyspnoea, also cause a cough and often haemoptysis. The latter is, however, never very severe.

6. Kidney function is affected and this leads to a diminished output of urine (oliguria).

7. Congestion of the stomach and the intestines produce symptoms of dyspepsia, such as nausea, heartburn and vomiting. Stretching of the liver capsule may produce abdominal discomfort and pain.

8. *Oedema*. Oedema means the presence of fluid in the tissues. In congestive heart failure the

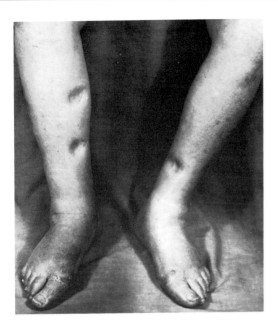

Fig. 5.18 Pitting oedema of the legs in a case of congestive heart failure.

fluid accumulates due to the increased pressure in the venous circulation which forces fluid from the capillaries into the tissues. As the pressure in the venous circulation is greatest in the lower part of the body, oedema is usually first noticed around the ankles when the patient is up and about. In the later stages, the fluid increases so that the legs become grossly swollen.

If the patient is in bed the oedema is usually most marked around the sacrum, producing the well-known sacral cushion or pad. This is because while the patient is in bed the sacral area becomes the lowest part of the body and the fluid first accumulates in this area.

The fluid may also accumulate in the different cavities of the body, such as the pleural cavity, producing what is known as a *pleural effusion*, and in the peritoneal cavity in the abdomen causing 'ascites'.

Increased venous pressure is thus an important factor in the causation of cardiac oedema. In addition, in cardiac failure the kidneys fail to excrete salt properly and this retention of salt in turn causes retention of water.

Treatment of congestive heart failure

Nursing The patient is nursed in a well supported upright position. Patients with heart failure are unable to lie flat as this increases the congestion of the lungs and so increases the dyspnoea. A bed-table on which the patient can lean is very useful. In many cases, however, the patient prefers to sit up in a chair so as to avoid the slipping down which may occur in bed. In addition, special beds known as cardiac beds, to keep the patient well propped up in a sitting position, are available.

Diet The diet must be light and easily digestible so as to avoid overloading the already congested gastrointestinal system. Restriction of added salt is advisable and fluids may also be restricted.

Bowels An aperient may be necessary to keep the bowels open and so prevent constipation and abdominal distension, with their added strain on the heart. The use of a commode at the bedside often causes less strain to patients than a bedpan.

Oxygen Oxygen is needed to improve the oxygen content of the blood and thereby relieve the cyanosis. It also, for the same reason, relieves the dyspnoea. The B.L.B. mask, the disposable plastic mask and the Venturi face-mask are all convenient and useful methods of administering oxygen, the last named having a flow meter to adjust the concentration of oxygen. It is most important that no open flame should come in contact with the oxygen due to the risk of fire. For this reason, smoking must be stopped and the patient warned about this danger. The concentration of oxygen must be carefully controlled in cases of chronic bronchitis.

Diuretics These compounds cause an increased output of salt and fluid by the kidneys and so relieve the oedema and circulatory congestion. They probably act by enhancing sodium excretion from the kidney tubules and this carries fluid with it. Potassium will also be lost, unless a potassium sparing diuretic is used. Several diuretics are now available:

1. *Frusemide* and related drugs. Intravenous preparations are available for urgent effect but usually they are given as tablets, preferably in the

Nursing care

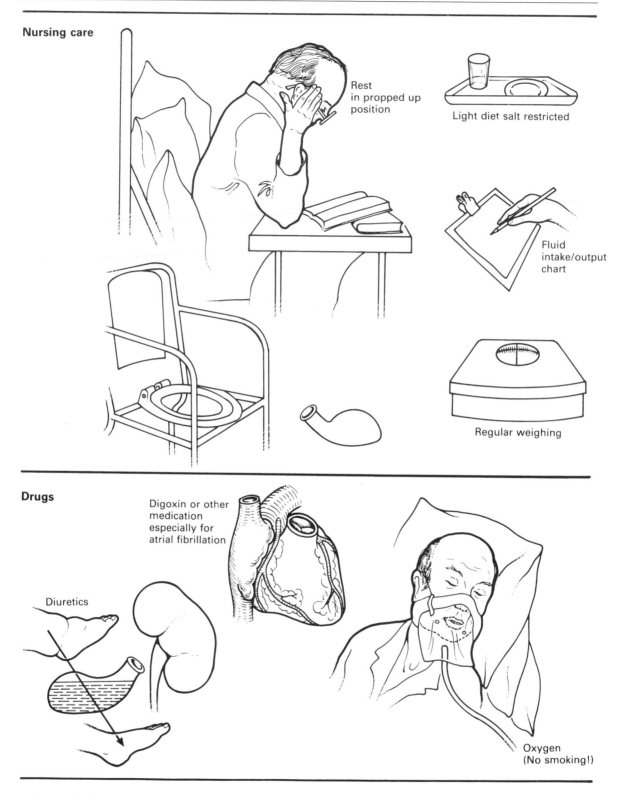

Rest
in propped up
position

Light diet salt restricted

Fluid
intake/output
chart

Regular weighing

Drugs

Diuretics

Digoxin or other
medication
especially for
atrial fibrillation

Oxygen
(No smoking!)

Fig. 5.19 Treatment of congestive heart failure.

morning to avoid nocturnal diuresis which might keep the patient awake. Where the oedema and congestion are severe, intravenous frusemide can be given until the condition has subsided. Thereafter, a smaller maintenance dose helps to keep the patient free from oedema. Potassium supplements such as potassium chloride or potassium effervescent tablets should be given.

2. *Chlorothiazide* compounds have effects other than diuresis. They help to bring down the blood pressure and are often prescribed with more powerful hypotensive agents in the treatment of hypertension. They enhance the effect of digitalis so that in patients taking digoxin the dose of digoxin may have to be reduced to avoid toxic effects. They also cause a rise in blood uric acid and in blood sugar so that prolonged usage of these diuretics may precipitate gout or lead to diabetes.

3. *Spironolactone* (Aldactone) antagonizes the hormone aldosterone and so causes loss of sodium and fluid from the kidneys. It has side effects such as gynaecomastia and hence is reserved for cases not responding to chlorothiazide. A useful means of telling when the patient is responding to diuretic therapy or, on the other hand, beginning to develop oedema, is regular weighing. As soon as they are fit, patients with heart failure should be weighed once or twice weekly.

Digoxin. This drug is of benefit in the treatment of congestive failure. As has been noted, digitalis is the specific drug used in controlling atrial fibrillation, and the most dramatic results are obtained in those cases of congestive failure accompanied by atrial fibrillation. Digoxin may be, however, also of value in those cases of failure not associated with atrial fibrillation.

Sedatives. Diamorphine may be given to severe cases to relieve breathlessness and ensure a good night's sleep and, thus, much needed rest. Most patients with heart failure before coming under treatment have probably lacked sleep for some time. In congestive failure due to chronic bronchitis and emphysema, morphine is best avoided, owing to its depressant action on the cough reflex.

Convalescence. When the oedema has subsided and the congestion in the lungs improved, a gradual return to a limited activity is started. With the treatment outlined above, the patient may be able to get about again and even do light work. However it is unfortunately likely that the patient will relapse, as in most cases the heart disease causing the failure cannot be cured.

PERICARDITIS

The pericardium is the outer covering of the heart and contains serous fluid which reduces friction when the heart contracts. Pericarditis (inflammation of the pericardium) can be due to infection or it can be associated with rheumatic fever, systemic lupus erythematosis or myocardial infarction. If there is excessive fluid in the pericardial sac (an effusion), it may impair heart function and require to be tapped and removed. This may be also done in some cases for diagnosis.

1. *Benign pericarditis* is due to a virus infection. It is manifested by fever, malaise, breathlessness and chest pain. There may be a pericardial effusion which makes the heart shadow on X-ray appear large and rounded. The disorder usually subsides without special treatment other than bed rest. Aspirin (300 mg every 4 hours) can be used until the pain has settled.

2. *Infective pericarditis* may be due to any bacterial infection including tuberculosis. It is associated with high fever, restlessness and dyspnoea. It responds to appropriate antibiotics.

3. Pericarditis sometimes follows myocardial infarction, giving rise to a rise in temperature and chest pain during the stage of recovery from the infarct. It is due to a non-infective inflammation and responds to steroid therapy.

4. *Constrictive pericarditis*. The pericardium becomes thickened and impairs the action of the heart beat by encasing it too tightly. This leads to breathlessness and congestion of the veins. Surgical removal of the constricting pericardium may become necessary. Constrictive pericarditis is often associated with previous tuberculous infection or malignant tumour infiltration.

DISEASES OF THE BLOOD VESSELS

The arteries

With increasing age, the arteries become thicker and less elastic, a condition known as *arteriosclerosis*. Arteries can be blocked by thrombosis or embolism and these disorders will now be described.

Arteriosclerosis

Causes Arteriosclerosis is a very common condition, most frequently found in middle-aged and elderly people. The exact cause of arteriosclerosis is unknown, but certain factors do appear to play an important role in the causation of the disease:

1. There is a strong hereditary basis.

2. Certain diseases predispose to this lesion, e.g. diabetes is very often associated with arteriosclerosis.

3. High blood pressure (hypertension). This common disease is distinct from arteriosclerosis, but there is some evidence that its presence aggravates or predisposes to the development of arteriosclerosis. Both conditions, however, may occur independently of each other.

4. The possible part played by the fat content of the diet in the causation of arteriosclerosis is now being investigated. It is believed that an excessive consumption of animal (saturated) fats (bacon, butter, cream, fat of meat) and a low intake of vegetable (unsaturated) fats may predispose to arteriosclerosis.

Pathology Arteriosclerosis is a degenerative disease and causes thickening and narrowing of the arteries owing to changes in the inner wall of the vessels. Localized deposits of fatty material appear on the inner surface of the arteries, forming large patches known as atheromatous plaques. These plaques narrow the smaller arteries and so they cause deficient blood supply to organs and tissues. Atheromatous plaques are also very liable to break down and form ulcers. Thrombosis may then develop as a result of the roughening and ulceration of the inner coat of the arteries. Arteriosclerotic changes commonly affect the aorta and spread to the aortic valve to cause an incompetence or stenosis of the valve.

The symptoms and signs caused by arteriosclerosis are due to:

1. the narrowing of small arteries which reduces the blood supply to the various organs and tissues

2. the thrombosis which is liable to occur in the diseased arteries.

Symptoms and signs In many arteries arteriosclerosis may have little effect, but in the following sites arteriosclerosis produces well-recognized diseases:

1. In the coronary arteries, where it causes (i) angina pectoris, (ii) coronary thrombosis

2. In the 'cerebral' arteries, where it causes cerebral thrombosis (one form of 'stroke')

3. In the leg arteries, where it causes (i) intermittent *claudication*, i.e. severe pain in the legs on exertion due to the diminished blood flow through narrowed arteries (ii) peripheral thrombosis with gangrene of the limb

4. Near the aortic valve, where it causes aortic incompetence or stenosis.

Treatment Since the cause of arteriosclerosis is obscure there is no known method of preventing its occurrence. Diets have been devised which employ substitutes, such as olive oil, to animal fats. Lack of exercise, obesity, cigarette smoking and nervous strain are all factors which seem to be associated with the early development of arteriosclerosis, and patients should be advised accordingly. Similarly, the early recognition and treatment of diabetes and hypertension is important in reducing the dangers of arteriosclerosis.

Thrombosis and embolism

Arterial thrombosis

Thrombosis is clotting in a blood vessel. Apart from certain special arterial cases, thrombosis is usually seen in the veins. The circulation in the arteries is normally too rapid for a clot to occur, but in the veins a sluggish circulation is not uncommon. However, when there is severe disease of an artery, particularly arteriosclerosis, thrombosis does occur; it is also found as a result of injury to an artery. The main types of arterial thrombosis are:

1. coronary thrombosis in arteriosclerotic coronary arteries
2. cerebral thrombosis in arteriosclerotic or, less often, syphilitic cerebral arteries
3. thrombosis in arteriosclerotic arteries of the lower limbs.

Coronary and cerebral thrombosis have already been fully described elsewhere; there remains for discussion thrombosis in peripheral limb arteries. In advanced cases of arteriosclerosis with gross narrowing of the arteries due to atheromatous plaques and roughening of the inner wall, thrombosis may supervene and completely obstruct the already partially blocked vessel. The signs and symptoms that follow will depend on the size of the artery which is obstructed and whether other blood vessels (the collateral circulation) can supply the area.

In a mild case, pain in the calves develops on walking any distance, a condition known as 'intermittent claudication'. Examination shows that the foot pulses cannot be felt and the feet feel cold. Usually these symptoms improve with time, partly because the collateral circulation improves and partly because the patient learns to avoid exertion which brings on the pain. When a major blood vessel is obstructed by a thrombus, gangrene may result. The foot becomes pulseless, cold and discoloured. Infection with gas gangrene may follow and endanger life. An arteriogram is an X-ray of the artery after a dye has been injected and will show where the artery has been occluded. Sometimes a surgical operation can be undertaken to bypass the blocked area. A vein is removed and inserted into the artery above and below the obstructing thrombus to allow the blood to flow freely again. Unfortunately, in many cases this repair operation is not possible and the leg has to be amputated.

Arterial embolism

Embolism in the arterial circulation is usually due to a clot becoming detached from the left side of the heart and travelling in the circulation, finally to lodge in an artery. There are three conditions which frequently give rise to a clot in the left side of the heart and so may cause arterial embolism:

1. In mitral stenosis with atrial fibrillation a clot (thrombus) may form in the left atrium.
2. In coronary thrombosis a clot may form on the endocardium of the heart over the damaged muscle (mural or wall thrombus).
3. In subacute bacterial endocarditis the large vegetations on the valves are easily and repeatedly dislodged to travel in the circulation. These small emboli may then lodge in the skin, kidneys, brain, etc. In the cases of (1) and (2) the embolus most frequently lodges in an artery in the brain, leg, kidneys, or mesentery. In the brain, it causes cerebral embolism with its consequential paralysis, usually in the form of a hemiplegia. In a peripheral artery of the leg, it completely cuts off the blood supply causing severe pain in the leg which becomes white, cold, paralysed and later gangrenous. The changes brought about by arterial thrombosis and embolism are essentially the same except that in embolism the changes are much more dramatic and usually more complete. Sometimes, surgical intervention can remove the clot from within the artery (embolectomy).

Thrombo-angiitis obliterans (Buerger's disease)

Thrombo-angiitis obliterans, although not as common as the arterial diseases already described, is not rare. For some unknown reason it rarely affects women. The exact cause is unknown and the only factor of established importance is that smoking appears to play a part. The underlying cause of the symptoms is the deficient blood supply to the affected limbs which is the result of the marked narrowing of the diseased arteries. The lower limbs are most commonly affected, the patient experiencing pain in the calves on exertion (intermittent claudication) which disappears with rest. (This pain is similar in type to that of angina pectoris, which is also due to deficient blood supply – *ischaemia*.) In the later stages gangrene sets in, usually starting in the toes. Gangrene is often precipitated by exposure to cold or to injury.

The treatment of thrombo-angiitis obliterans is

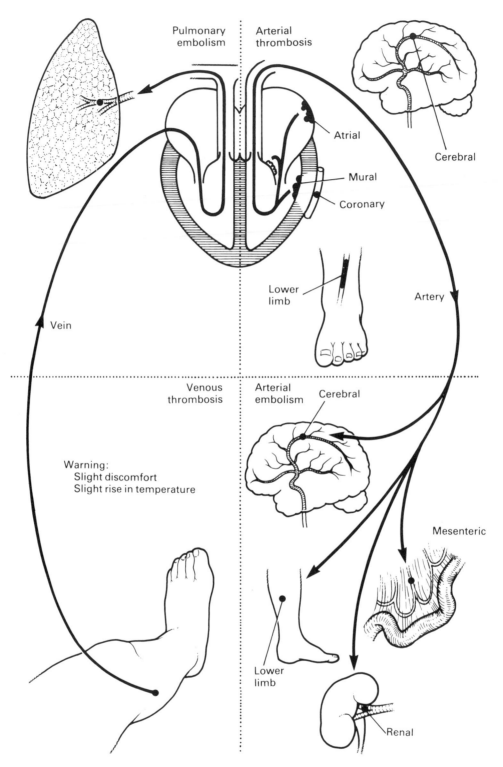

Pulmonary embolism

Arterial thrombosis

Atrial

Mural

Coronary

Cerebral

Lower limb

Artery

Vein

Venous thrombosis

Arterial embolism

Cerebral

Warning:
  Slight discomfort
  Slight rise in temperature

Mesenteric

Lower limb

Renal

Fig. 5.20 Thrombosis and embolism.

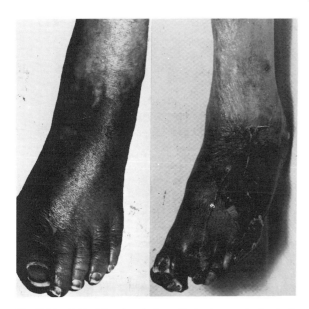

Fig. 5.21 **A.** Peripheral embolism. Early changes in the foot due to an embolus lodging in the popliteal artery. The foot is mottled blue and dead cold and the patient is unable to move it. The onset is marked by extreme pain. In this case the arterial embolus was dislodged from the heart, the patient having had a coronary thrombosis 12 days before. **B.** A later stage of arterial embolism of the leg showing advanced gangrene. The foot is black and necrotic.

unsatisfactory as there is no specific cure. The patient must stop smoking and take great care to avoid both the slightest injury to the feet and exposure to cold. Scrupulous attention to keeping the feet dry, warm and clean is essential. The nails must be trimmed with extreme care to avoid the slightest cut. If the patient is confined to bed special care must be taken to avoid pressure sores.

Regular leg exercises (Buerger's exercises) should be performed to improve the collateral circulation. The patient lies on a couch and the legs are supported 45 degrees above the horizontal until the feet blanch, usually after a few minutes. The legs are then lowered over the side until the feet flush pink. After a rest in the horizontal position the cycle is then repeated.

The operation of lumbar sympathectomy to cut the sympathetic nerves is of value in early cases. When gangrene occurs a high amputation is usually necessary. For the relief of pain analgesics such as codeine or aspirin are needed.

Raynaud's disease

In contrast to thrombo-angiitis obliterans, Raynaud's disease is usually seen in women and very rarely in men. Furthermore, it usually affects the fingers and seldom the feet, whereas the effect of thrombo-angiitis obliterans is precisely the opposite. Raynaud's disease is due to spasm of the arteries of the fingers and hands, causing deficient circulation. The hands first go blue and then dead white and feel numb. Exposure to cold is the usual cause of these symptoms. In severe cases gangrene may develop, but it is not as common a complication as in thrombo-angiitis obliterans. In the treatment of Raynaud's disease, protection from cold is most important. In severe cases sympathectomy may result in marked improvement. Vasodilator drugs and calcium antagonists (e.g. nifedipine) are said to relieve constriction of the arteries but in practice do not seem to be very effective.

The veins

Phlebitis

Phlebitis, or inflammation of a vein, is a very common condition, especially in the lower limbs. Apart from the cases in which it occurs for no obvious reason, phlebitis frequently arises during prolonged serious infections such as typhoid fever, as a result of injury to a vein (such as may occur during an operation), and during the puerperium.

If a superficial vein is affected it produces localized swelling, redness and pain. In the case of a deep-seated vein, marked oedema or swelling of the affected area and pain are the most prominent features. The chief danger in a deep venous phlebitis is the likelihood of a clot forming in the inflamed vein, whereupon the condition of 'thrombophlebitis' arises. If this happens, i.e. if a thrombus forms in cases of phlebitis, there is a small risk that the clot may become dislodged, travel through the venous system, and lodge in the lungs, so causing pulmonary embolism.

Venous thrombosis

Thrombosis frequently complicates a phlebitis

but it may also arise of its own accord. Any condition that produces a slowing of the venous circulation creates a predisposition to the formation of a clot in the veins. Such slowing of the venous circulation is frequently seen in patients who are confined to bed for a long time, particularly if they do not move about in bed. It is for this reason that venous thrombosis often develops in patients after major operations, especially in elderly people who are more reluctant to alter their position in bed.

Women taking the contraceptive pill have an increased liability to deep-vein thrombosis, probably because the pill contains oestrogens which disturb the normal clotting mechanism. Pregnancy is another common cause of venous thrombosis.

Congestive heart failure, because of the resultant slowing of the venous circulation, also predisposes to venous thrombosis.

In many cases of venous thrombosis, especially where there is no evidence of phlebitis, the symptoms and signs may be so slight that the first indication of the condition may be the occurrence of pulmonary embolism, the clot having become detached and travelled to the lungs. In the postoperative cases, the thrombus most commonly forms in the deep calf or pelvic veins. As a result, the patient may notice a sense of heaviness or slight pain in the calf, whilst slight swelling may be present. It is important to realize that the pain and swelling may be minimal even though a potentially dangerous thrombosis is present. Due weight should therefore be given to these slight signs. In these patients, a low-grade fever is also often present; after operation the presence of a slightly raised temperature for no obvious reason should arouse suspicion of a deep venous thrombosis.

Prevention and treatment of phlebitis and thrombosis Preventative treatment in those conditions likely to cause a venous thrombosis is most important. Early movement of the lower limbs combined with massage, to prevent undue slowing of the circulation, is desirable. Tight elastic stockings help reduce the risk of this condition. Early ambulation after operation also reduces the risk of thrombosis and embolism.

In the case of a superficial phlebitis, the danger of pulmonary embolism is rare. In mild cases a supportive elastic dressing may be all that is required. In the cases of deep venous thrombosis, usually confirmed by radiological methods, there is a very definite danger of embolism, and complete rest to the affected limb is essential; a splint or sandbags are useful means of immobilizing the limb, and a bed-cradle to take the weight of the clothes off the affected limb is advisable. Anticoagulant drugs are given to lessen the clotting of the blood, thus, by preventing the further spread of the thrombosis, reducing the risk of embolism. Heparin and warfarin are the most useful anticoagulant drugs for this purpose (see Table 5.1).

When deep vein thrombosis leads to repeated attacks of emboli, surgical intervention must be considered. X-rays of the veins after injections of dye (*venogram*) will reveal the full extent of the thrombus and the surgeon may either remove the clot or tie off the vein above it to prevent further emboli.

6

Diseases of the respiratory system

The respiratory system can be described in two parts. The upper respiratory tract consists of the nose, air sinuses, pharynx and larynx. The lower respiratory tract comprises the trachea, bronchi and lungs. During breathing, air enters from the nose and mouth through the larynx and trachea and thence to the two main bronchi. The bronchi divide into smaller bronchioles and these open into the pulmonary alveoli (Fig. 6.1).

The alveoli are large air sacs lined by thin flat cells and surrounded by capillary networks derived from the pulmonary arteries. It is in these alveoli that the interchange of gases takes place. The blood in the capillary network gives off carbon dioxide and exchanges it for the oxygen in the air freshly breathed into the alveoli. With each inspiration fresh oxygen is brought into the

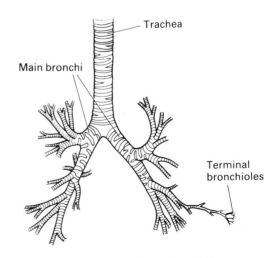

Fig. 6.1 Trachea, main bronchi and bronchioles.

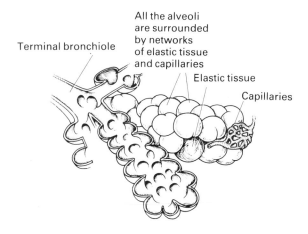

Terminal bronchiole

All the alveoli are surrounded by networks of elastic tissue and capillaries

Elastic tissue

Capillaries

Fig. 6.2 Bronchiole and alveoli.

alveoli and with each expiration carbon dioxide is exhaled. In this way the blood circulating through the lungs replenishes its oxygen supply in exchange for its waste carbon dioxide.

THE MECHANISM OF RESPIRATION

Air is drawn into the lungs by the act of inspiration. During inspiration the chest cavity is inflated by contractions of the respiratory muscles attached to the bony cage of the chest (intercostal muscles), which pull out the ribs. The diaphragm descends during inspiration, and this further helps to enlarge the chest cavity and so inflate the lungs. The lungs, in expanding, suck in air through the respiratory passages into each alveolus, and so allow the oxygen to be taken up and the waste product, carbon dioxide, to be given off. At the end of inspiration the intercostal muscles and diaphragm relax and allow the chest wall to fall back, thus deflating the lungs. In addition, the elasticity of the lungs themselves, by exerting a pull on the chest wall, also plays an important role in expelling the air. This expulsion of air from the lungs is known as expiration.

CONTROL OF RESPIRATION

Respiration is controlled through the respiratory centre in the medulla of the brainstem, which, through its influence on the nerves supplying the respiratory muscles and the diaphragm, can in-

crease or decrease the act of respiration. Diseases that involve the respiratory centre may affect the rate or depth of respiration. Furthermore, for the normal control of respiration the amount of carbon dioxide in the blood is most important. Even a slight increase in carbon dioxide stimulates the respiratory centre to increase the rate and depth of the respirations. A marked reduction in the oxygen content of the blood also stimulates respiration.

INVESTIGATION OF CHEST DISEASES

Chest X-ray

A chest X-ray (radiograph) is undoubtedly the single most important investigation in every patient suspected of a chest disorder. It provides essential information not only of the lungs but also of the heart, the aorta, the pulmonary vessels and the hilar lymph nodes.

A tomograph is an X-ray focused on a selective plane of the lungs and helps to identify smaller shadows more accurately.

Computed tomography (CT scans) and magnetic resonance imaging (MRI) are more sophisticated imaging techniques that allow fine structural detail to be seen. A bronchogram is an X-ray taken after an opaque fluid has been instilled into the trachea, so outlining with clarity the bronchi and the bronchioles.

Bronchoscopy

The bronchoscope is an illuminated tube, which, when passed into the bronchus, allows the operator to inspect the lining of the bronchus and to take a *biopsy* or cutting of any suspicious area for examination under the microscope. Its main value is in the diagnosis of lung cancer. With the invention of a flexible bronchoscope, the smaller bronchi have become accessible to inspection and a biopsy can be taken under direct vision. Examination of sterile saline instilled into an area of lung and aspirated back using the bronchoscope (bronchoalveolar lavage) can be useful in the detection of some conditions, particularly atypical infections and tumours that cannot be reached

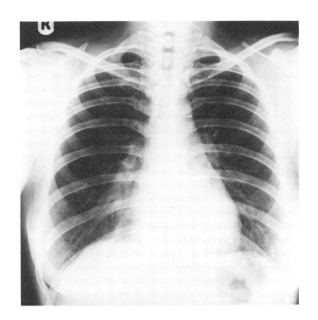

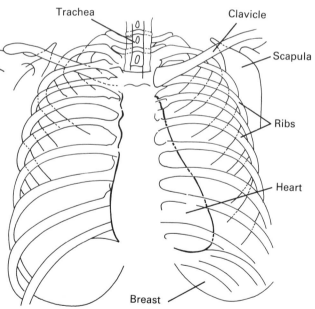

Fig. 6.3 X-ray of normal female chest.

using the bronchoscope.

Pleural and lung biopsy

A biopsy of pleura or lung may be obtained by penetrating through the chest wall with a special needle. Sometimes this is done with the aid of ultrasound or CT scanning, to localize accurately the area to be biopsied.

Tests of lung function

Various simple tests are available to test the functional capacity of the lungs and are valuable in assessing the results of treatment to see if there is a measurable improvement. A spirometer is an apparatus for measuring the amount of air breathed into it. The patient is asked to take in as deep a breath as possible and then to blow it out into the spirometer as fully and quickly as possible. This gives the forced vital capacity (FVC). The volume expired in one second is known as the forced expiratory volume (FEV_1). Normally, about three quarters of the vital capacity can be blown out in one second. This can be written as FEV/FVC = 75%.

In conditions such as asthma or bronchitis, the air passages are obstructed and expiration is delayed. Therefore, the FEV/FVC ratio may only be 40%. These disorders are called obstructive airway diseases. Measurements of the peak air flow during forced expiration are particularly useful in monitoring the severity and response to treatment of these conditions.

In chest ailments where the whole chest movement is restricted both FEV and FVC are greatly reduced but the ratio may remain normal. These disorders are known as restrictive airway diseases.

Blood gas analysis

The efficiency of the alveoli in exchanging gases can be assessed by measuring how much oxygen and how much carbon dioxide is present in arterial blood. Normally the pressure of oxygen in arterial blood is 13.3 kilopascals (expressed as P_{O_2} = 13.3 kPa) while the pressure of CO_2 is 5.3 kilopascals (P_{CO_2} = 5.3 kPa).

Different respiratory disorders may affect the blood gases in different ways. For example, in pneumonia, gas exchange is impaired and the oxygen in the blood falls (perhaps as low as 6 kPa). The carbon dioxide concentration is usually normal in these patients. As the red cells in the

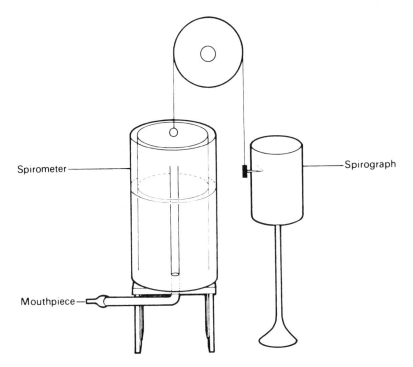

Fig. 6.4 Spirometer.

blood no longer contain sufficient oxygen the blood becomes less red and more blue in colour and the patient is said to be cyanosed; severe cyanosis may result in confusion. Giving oxygen in high concentrations is important in this situation.

In patients with chronic chest disease, there may be retention of CO_2 as well as inadequate oxygen. Pco_2 may rise above 13.3 kPa and this degree of carbon dioxide retention will lead to mental confusion. Since the arterial oxygen falls correspondingly, it may seem reasonable to give the patient pure oxygen to breathe, but this may do more harm than good. These patients have become used to having high concentrations of CO_2, and the respiratory centre is now dependent on low oxygen to stimulate breathing. Therefore oxygen should be given at a low concentration (28%) by a special mask so that the Po_2 does not exceed 50 mmHg. If the oxygen content rises above this, the stimulus to breathe is diminished and more carbon dioxide is retained.

COMMON SYMPTOMS OF RESPIRATORY DISORDERS

Cough

A cough is an explosive expiration against a closed glottis. It is a reflex action produced by stimulation of nerve endings in the membranes lining the air passages. These nerve endings are sensitive to foreign particles inhaled from the air and to collections of mucus formed because of infection. Consequently, coughing is a response to these stimuli and helps to clear the air passages of unwanted material.

In many mild disorders of the respiratory tract and in the early stages of infection or of bronchial carcinoma, no mucus has formed and the cough is dry and *unproductive*. Some drugs can cause a dry cough, notably ACE inhibitors used in the treatment of high blood pressure and heart failure.

A *productive* cough is one that produces sputum and so helps to clear the air passages.

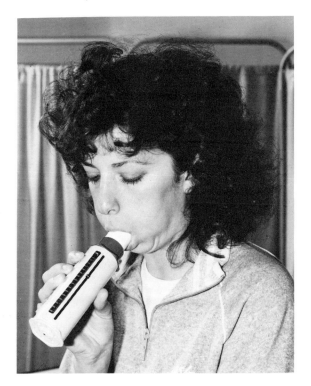

Fig. 6.5 Peak flow meter.

Sputum or phlegm

Sputum is an excretion from the lining mucous membrane of the respiratory passages. According to the nature and extent of the disease the sputum varies in amount and character. In the early stages of disease sputum may be absent, appearing later when the lesion in the respiratory tract has progressed. The sputum may be a clear white colour, when it is called mucoid. In such cases the sputum is usually the result of minor irritation of the respiratory passages. In more severe lesions, especially inflammatory diseases due to infection, the sputum is frankly purulent. Where actual destruction of tissue is present, the sputum may be bloodstained owing to erosion of a blood vessel.

Some diseases of the lungs are associated with chronic widespread damage to the lung tissue, and in these cases abundant purulent sputum, often offensive and bloodstained, is present. Such diseases are bronchiectasis, lung abscess, lung cancer and advanced tuberculosis.

Dyspnoea

Dyspnoea means difficulty in breathing or, as it is most usually called, breathlessness. The underlying cause is usually a deficiency of oxygen. Any disease that interferes with the proper uptake of oxygen stimulates the respiratory centre, so that an increase in the respirations occurs to try to overcome this oxygen deficiency. Apart from diseases primarily involving the lungs, other diseases, especially heart failure, can cause dyspnoea. In heart failure, owing to the impaired action of the heart, the circulation through the lungs becomes slower so that congestion of the lungs results and seriously interferes with the proper uptake of oxygen. In addition, any disease that makes the respiratory act painful may cause dyspnoea.

Cyanosis

When the oxygen content of the blood falls, the blood in the skin capillaries takes on a bluish colour, known as cyanosis. Cyanosis usually denotes a severe degree of involvement of the respiratory system.

Pain

This is usually due to the pleurisy (inflammation of the pleura) which accompanies many forms of chest disease. When the inflamed surfaces of the pleura are rubbed together during respiration, this causes pain. It is important to remember that other conditions such as angina, a heart attack or a pulmonary embolus may cause severe chest pain. Localized pain may occur in the chest wall, for example from a fractured rib.

Haemoptysis

Coughing up blood is called *haemoptysis* and may vary from mere staining of the sputum, as mentioned above, to frank blood. The coughing up of blood is a most important sign, and usually denotes a serious chest disease, especially pulmonary tuberculosis and lung cancer.

Causes of haemoptysis

1. Pulmonary tuberculosis

2. Congestion of the lungs as seen in congestive heart failure, particularly in cases of mitral stenosis
3. Carcinoma of the bronchus; this is the most frequent cause of haemoptysis in older people
4. Bronchiectasis
5. Certain acute chest diseases, such as pneumonia (rusty sputum) and pulmonary embolism.

Haemoptysis has to be distinguished from haematemesis, which is the vomiting of blood.

Many patients find it difficult to be sure whether they actually cough or vomit the blood. Table 6.1 is of help in distinguishing between the two.

If the exact diagnosis is not obvious from the history or physical findings, an X-ray of the chest may suggest the cause. The next investigation is usually bronchoscopy, but even then sometimes no cause for the haemoptysis can be found.

Table 6.1 Distinguishing between haemoptysis and haematemesis

Haemoptysis	Haematemesis
The blood is thick, frothy, bright red and is coughed up	The blood is dark, is usually mixed with food, and is vomited up
There is a tendency to spit up small amounts of blood, often mixed with sputum, for several days after the initial haemorrhage	It is usually vomited up all at once or in several large amounts
There may be signs of chest disease or mitral stenosis	There may be a history of indigestion, peptic ulcer, or other diseases of the stomach

Treatment of haemoptysis

1. A slight degree of haemoptysis does not call for any treatment other than that of the causative disease.

2. Severe haemoptysis. Complete bed rest is recommended if the patient has a large haemorrhage.

Fluids only will be wanted in the early stages; later, a light diet is given as the general condition improves.

Most patients are best nursed in the semi-propped-up position as this is the most comfortable for them.

Haemoptysis is very rarely fatal in itself but nevertheless can be very frightening, so the patients will need comfort and reassurance.

Sedatives may be needed to allay anxiety and give the patient must needed rest. Morphine is best avoided as it depresses the cough reflex and respiration and may allow the lungs to become filled with blood. On the other hand, excessive coughing is also harmful as it can prolong haemorrhage, and so a mild sedative to reduce coughing, such as codeine sulphate (60 mg), is useful.

DISEASES OF THE UPPER RESPIRATORY TRACT

The upper respiratory tract is usually taken to include the nose, sinuses, pharynx and trachea. Diseases affecting this part of the respiratory tract are extremely common, and many of them are described in textbooks on surgery. For instance, chronic enlargement of the tonsils and adenoids, sinusitis, etc. are not discussed here. Many infectious diseases which may affect the upper respiratory tract are dealt with in the chapter on infectious disease.

The common medical diseases which affect the upper respiratory tract include the following:

1. acute coryza
2. acute tonsillitis
3. acute tracheitis
4. laryngitis
5. hay fever.

Acute coryza (the common cold)

This is caused by a virus which is very infectious and spreads rapidly from person to person. One attack produces no immunity or resistance in the body, so that further attacks can and, of course, do occur.

Symptoms and signs

These will already be familiar and need little description. The essential feature is an inflammation of the nasal passages, known as rhinitis, which produces a running nose and sneezing. Running eyes are also common and, perhaps, mild conjunctivitis. The inflammation often spreads to involve the pharynx and trachea. This results in pharyngitis and tracheitis with resulting huskiness, sore throat and cough.

Course and prognosis

Most cases clear up within a few days and the only danger is that infection may spread down to affect the lungs and thus cause bronchitis. This is likely to occur only in patients in debilitated states, especially elderly people and infants.

Treatment

A day or two at home helps to limit the spread of infection to others. Treatment is symptomatic.

Acute tonsillitis (acute streptococcal throat)

This is a very common infection, especially in any institution where large numbers of people are closeted together. The cause is most often the haemolytic streptococcus, but other organisms, particularly viruses, can cause an acute tonsillitis.

Symptoms and signs

1. The onset is usually sudden, with a general feeling of malaise, fever and headache.
2. The patient complains of a sore throat and difficulty in swallowing. The throat is often described as feeling very dry.
3. When the throat is examined it will be found to be inflamed and red and usually white spots (exudate) are present on both tonsils.
4. Occasionally a peritonsillar abscess forms which produces a large and very painful swelling in the mouth. 'Quinsy' is a frequently used name for a peritonsillar abscess.

Diagnosis

This is usually fairly obvious because of the presenting complaint of a sore throat. Difficulties,

however, often arise in infants and young children. Here, even with children old enough to give an account of their symptoms, a soreness of the throat is seldom complained of. The presenting symptoms in young children are usually fever, malaise and abdominal colic; the last may give rise to a mistaken diagnosis of acute appendicitis.

Examination of the throat in sick children is therefore most important as a routine, whether or not a sore throat is complained of. The nurse should have readily available a spatula and suitable illumination (torch) for the doctor when he is examining all sick children. The ears are always examined as a routine in all sick children. An auriscope of suitable size should therefore also be to hand.

Treatment

Bed rest is advised and a throat swab can be taken to find the causative organism. In cases which do not improve rapidly, appropriate antibiotics may be administered. Diet has to be light, with plenty of hot drinks, which are soothing to the throat. If the throat is very painful, especially in cases of peritonsillar abscess, analgesia with paracetamol is appropriate, and these drugs have the additional benefit of reducing fever.

If a peritonsillar abscess is present and does not subside rapidly on the above treatment it will need to be opened. This is done under local anaesthetic by means of sharp-pointed sinus forceps or a short-bladed knife.

There are two other diseases that give rise to sore throats and symptoms like those in acute streptococcal sore throat and it is important to differentiate between them: diphtheria and glandular fever. *Diphtheria* is now a rare disease because of vaccination. Here, the symptoms are very similar except that the patient is usually more ill and toxic, and the pulse is more rapid. There is also the characteristic membrane in the throat, which does not occur in most cases of acute tonsillitis. A throat swab will reveal the diphtheria bacilli.

Glandular fever produces a sore throat with greyish ulceration on the tonsils. Enlargement of the lymph nodes in the neck, mild fever and malaise are frequently present. A rash may occur, particularly if the patient has been treated with antibiotics. The infecting organism is the Epstein–Barr virus, and a blood test (monospot) is required to make the diagnosis. Treatment is symptomatic, and recovery usually occurs in 2–3 weeks.

Acute tracheitis

Inflammation of the trachea may occur:

1. in association with certain of the infectious fevers, such as measles or influenza
2. with the common cold
3. as a primary infection in itself.

Symptoms and signs

The general signs of infection, including fever, malaise and headache, are present. In addition, the patient complains of a typical sore feeling behind the sternum. A dry or slightly moist cough is also common.

Treatment

Steam inhalations or a cough linctus may be advised. Simple analgesia with paracetamol is appropriate.

Laryngitis

Acute laryngitis

Causes: (i) acute infectious fevers, particularly measles, diphtheria and influenza; (ii) the common cold, acute tracheitis, or acute bronchitis may all be associated with acute laryngitis.

Symptoms and signs Besides the general signs of infection, including malaise, fever and headache, there is the characteristic huskiness of voice and hoarseness. Sometimes there may be almost complete loss of voice. The throat is sore and there is an accompanying dry cough.

Diagnosis The diagnosis of laryngitis is usually obvious, but it is important to distinguish those cases that are due to measles and diphtheria. The examination of the mouth will show any Koplik's spots, thus identifying the case as one of measles, as also would, of course, the presence of a morbilliform rash. In diphtheria there is usually the characteristic membrane present in the throat, but in a few patients this may be absent. If there is any suspicion that the laryngitis might be due to diphtheria the case is treated as such till a definite diagnosis is made. In doubtful cases a throat swab should be taken and sent to the laboratory for culture.

Treatment of acute laryngitis The patient is nursed in bed in a well-ventilated atmosphere, but avoiding draughts. If it is thought that the laryngitis may be due to measles, diphtheria or any other infectious fever, then proper isolation precautions are taken and, in addition, any specific treatment, e.g. diphtheria antitoxin, given.

The diet should be light, with plenty of fluids. Some patients with laryngitis find a steamy atmosphere soothing and inhalations from an inhaler or a steam tent may be used.

Since most cases are due to a virus infection, there is no specific treatment and most cases settle in a few days. If the case is a severe one, with high temperature and signs of toxicity, penicillin or another antibiotic may be given for the possibility of a secondary bacterial infection.

Chronic laryngitis

Causes: (i) prolonged overuse of the voice as in singers or auctioneers; (ii) cigarette smoking; (iii) tuberculous laryngitis; (iv) malignant disease of the larynx.

Symptoms and treatment The predominating complaint is one of chronic progressive hoarseness, eventually leading to loss of voice. In all cases of chronic hoarseness an examination of the throat and vocal cords will be made by means of a laryngoscope and a biopsy taken for histological examination to exclude malignant disease. By this means the exact nature and cause of the laryngitis can usually be identified.

The treatment will naturally vary according to the cause. In those cases due to overuse of the voice, prolonged rest is usually sufficient. In tuberculous patients there is usually an advanced pulmonary tuberculous lesion as well, which requires the appropriate treatment as outlined on page 134. Analgesia may be given for the pain.

In malignant disease of the larynx, operation or radiotherapy is carried out unless the disease has spread too far, in which case only palliative treatment can be given.

Hay fever

Hay fever is an allergic disease, like many cases of asthma and urticaria. In hay fever the patients are sensitive to grass or tree pollens and when they come in contact with them the typical symptoms of hay fever develop. Similar symptoms may occur as a result of other allergies, for example to house dust mites or animal fur.

Symptoms and signs

1. The onset is often at a specific time of the year, which may vary according to the particular allergen.
2. Paroxysmal attacks of sneezing, associated with a running nose and running eyes, occur. The bouts of sneezing may last in some cases for hours on end. There is usually severe congestion of the nasal passages and eyes.

Treatment

Symptoms can often be controlled with antihistamines, with newer agents such as terfenadine being less likely to cause sedation than older drugs. Anticongestant sprays may appear helpful, but are not usually recommended as they may cause worse congestion (rebound congestion) when they are stopped. Steroid or sodium cromoglycate nasal sprays are helpful in preventing attacks, but have to be taken for several days before they are effective.

DISEASES OF THE LOWER RESPIRATORY TRACT

Acute bronchitis

This is a common condition often initiated by a viral infection of the upper respiratory tract with secondary bacterial infection with *Haemophilus influenzae* or haemolytic streptococci. It is commoner in the winter months and particularly in smokers, the elderly, the frail or in those with a chronic chest disorder.

Bronchitis often occurs in children with infectious fevers, especially measles, influenza and whooping cough.

Symptoms and signs

1. There are the symptoms of a mild fever such as malaise, headache and loss of appetite.
2. A cough is an early symptom and is associated with a moderate amount of mucoid or purulent sputum.
3. There may be soreness or pain beneath the sternum caused by an accompanying tracheitis.
4. The respirations are usually a little fast and somewhat laboured, but except in serious cases there is no severe dyspnoea or cyanosis.

Course

The disease usually subsides fairly rapidly in a few days, and is serious only in young children and elderly people where the inflammation may spread and cause bronchopneumonia. Repeated attacks of acute bronchitis may, however, give rise to chronic bronchitis with much more serious consequences.

Treatment of acute bronchitis

The patient is put to bed and kept warm in a well-ventilated atmosphere. Light diet is given with plenty of drinks. Aspirin or paracetamol will probably be found useful (aspirin should not be given to children under the age of 12), and on this treatment most cases will subside rapidly. More serious cases will need treatment as discussed under acute exacerbation of chronic bronchitis.

Pneumonia

Pneumonia is an inflammatory condition of the lung caused by infection, usually bacterial or

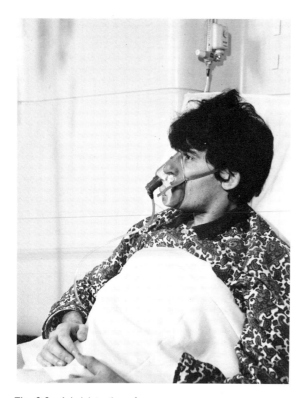

Fig. 6.6 Administration of oxygen.

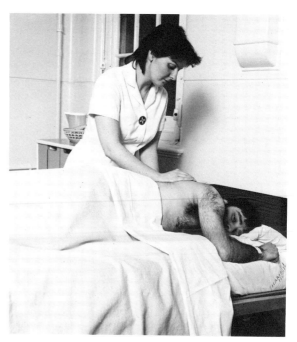

Fig. 6.7 Physiotherapy.

viral. As a result of infection, the alveoli become filled with serous fluid and inflammatory cells: the area of lung involved is said to have undergone consolidation. As recovery takes place, the alveolar inflammatory material is coughed up: in the early stages this sputum often contains many red cells and is rusty in appearance. Later, as the white cells invade the alveolar exudation, the sputum becomes yellow and purulent.

It is helpful in the diagnosis and treatment of pneumonia to distinguish between infections acquired in the community, and those which develop in hospitalized patients. Further categories include pneumonia in patients with a defective immune system (particularly AIDS) and aspiration pneumonia.

Community-acquired pneumonia

Most cases are due to pneumococcal infection which causes the classical pneumonic consolidation involving one or more lobes of the lung.

Consolidation involving patches of lung tissues, usually affecting both lungs in different areas and not confined to any one lobe is also common. This generalized pneumonia (sometimes called *bronchopneumonia*), may be due to bacterial invasion by organisms such as *Branhamella catarrhalis* or *Haemophilus influenzae*. Staphylococcal infection may occur following infection with influenza, particularly in the frail and elderly. Pneumonia may also be caused by virus infections or by *Mycoplasma pneumoniae*. *Mycoplasma* is a bacterium which lacks a cell wall but it is, however, sensitive to some antibiotics such as erythromycin. Rare but important causes of pneumonia in this category include *Legionella* infection, which may occur in patients exposed to a contaminated water supply. Outbreaks have often been associated with hotels, or even hospitals. Q fever is an infection often present in animals such as sheep, cows and goats. Man becomes infected by drinking milk or inhaling dust containing the organism. It can cause pneumonia and sometimes affects the heart as well. The diagnosis is made by finding antibodies to the organism in the blood and treatment is tetracycline. Psittacosis (ornithosis) is an infection caused by the bacterium *Chlamydia psittaci* which is caught from parrots, canaries and budgerigars and can lead to generalized patchy pneumonia. The onset is gradual with general malaise, a raised temperature, headache and cough. It is diagnosed by testing the blood for antibodies and usually responds to treatment with tetracycline.

Pneumonia can occur in a previously healthy person due to an overwhelming infection. However, many conditions may predispose to the development of pneumonia:

1. Any chest diseases already present, such as chronic bronchitis and emphysema, lung cancer or bronchiectasis.

2. Especially in the winter months, the old and the frail are liable to respiratory infections leading to pneumonia.

3. Alcoholism and malnutrition dispose to chest infections.

4. In babies and small children, infectious fevers such as whooping cough and measles can lead to pneumonia.

5. Aspiration of infected mucus from the nose or the sinuses following a simple infection of the upper respiratory tract may lead to areas of bronchopneumonia.

Clinical features The clinical features will depend on the type of infection causing the pneumonia (bacterial, viral or mycoplasmal) and on whether it supervenes on a chest disease already present.

Lobar pneumonia

1. The onset is sudden, with a high fever (often 102° to 104°F) (39° to 40°C), and is often accompanied by shivering attacks (*rigors*). A severe pain in the chest over the affected lobe of the lung may be present owing to the frequently accompanying pleurisy. This pain characteristically catches the breathing so that the patient is nervous of taking a deep breath. For this reason also the cough, which is usually present, is short and suppressed. The pulse and respirations are usually rapid.

2. The face is flushed and herpes labialis (*cold sore*) is very commonly present on the lips and cheek. This is a small group of vesicles clustered together which after a few days crust and resolve. Herpes labialis is most commonly associated with lobar pneumonia or the common cold.

3. After a day or so the cough becomes moist with the typical rusty sputum, the colour being due to altered blood. The sputum is very thick and tenacious and often adheres to the side of the sputum carton.

4. In severe cases the breathing may be very distressed and cyanosis is present. In these severe attacks delerium may also occur.

Pneumonia due to viruses, mycoplasma and atypical organisms

This type of pneumonia varies considerably in severity. The onset is usually characterized by constitutional symptoms such as general malaise, headache, sore throat, loss of appetite and temperature. These features may persist for several days before chest symptoms of cough, pleuritic pain and breathlessness become apparent.

Diagnosis When the doctor examines the chest with a stethoscope, typical alterations in the breath sounds over a consolidated lobe may be heard which, with the above symptoms, allow a ready diagnosis of lobar pneumonia to be made. More frequently, however, the signs are less clear, and X-ray examination of the chest should be carried out to confirm the diagnosis and to watch the resolution of the pneumonia. The solid lobe shows up on X-ray as a dense shadow. Blood and sputum samples are taken for culture to identify the organism involved. Blood gas estimation is also important as this can suggest the severity of the infection, and may indicate the need for oxygen.

Most cases respond rapidly to treatment with appropriate antibiotics. The temperature falls after a few days, the breathing becomes comfortable and the cough becomes productive of purulent sputum. The antibiotic most likely to be successful in pneumococcal pneumonia is penicillin and this should be given by injection. In less severe cases, ampicillin or amoxycillin may be prescribed in capsule form by mouth. If, as is usually the case, the infective organism is not known, more than one antibiotic will be prescribed to cover the most likely infecting organisms – for example ampicillin plus erythromycin.

Pneumonia due to the bacterium *Klebsiella* often leads to abscess formation in the lung. It does not respond to penicillin but usually does so to gentamicin or cotrimoxazole.

Staphylococcal pneumonia sometimes follows a staphylococcal infection elsewhere in the body, such as a carbuncle or osteomyelitis. It may be resistant to penicillin and the choice of antibiotic may be decided by the sensitivity of the bacteria to various antibiotics after blood culture.

Mycoplasma pneumonia tends to run a slow course even when treated, and cough and X-ray shadows may persist for several weeks before complete resolution and recovery.

Mycoplasma infections respond well to erythromycin or tetracycline.

Although virus infections are not sensitive to antibiotics, they are often prescribed partly because the diagnosis may be in doubt, and partly because viral pneumonias may be complicated by bacterial infection.

Patients who do not get better as expected may need a change of treatment because the infection is resistant to the antibiotic being used. Other complications may be present, particularly:

1. An empyema may have formed. This is a purulent effusion in the pleural cavity.
2. There may be underlying lung cancer or pulmonary tuberculosis.

Treatment Treatment is as follows:

1. The patient should be propped up in bed in a comfortable upright position and encouraged to cough up sputum. When breathing is made difficult by pleuritic pain, non-steroidal anti-inflammatory drugs such as ibuprofen may be helpful, but occasionally diamorphine may be needed despite its property of depressing the respiratory centre.
2. Appropriate antibiotics should be given (intravenously if the patient is seriously ill) as discussed above.
3. In the acute phase, if breathing is difficult and the patient cyanosed, oxygen may be helpful

by oxygen mask. A nervous patient will need reassurance and explanation before the mask is applied.
4. Especially in the elderly, the physiotherapist is invaluable in helping the patient to cough up sputum and to move his or her legs to help prevent a deep venous thrombosis developing.

Hospital-acquired pneumonia

This is defined as pneumonia occurring 2 days or more after hospital admission. Pneumonia occurring in hospitalized patients is often more severe and is often difficult to diagnose and treat for several reasons:

1. Patients are often debilitated from other illnesses (e.g. chronic chest disease, stroke, diabetes mellitus). Aspiration of stomach contents may cause an associated chemical pneumonitis.
2. Patients may have undergone recent surgery.
3. The widespread use of antibiotics in hospitals means that organisms may be resistant to commonly used antibiotics.

Diagnosis is often difficult, as the patient may not complain of typical symptoms or even develop a fever. Mental confusion may be the only sign that all is not well. Blood and sputum cultures are routinely taken, but only provide a definitive diagnosis in 25% of cases. *Legionella* infection should be considered and can be diagnosed by looking for antibodies in the blood.

The usual treatment of hospital-acquired pneumonia is with high-dose, broad-spectrum, intravenous antibiotics. Other measures as described above are of course essential. Respiratory failure may occur and the patient may have to be managed on an intensive care unit.

Pneumonia in immunocompromized patients

The groups of patients discussed here are those who have a defective immune system, either because of radiotherapy or chemotherapy (e.g. for cancer or in transplant recipients), or because they have the acquired immune deficiency syndrome (AIDS).

When the body's immune defence mechanisms are inadequate the lungs frequently become infected with unusual or opportunistic organisms: these may be bacteria, viruses or fungi. The commonest organisms are:

1. *Pneumocystis carinii.* This is particularly common in AIDS. Typically, there is a dry cough and dyspnoea. Fever is often present. Patients may have other features of HIV infection such as weight loss, fatigue and oral candidiasis. A chest X-ray may suggest the diagnosis (Fig. 6.8), but definitive diagnosis is from sputum or broncho-alveolar lavage. Most cases respond well to cotrimoxazole.

2. Cytomegalovirus (CMV). This virus frequently causes pneumonia in transplant patients, but rarely in AIDS (although generalized CMV infection is common in AIDS). Patients usually present with fever, dry cough and muscle and joint pains. Treatment is with the antiviral drug ganciclovir.

3. *Aspergillus.* Infection by this fungus is par-

ticularly common in patients treated for acute leukaemia. This is a severe infection with high mortality. Treatment is with amphotericin B.

4. *Candida.* This fungus is the cause of oral or vaginal thrush, but may spread to the lungs in immunocompromized patients. Another source is the skin, and infection may spread from an intravenous cannula. Again this is a severe infection. Amphotericin B is used as treatment.

5. Others. Tuberculosis and typical bacterial pneumonias are common in immunocompromized patients, and should always be considered.

Bronchiectasis

Bronchiectasis is a disorder characterized by widening and dilatation of the bronchi: these become infected and form sumps of purulent phlegm. The cause is usually unknown but may follow pneumonia or whooping cough in childhood. Other cases of bronchiectasis are due to inherited diseases, particularly cystic fibrosis.

Clinical features

The characteristic features of bronchiectasis are cough with the production of large quantities of purulent sputum. Often the cough occurs in paroxysms and is worse in the early mornings.

There may be haemoptysis, breathlessness and loss of weight. Where the chest infection is severe, clubbing of the fingers may occur.

Diagnosis

In the early dry stage the diagnosis can be confirmed by CT or MRI scanning, but the best technique is X-ray examination of the chest after inserting an opaque oil into the bronchi (*bronchogram*). The bronchi can then be outlined and if they are dilated and widened above the normal the diagnosis of bronchiectasis is confirmed. For the more advanced cases the diagnosis is usually obvious, owing to the typical symptoms and signs, especially the chronic cough, copious sputum and the clubbing of the fingers.

Complications

Bronchopneumonia. This is the most common

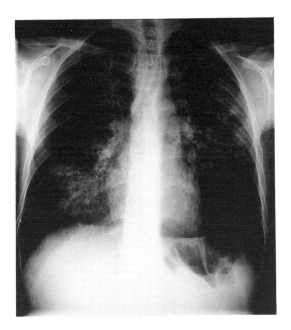

Fig. 6.8 Chest X-ray in patient with pneumocystis carinii infection in association with HIV infection. Diffuse bilateral shadowing as seen here is common in this condition, but the chest X-ray may be entirely normal. X-ray courtesy of Dr Walter Curate, Consultant Radiologist, Hammersmith Hospital.

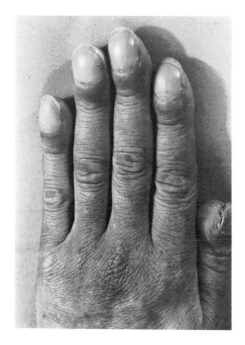

Fig. 6.9 Clubbing.

complication, and is usually recurrent.

Cerebral abscess. Septic emboli may travel from the lungs into the arteries and to the brain to cause a cerebral abscess.

Treatment of bronchiectasis

Repeated courses of antibiotics such as ampicillin help to keep the sputum from becoming profuse and purulent.

Postural drainage is effective in preventing sputum from collecting in the dilated bronchi. If, for instance, the lower parts of the lungs are affected, then the patient is 'tipped up' so that the foul sputum is brought up more easily on coughing. The patient can be tipped up by elevating the foot of the bed with the patient lying flat on the bed, or else by the patient leaning forward over the edge. Special beds are available which allow easy posturing of the patient. Patients and their families can be taught these techniques by the physiotherapist.

If the bronchogram reveals that only one segment of the lung is involved and the condition continues to be troublesome despite postural drainage, particularly if haemoptysis is present,

surgical resection of the affected segment of the lung can be undertaken.

Lung abscess

Abscess of the lung is an uncommon condition but is seen in the following circumstances:

1. following the inhalation of a foreign body into the lungs
2. due to inhalation of septic matter from the nose or throat following operations on these parts.

Symptoms and signs

There are usually signs of infection, with swinging fever, sweating and general malaise. With these symptoms there are usually a persistent cough and sputum which is characteristically foul, copious, and may be bloodstained. If the condition is allowed to become chronic, signs of bronchiectasis with clubbing of the fingers may occur.

Diagnosis

Following the inhalation of a foreign body, or after an operation on the nose, the presence of a persistent cough and foul sputum will inevitably lead to a chest X-ray being taken. The abscess cavity will then be seen.

Treatment

Any foreign body should be removed by bronchoscopy. Penicillin is the drug most commonly used in lung abscess, often with very good results. Postural drainage for more chronic cases may also be very useful. If the condition does not respond to the above measures, surgical treatment to drain the lung abscess may be necessary.

Pulmonary tuberculosis

Tuberculosis is the name given to the illness caused by infection with the tubercle bacillus (*Mycobacterium tuberculosis*). There are two main types of tubercle bacillus, the human and the

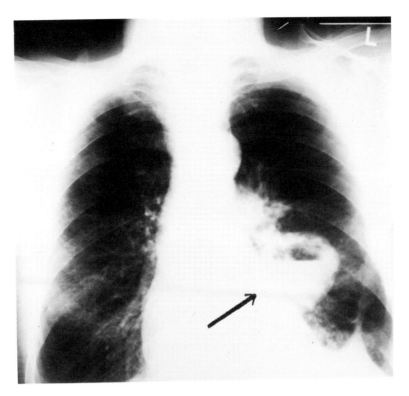

Fig. 6.10 Lung abscess.

bovine. Human tuberculosis is spread from person to person, mainly by droplet infection. Bovine tuberculosis occurs in cattle but can spread to man by drinking infected milk.

Tuberculosis can affect many parts of the body. The lungs are the organs most commonly involved, but tuberculosis can also affect the glands, the meninges, the bones, the kidneys, and the joints.

Tuberculosis was a widespread disorder in the last century and was a prominent cause of death in children and young adults. There are many reasons why it is now comparatively uncommon in developed countries:

1. Tuberculosis thrives when there is dirt, overcrowding, and malnourishment. Better sanitation and a better standard of living have contributed greatly to overcoming the spread of tuberculosis.

2. Tuberculosis used to affect cows and this led to milk infected with bovine tuberculosis. Today, all dairy herds in Britain are free from tuberculosis, and pasteurization of milk (heating to a temperature lethal to bacteria) provides an additional safeguard.

3. Easy availability of chest X-rays uncovers cases of unsuspected pulmonary tuberculosis. Routine chest X-rays should be taken:
   a. in those most likely to acquire tuberculosis, such as certain immigrant groups or those living in lodging houses
   b. in those most exposed to the disease such as nurses and hospital workers, and
   c. those likely to spread the ailment – such as schoolteachers or waiters.

4. Immunization by BCG vaccine protects against tuberculosis.

5. Effective chemotherapy is available for patients who have contracted pulmonary tuberculosis.

Pathology

The tubercle bacillus is an *acid-fast* bacillus. When specimens of sputum or other material are

Spread

Primary infection
Most children combat
the disease and acquire
immunity

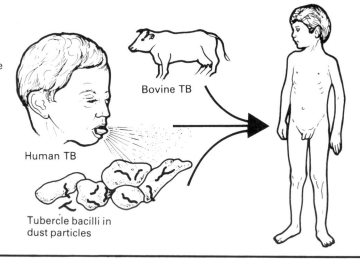

Bovine TB

Human TB

Tubercle bacilli in
dust particles

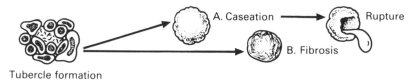

Tubercle formation

A. Caseation ⟶ Rupture

B. Fibrosis

Diagnosis

Tuberculin test

Microscopy

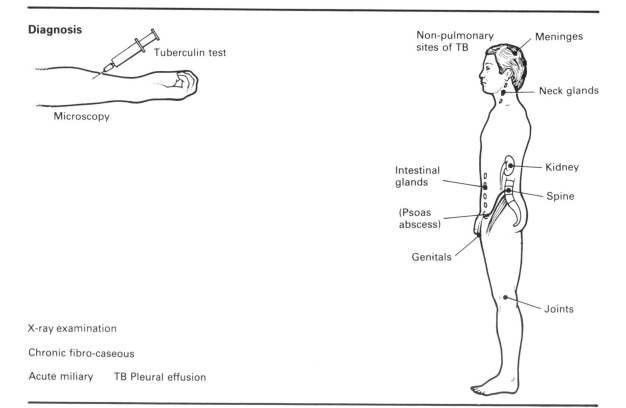

Non-pulmonary
sites of TB

Meninges

Neck glands

Intestinal
glands

Kidney

Spine

(Psoas
abscess)

Genitals

Joints

X-ray examination

Chronic fibro-caseous

Acute miliary   TB Pleural effusion

Fig. 6.11 Spread of tuberculosis.

stained with dyes to show up bacteria under the microscope, unlike most bacilli, the tubercle bacilli do not lose colour when acid is added. This is a valuable method of identification, as culture of the tubercle bacillus can take 6 weeks.

Tubercle formation

The tubercle bacillus is so called because it leads to the formation of a small rounded area or *tubercle*. The tubercle is a collection of small endothelial cells and lymphocytes around the bacilli. 'Giant' cells typical of tuberculosis occur. These tubercles can merge so that a wide area of tissue may be affected, and this process may then be followed by caseation and fibrosis.

Caseation

This is a breaking down, or necrosis, of the tubercles into a soft cheesy mass which may liquify to form tuberculous pus. What happens next depends on where the lesion is; for example, if it is in the lungs it can rupture into a bronchus and leave behind a cavity; if in a lymph gland it can produce ulceration with discharge of tuberculous pus, forming a sinus.

Fibrosis

Active fibrous tissue formation can occur around the tubercles. The fibrous tissue is an attempt by the body to wall off the infection and heal the lesion by scar-tissue formation.

Usually caseation and fibrosis are present together. Marked caseation and slight fibrosis are evidence of severe infection and little effort on the part of the body to heal. Alternatively, when fibrosis is marked, then the disease is usually arrested or limited. Sometimes calcium is deposited in the caseated mass, and this calcified lesion is also usually arrested or healed.

The commonest entry of tubercle bacilli is by inhalation. When sputum is expectorated from someone with pulmonary tuberculosis, the tubercle bacilli can survive for many months. Infection can occur by inhaling dust which contains the bacilli or by direct droplet infection. The respiratory tract can be affected in different ways:

1. Pulmonary tuberculosis. The upper lobes of the lungs are particularly liable to be involved with infiltration and spread of the disorder to other parts of the lung. Caseation may occur with formation of cavities.

2. Infection of the pleura leads to pleurisy and pleural effusion.

3. Miliary tuberculosis. The bacteria invade the blood stream and small tubercles appear throughout the lungs and many other organs as well, especially the liver.

Primary tuberculosis

Many children or young adults are infected with tubercle bacilli without any symptoms or obvious illness. There is normally only a small area of lung or pleura involved, with enlargement of hilar glands. Healing occurs in most cases without trouble, often followed by calcification. Therefore it is not uncommon in routine chest X-rays of the healthy population to find evidence of a healed primary infection in the form of a calcified focus.

Further evidence that there has been a previous primary infection with tuberculosis is provided by the *tuberculin test (Mantoux reaction)*. Tuberculin is a purified protein derived from tubercle bacilli and available in different strengths.

Tuberculin is injected intradermally, starting with a low strength. In those who have previously been infected, a red raised area appears at the site of the injection: these subjects are designated *tuberculin–positive*. Those who do not react in this way are *tuberculin–negative*. The Heaf test is a similar test using a drop of tuberculin placed on the skin through which six needle punctures are subsequently made with a special needle holder.

Routine tuberculin testing of school children aged about 13 shows about one in ten to be tuberculin positive. If they have X-ray evidence of lung involvement, they may need active treatment with chemotherapy.

In children who are tuberculin-negative, BCG vaccination is undertaken.

Prevention

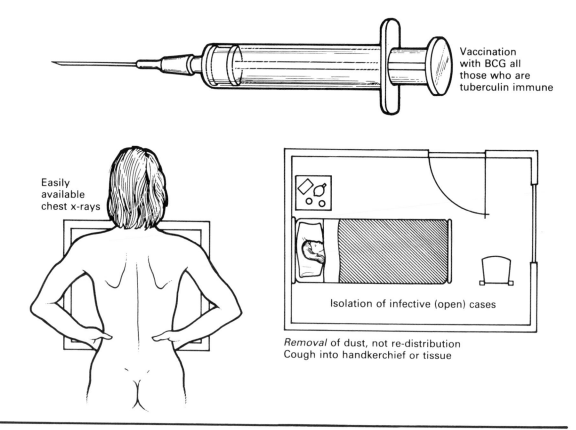

Vaccination with BCG all those who are tuberculin immune

Easily available chest x-rays

Isolation of infective (open) cases

Removal of dust, not re-distribution
Cough into handkerchief or tissue

Treatment

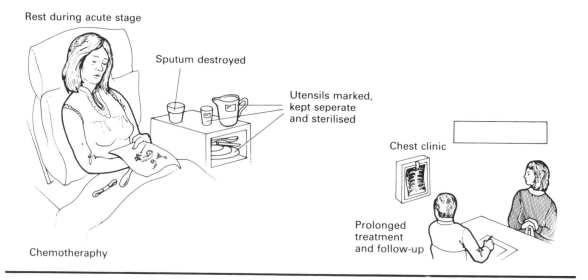

Rest during acute stage

Sputum destroyed

Utensils marked, kept seperate and sterilised

Chest clinic

Prolonged treatment and follow-up

Chemotheraphy

Fig. 6.12 Prevention of tuberculosis.

BCG vaccination BCG (Bacillus Calmette Guérin) is a harmless bacillus which resembles the tubercle bacillus. When BCG is inoculated it stimulates antibody formation and so protects against tuberculosis for at least 15 years.

BCG is given routinely with parental consent to tuberculin-negative school children aged 13–15; it is given in the neonatal period in high-risk populations. It is also given to those who are tuberculin-negative and at special risk, for example nurses and doctors working in chest units.

Postprimary pulmonary tuberculosis

This is a progressive tuberculous involvement of the lungs, sometimes occurring many years after the primary infection. It may present in a variety of ways:

1. Clinical features of a constitutional disorder with loss of weight, loss of appetite, malaise, low-grade fever, night sweats and fatigue.

2. A persistent cough, often attributed to cigarettes, may be the first symptom of pulmonary tuberculosis.

3. Haemoptysis. There may be bloodstained sputum or the sudden coughing up of bright red blood. When an erosion of an artery in a cavity occurs, the haemoptysis may be profuse and recurrent.

4. Patients who present with pneumonia but fail to respond completely to antibiotics may have underlying chronic pulmonary tuberculosis.

5. Routine chest X-rays frequently reveal the presence of unexpected pulmonary tuberculosis. It is for this reason that a chest X-ray is always taken in anybody who has lost weight for no known reason or has shown deterioration in general health.

Pleural effusion due to tuberculosis usually comes after the primary infection in young people. The early symptoms include (i) chest pain made worse by coughing or deep breathing; (ii) general malaise and a raised temperature; (iii) increasing breathlessness.

Miliary tuberculosis

This is due to widespread dissemination of small tubercles through the bloodstream. The onset is usually insidious with lassitude, pyrexia, sweats and loss of weight. Tuberculous meningitis may cause headaches and drowsiness.

Diagnosis of pulmonary tuberculosis

X-ray of the chest may suggest the diagnosis but this can be confirmed only by the finding of acid-fast bacilli in the sputum. Patients must be encouraged to cough up their sputum into a disposable carton and this is then taken to the laboratory for special staining (*Ziehl–Neelsen technique*) and examination under the microscope.

The sputum will also be cultured for growth of the bacilli.

When it is not possible to obtain sputum because the patient swallows it, gastric washings should be obtained. This is best obtained in the early morning. A nasogastric tube is passed through the nose or mouth into the stomach, 10 ml of saline is injected through the tube with a syringe, and all the stomach fluid withdrawn for transmission to the laboratory.

Investigation of a pleural effusion requires aspiration of the chest and a pleural biopsy. The simplest apparatus for aspiration is a syringe with a two-way tap, one way allowing fluid to be sucked into the syringe from the chest and the other allowing the fluid to be ejected from the syringe into a bottle. The fluid is sent to the laboratory for examination of white cells (in tuberculosis they are mainly lymphocytes) and for culture to grow and identify the tubercle bacilli. A biopsy of the pleura can be obtained by the insertion of a special needle into the chest which cuts off a small piece of pleura when it is being withdrawn. The pleura examined under the microscope may show inflammatory cells characteristic of a tuberculosis infection.

The tuberculin test may be used as a confirmatory test in doubtful cases since it will be strongly positive in the presence of active tuberculosis. If the test is negative, it makes the diagnosis unlikely.

Management of tuberculosis

Chemotherapy successfully cures pulmonary tuberculosis and hospital treatment is usually only advised for the first week or so to make sure that the patient understands fully the details of the treatment and how and when to take the appropriate drugs. Hospital in patient treatment is also advised:

1. in all patients with miliary tuberculosis or pleural effusion until recovery is complete
2. in ill, poorly nourished or elderly patients requiring rest and general care
3. patients with infected sputum, especially if they have children in the family at home
4. uncooperative patients with a poor social background, perhaps living in a hostel or with a history of alcoholism
5. patients who have developed side-effects with the drug treatment.

Chemotherapy

Since the tubercle bacillus develops resistance to most of the antituberculous drugs given on their own, at least two drugs must be given together. In the initial treatment quadruple or triple therapy is prescribed. Five drugs are in common use:

1. *Isoniazid*. This drug is safe, effective and inexpensive. It seldom gives rise to toxic effects. Its disadvantage is that occasionally the tubercle bacilli become resistant to it. It is usually given as a single dose of 300 mg each day.
2. *Rifampicin*. This antibiotic is bactericidal for the tubercle bacilli but can have toxic effects on the liver. If given alone, it can lose its effect after a time because the bacilli become resistant to its action. It is expensive. It should be given as a single dose of about 450 mg each morning on an empty stomach.
3. *Ethambutol*. This is usually given with the other two drugs as initial treatment as a single morning dose of about 800 mg each morning.
4. *Streptomycin* has to be given by intramuscular injection and can have toxic effects on the vestibular system, causing vertigo and deafness if given in excess.
5. *Pyrazinamide*. This drug has enabled the total treatment time to be reduced from the traditional 9 months to 6 months. Side-effects include hepatitis and rashes.

The guiding principles of treatment are:

1. The nature of the ailment must be explained to the patient so that his full cooperation is obtained. A successful cure depends on the patient following the treatment and attending regularly, usually at a chest clinic, for supervision and advice.
2. Treatment begins with four drugs, usually isoniazid, rifampicin, pyrazinamide and ethambutol, all given each morning as a single dose and maintained for 2 months.
3. Treatment is then maintained with two drugs, isoniazid and rifampicin, for a further 4 months, making 6 months continuous daily treatment in all.
4. Long-term supervision, perhaps annually, is sometimes advised by the chest clinic to make sure that there is no relapse.

Social aspects

Tuberculosis is a notifiable disease. Once notification has been made:

1. Examination is made of those who have been in contact with the patient at home and at work. This may necessitate doing a tuberculin reaction and a chest X-ray.
2. The health visitor will be informed and may visit the patient's home to see if help is needed and if the diet is adequate.
3. Housing and sanitation facilities will be inspected.
4. Special financial grants are available to help the patient find more suitable employment if that is necessary.

Diseases of the pleura

The pleura is a membrane covering the lungs (the *visceral pleura*) and lining the inner side of the chest wall and diaphragm (the *parietal pleura*). Normally the visceral and parietal pleura are in smooth contact with each other, lubricated by a thin film of serous fluid. When the chest moves with respiration, this fluid prevents friction between the two layers of pleura.

Pleurisy

Inflammation of the pleura (*pleurisy*) may cause friction or adhesions between the two layers. This is due to a bacterial or viral infection, and although this can occur on its own, pleurisy is commonly associated with pneumonia or with pulmonary tuberculosis.

Clinical features are as follows:

1. The onset is often abrupt with raised temperature, headache and general malaise.

2. The breathing is rapid and shallow because deep inspiration leads to severe chest pain due to stretching of the inflamed pleura. The patient may be in obvious distress and may grunt with each breath.

3. Coughing causes pain and so the cough is short and barking in character.

The diagnosis may be confirmed by hearing a pleural rub with the stethoscope. This is a grating sound heard over the chest and caused by friction between the inflammed layers of pleura.

Treatment The treatment will depend on the cause. If it is bacterial, appropriate antibiotics may be prescribed. Analgesics may be necessary to relieve the discomfort. Non-steroidal anti-inflammatory drugs combined with codeine are particularly useful. If the pain is severe, pethidine or diamorphine may be advised, though these have the danger of depressing respiration. Sometimes the application of heat in the form of a hot water bottle or electric heating pad offers comfort when placed on the chest.

Pleural effusion

Sometimes pleurisy may lead to a considerable increase of the fluid between the two layers of pleura. This *pleural effusion* may be large enough to compress the lung and cause difficulty in breathing. This can occur when pleurisy is associated with pneumonia and particularly when the pleurisy is due to pulmonary tuberculosis (see p. 131).

Carcinoma of the bronchus can invade the pleura and can cause a pleural effusion which is often bloodstained.

A pleural effusion can be part of general retention of fluid due to chronic nephritis, cirrho-sis of the liver, or congestive heart failure. Oedema of the legs and ascites may also be present.

Clinical features A pleural effusion usually causes breathlessness on exertion and if it is due to infection, there may be general features of a raised temperature and malaise as well. When the chest is examined by the physician, on tapping with the finger the percussion note sounds dull instead of resonant. An X-ray of the chest will reveal the presence of fluid.

If the nature of the effusion is in doubt, aspiration of the fluid can be undertaken. A needle is inserted through the chest wall and some fluid is withdrawn for examination and culture in the laboratory. Repeated aspirations may be necessary to relieve breathlessness. In some cases of recurrent pleural effusion due to a tumour, injection of an irritant such as talc into the pleural space may be tried in the hope of causing the two layers of pleura to fuse. This will prevent the effusion from returning.

Empyema

This term is used to describe a pleural effusion that has become infected and purulent. It is a localized collection of pus in the pleural space and is most commonly associated with pneumococcal or staphylococcal pneumonia. The empyema usually develops a week or two after the onset of pneumonia. As a rule, the patient has not been responding well to treatment. The temperature starts to rise again and the patient becomes more ill, with sweating and breathlessness. The diagnosis is suspected when the chest is examined. An X-ray confirms the presence of a pleural effusion. Aspiration must be undertaken and turbid purulent fluid will be withdrawn and sent for examination.

Treatment Appropriate antibiotics, usually penicillin and flucloxacillin, must be given which will destroy the bacteria causing the infection. In addition, antibiotics such as penicillin may be injected into the pleural cavity. It may be necessary to repeat the aspirations and pleural injections of penicillin on several occasions before the empyema subsides. In some cases where this treatment is not successful, surgical intervention may be necessary. Part of a rib is resected under anaesthetic, and a large chest drain inserted to allow drainage of the purulent material.

Pneumothorax

A small tear in the visceral pleura can allow air to escape from the alveoli into the pleural space. This is known as a *pneumothorax*. Sometimes, a flap is formed which allows air to enter the pleural cavity but prevents its escape. If the patient coughs a lot, more and more air is forced into the pleural space and the pressure increases. This is known as a tension pneumothorax and can cause considerable compression of the lung.

A pneumothorax can occur spontaneously in young people, probably due to the bursting of a small blister on the visceral pleura. Pneumothorax can complicate an established chest disorder such as emphysema, asthma or pulmonary tuberculosis. It is also an important complication of chest injury.

Clinical features Often the only symptom is that of mild breathlessness on effort and there are no constitutional symptoms. Sometimes the onset is marked by sudden pain in the chest and steadily increasing breathlessness. When there is a ten-

sion pneumothorax, the patient may be very breathless, cyanosed and distressed.

The diagnosis is usually suspected when the chest is examined by the physician and confirmed when a chest X-ray is taken. Air in the pleural space can be seen to compress the lung. The heart and the mediastinum may be pushed across (mediastinal shift) by the pressure of air in the pneumothorax.

Treatment The patient is best supervized in hospital, but in most cases where the symptoms are not severe, the pleural tear seals off on its own and the air is gradually absorbed through the pleura. The lung soon expands again and no further treatment is needed.

In more severe cases, and especially in a tension pneumothorax, which is a medical emergency, a chest drain must be inserted into the pleural space to relieve the pressure by releasing the trapped air. This usually consists of a trocar introducer and a rubber tube, and is inserted between the ribs after infiltration with local anaesthetic. The other end of the tube lies under water in a container to prevent air returning into the chest. When the patient coughs, air is expelled as bubbles into the water, sometimes gentle suction will need to be applied.

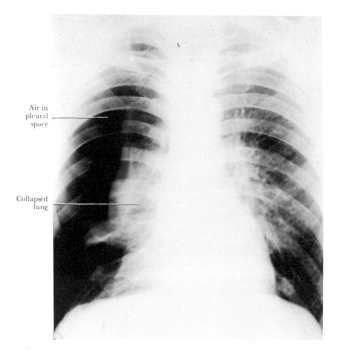

Air in
pleural
space

Collapsed
lung

Fig. 6.13 Pneumothorax.

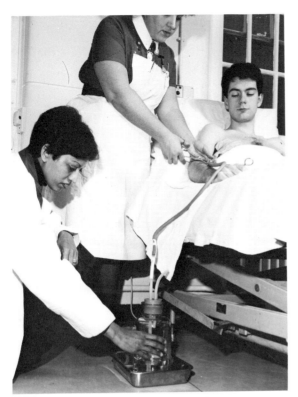

Fig. 6.14 Insertion of a chest drain in the treatment of pneumothorax.

Usually, the pleural flap heals over after some days and the catheter can be withdrawn. The wound is closed using a purse string suture. Very occasionally surgical intervention is necessary to seal the pleural tear when natural healing does not occur and the pneumothorax persists or recurs.

Obstructive lung disorders

Chronic bronchitis and emphysema (chronic obstructive airway disease)

These are two disorders which frequently exist together to a lesser or greater degree. In chronic bronchitis, there is swelling and thickening of the lining of the bronchial tree and obstruction to air entry is made worse by the presence of thick mucus. Emphysema is characterized by distension and damage of the alveolar air sacs: there is a loss of elasticity in the lungs as a whole. Chronic bronchitis and emphysema can lead to progressive disablement of the sufferer, the so called respiratory cripple, breathless and incapacitated.

Chronic bronchitis is a serious cause of disability and death, more common in men than women and usually becoming manifest in middle age. Cigarette smoking is the most important single cause, though air pollution by smoke and sulphur dioxide or working in a dusty atmosphere (e.g. coal miners) could be contributory causes.

Clinical features The onset of chronic bronchitis is usually insidious, and heralded by a morning cough (the so called 'smokers cough'), expectoration of mucoid sputum and breathlessness on exertion. These symptoms get worse over the winter months, particularly after an upper respiratory tract infection. Gradually the cough becomes more persistent, the sputum frequently purulent, and the breathing more wheezy and difficult.

As the years go by, particularly if smoking is not discontinued, the disability slowly gets worse. As the airway obstruction increases, the colour becomes more cyanosed and the strain on the right ventricle of the heart may lead to congestive heart failure, often termed *cor pulmonale*. The patient is now breathless even at rest, the sputum more frequent and purulent, the face is cyanosed and suffused and the legs oedematous.

Acute exacerbations are caused by episodes of infective bronchitis, leading to respiratory failure. The oxygen content of the blood becomes seriously depleted and there is a dangerous retention of waste carbon dioxide. This leads to deep cyanosis and mental confusion or coma. Unless vigorous measures are adopted to clear the airways and oxygenate the lungs, death will follow. In the early stages:

1. Every effort must be used to persuade the patient to give up cigarette smoking entirely. Smoky atmospheres should be avoided where feasible and a dusty occupation may have to be changed.

2. Antibiotics such as amoxycillin or cotrimoxazole should be given two or three times daily and continued for 10 days at the first sign of a chest infection or when the sputum becomes purulent.

3. Where wheeziness is present, bronchodilators may be helpful. Salbutamol is most effective,

usually by inhaler. Nebulized bronchodilators may be used during exacerbations, or even by patients at home in severe cases. Wheeziness suggests an allergic response (see asthma) and in some cases steroids are helpful, usually as a beclomethasone inhaler. Before prescribing steroid therapy, it is usual to perform lung function tests before and after a trial period: there is no point in giving steroids for a long term if the response to a trial does not lead to measurable improvement.

Cor pulmonale

1. Treatment may need to be maintained throughout the winter months and perhaps even in the summer as well. This is because the patient's resistance to respiratory infections is very low at this stage and because when there is so little functional respiratory reserve, even a minor chest infection can be dangerous.

2. Diuretics. Diuretics help to relieve systemic and pulmonary oedema induced by strain on the right ventricle of the heart. Bendrofluazide or frusemide are two useful diuretics in this respect. They relieve oedema of the legs and ease the breathing.

3. Oxygen. Oxygen increases the oxygen content of the blood and gives symptomatic relief.

Where there is excessive carbon dioxide retention, too high an increase of blood oxygen may depress respiratory function and so lead to further CO_2 retention. Therefore oxygen should be given by a Venturi mask which provides oxygen in a concentration of 28%: the concentration of oxygen in air is only 21%. Long-term oxygen (at least 16 hours per day) has been shown to improve survival in patients with chronic obstructive airways disease. This can be provided at home in cylinders or as a machine that concentrates oxygen from the air.

Respiratory failure

A patient may become acutely unwell with severe cyanosis and confusion or unconsciousness. The first essential is to ensure a clear airway. The patient is encouraged, if he is able, to cough up sputum. Physiotherapy can be invaluable in this respect. If this fails to lead to an improvement, a cuffed endotracheal tube can be passed into the trachea and attached to a mechanical ventilator. By this means, the mucous secretions can be sucked out of the air passages and a mixture of air and oxygen transmitted into the lungs by the ventilator. The ventilator provides a positive pressure intermittently to mimic normal breathing and this is known as intermittent positive pressure ventilation (IPPV). Patients in respiratory failure need continuous supervision and nursing and are often cared for in an Intensive Care Unit. The prognosis for patients with chronic obstructive airways disease who reach this stage is often very poor.

Emphysema

Whereas inspiration is an active process brought about by contraction of the chest muscles, expiration is a passive movement caused by the elastic recoil of the lungs as the chest muscles relax. In emphysema, the alveolar air spaces are distended and enlarged and the lungs lose their elasticity. Consequently, the chest moves poorly and expiration is prolonged and difficult.

Emphysema is often associated with chronic bronchitis and is due to much the same causes. However, in some patients there is a deficiency of an enzyme (alpha-l-antitrypsin) which normally protects the structure of the alveolar walls.

Clinical features The salient symptom of emphysema is breathlessness, gradually over the years becoming more incapacitating. Cough and sputum are not troublesome unless chronic bronchitis is present as well. The chest moves poorly, the respiration rate is rapid and expiration is laboured and prolonged. Often the colour is good and the patient is not cyanosed.

Treatment is mainly that of associated chronic bronchitis or the complications already discussed.

Interstitial lung diseases

This group of disorders includes conditions where there is infiltration or fibrosis of the lung tissue, and includes sarcoidosis, pulmonary fibrosis and the pneumoconioses. Fibrosis of the

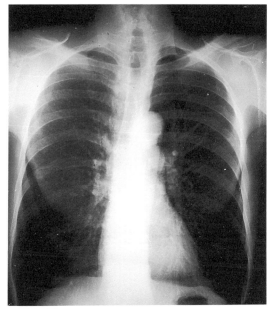

A

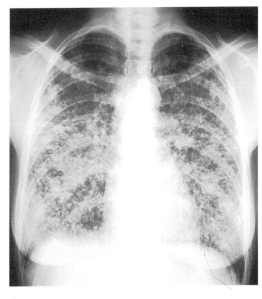

B

Fig. 6.15 Chest X-rays of (**A**) obstructive lung disease in a patient with emphysema - note increased apparent size of lungs due to air trapping, and (**B**) restrictive lung disorder - sarcoidosis. X-rays courtesy of Dr Walter Curate, consultant Radiologist, Hammersmith Hospital.

lungs, like fibrosis in any tissue or organ, is a response to injury and is the predominant change occurring in chronic inflammations. Fibrosis of the lungs is seen in many chronic inflammatory chest diseases, especially in tuberculosis (fibro-caseous type) and bronchiectasis.

Sarcoidosis

Sarcoidosis is a disease which resembles tuberculosis in that tissue affected by sarcoid appears under the microscope to contain tubercles (or granulomas) but tubercle bacilli are not found. The cause is still unknown. It affects many organs and systems but the lungs, lymph glands and skin are frequently involved. Sarcoid is usually not as serious as tuberculosis and tends to get better without treatment. The tuberculin test is negative unless as sometimes happens tuberculosis itself supervenes. It tends to affect adults between the ages of 20 and 40.

Lungs. The commonest symptoms are breath-lessness and cough. X-ray shows a diffuse mottling of the lungs, resembling miliary tuberculosis. The condition usually improves over several months, but sometimes cortisone (or another steroid) is necessary when progress is slow.

Skin. Pinkish nodules may appear on the face and chest. Apart from this, erythema nodosum is a common manifestation of sarcoidosis. Raised red painful areas appear on the shins and sometimes on the forearms; these may persist for several weeks before subsiding, and are sometimes associated with pyrexia and malaise.

Glands. Enlargement of the lymph nodes in the neck and in the mediastinum may occur but in contrast to tuberculosis, these glands do not suppurate.

Inflammation of the eyes (iritis) and of the salivary glands may also occur. The bones may be affected and so excess calcium appears in the urine.

Course and treatment The disease runs a variable course, but after many months or even years the majority of patients show spontaneous recovery. Steroids may be helpful in stubborn cases, and where tuberculosis occurs specific treatment, as mentioned earlier, must be used.

Cryptogenic fibrosing alveolitis

This is a fibrosing lung condition of unknown cause, although it is sometimes associated with autoimmune diseases. The patient typically presents with progressively worsening breathlessness on exertion. Clubbing of the fingers may occur. Examination of the chest reveals fine crackles at the bases of the lungs, and the chest X-ray shows shadowing at the lung bases. The diagnosis may have to be confirmed by lung biopsy. Treatment of this condition is difficult. Steroids or cytotoxic drugs are used and are sometimes effective, but the prognosis is often poor, with progression to respiratory failure. Some patients have been successfully treated by single lung transplantation.

Extrinsic allergic alveolitis

This group of conditions are distinct from asthma (which is a disease of the airways), and are due to an allergic response in the alveoli. They can take either an acute or a chronic form. A very wide range of allergens may be responsible; some of the commonest are:

1. fungi from rotting compost (farmers' lung)
2. birds (bird fanciers' lung)
3. fungi from wood pulp (wood pulp workers' lung).

In the acute form of the disease there are typically flu-like symptoms a few hours after exposure to the allergen, which is associated with cough and shortness of breath. Usually the symptoms resolve spontaneously over a few days. If exposure continues and recurrent attacks occur (which may not all be noticed), the disease takes on a chronic form with worsening dyspnoea due to progressive and irreversible pulmonary fibrosis.

Investigation is with lung function tests which show a restrictive pattern (see p. 117) and a chest X-ray, along with identification of the causative agent. Treatment is primarily avoidance of the allergen, but such a patient may have difficulty coming to terms with this, particularly if their hobby or livelihood is threatened. Corticosteroids are of some benefit in prevention of acute attacks and in the treatment of the chronic form.

Pneumoconiosis

Prolonged exposure to certain types of dust may cause irritation of the lungs from constant inhalation of the fine particles of dust. The result is a dense diffuse fibrosis throughout the lungs which is termed *pneumoconiosis*. The people who may develop pneumoconiosis are:

1. anthracite coal miners (anthracosis)
2. stone workers, gold miners and potters (silicosis)
3. steel workers; tin, lead and iron miners (siderosis)
4. asbestos workers (asbestosis).

In all these occupations there is a very definite liability to develop dust disease of the lungs. This causes gradually increasing dyspnoea with chronic cough and sputum. X-ray examination of the lungs reveals a typical picture of diffuse fine mottling.

Treatment Prophylactic measures to render the dust as harmless as possible are most important. Moistening the atmosphere with sprays, and full ventilation, with fans if necessary, are most valuable. Respirators should be worn wherever practicable. Once the condition has arisen the patient must change his occupation or else the disease will progress, with a great risk of tuberculosis or bronchiectasis, and eventual heart failure.

Asthma

Asthma is a disorder characterized by attacks of wheezing and difficulty in breathing, and due to reversible narrowing of the airways. This restriction of the airway is not permanent and is due to:

1. Bronchospasm. This is spasm due to tightening of the constricting muscles of the smaller bronchi.

2. Congestion and thickening of the lining of the bronchial tree.

3. Accumulation of mucus and phlegm in the smaller bronchi.

There are many factors which can cause or precipitate an attack of asthma.

Heredity. Especially in childhood, asthma is likely to be associated with other allergic disorders such as hay fever or urticaria. Allergic susceptibility commonly occurs in more than one member of the family, suggesting a hereditary tendency. Allergy means an excessive reaction to certain environmental substances. These include pollen, plant spores, moulds, animal hairs, house dust containing mites and even certain foods. When these are inhaled by sensitive subjects, they cause spasm and swelling of the smaller bronchi.

Infection. Any upper respiratory tract infection, even a heavy cold, can set off an attack in an asthmatic subject.

Other factors may dispose to attacks in some asthmatics. These include sudden exposure to cold air; undue physical exercise; eating foods such as shellfish, chocolates or eggs, and taking certain drugs such as beta-blockers or aspirin.

Unknown factors. Asthma can begin later in life and is sometimes called *intrinsic asthma.* In these cases, allergy does not seem to be responsible and no reason can be found for the attacks.

Clinical features

An attack of asthma usually begins fairly suddenly with wheezy respiration and a sense of tightness in the chest. When the attack is mild, the subject can usually manage to keep going, though with difficulty. When the attack is more severe, unless there is recourse to treatment, rest is essential. The duration of the attacks varies considerably, usually for a few hours.

As a rule, when asthma occurs in childhood the attacks get less frequent as the child gets older, but this is not always so. In some, the attacks may be frequent and some wheeziness on expiration is always present.

Status asthmaticus

This is the term used to describe a severe and per-sistent attack of asthma sometimes continuing for many hours or even days. The patient becomes exhausted and demoralized due to lack of sleep and the physical effort of breathing. There is often a cough productive of sticky mucoid phlegm. A patient admitted to hospital in status asthmaticus is cyanosed and sweating with a rapid pulse rate and sometimes a low blood pressure. This can lead to mental confusion due to lack of oxygen or even to coma with a fatal outcome.

Management of asthma: preventive measures

Education It is important that patients with asthma are taught to understand and manage their own disease. This should include use of a home peak flow meter to monitor the disease, with clear instructions about what action to take in which circumstances, particularly when hospital treatment is necessary. Inhaler technique must be taught and checked on frequently. Many patients (particularly children) with asthma may experience psychological problems. Giving them the knowledge and means to control their asthma is an important part of the management of this aspect of the condition.

Allergy Careful questioning of the patient is the best way of finding out what factors bring on attacks and consequently how to avoid them. For example, if attacks occur in the spring or early summer it is likely that pollen is responsible. If they come on at night on going to bed, it might be house dust or a feather pillow. Questions should be answered from a prepared list about food, drugs, household pets and other possible provocative agents.

Skin tests seldom do more than confirm the significance of the possible factors involved. A drop each of various solutions containing the suspected provocative factor (allergen) is placed on the skin and a superficial scratch made through it. A raised weal appears within 15 minutes if the subject is sensitive to the particular allergen.

Sometimes the asthmatic subject can avoid substances known to provoke the attacks, for example, foods, drugs, dogs or cats. Feather pillows can be changed for sorbo rubber. The bedroom should be kept clear of dust by repeated vacuum cleaning.

Infections Although viral infections may precipitate asthma, there is often little evidence of bacterial infection. Antibiotics should be reserved for proven cases of bacterial infection.

Smoking. This should be strongly discouraged.

Management of asthma: treatment for attacks

Drugs Bronchodilators are drugs which relieve bronchial spasm and are most commonly given using inhalers. Salbutamol (Ventolin) is supplied by a pressurised aerosol: after breathing out completely the vapour is inhaled from the aerosol and the breath held for a moment to allow full absorption to take place. This leads to quick relief of wheeziness, but the benefits do not last long. The inhaler can be used four times a day. These drugs can also be given in dry powder inhalers (e.g. turbohaler) via a spacing device or via a nebulizer.

Steroid inhalations relieve the congestion of the bronchial mucosa (lining) and have a longer effect than the bronchodilators. Given as aerosols containing beclomethasone (Becotide) or betamethasone they act only on the bronchi and do not have the disadvantages of cortisone given by mouth or injection (see p. 330). It is important to remember that steroid inhalers have no benefit in the acute attack, their main role being in the prevention of future attacks. Sodium cromoglycate is also useful in the prevention of attacks, particularly in children.

Theophyllines The main role for these drugs is in the management of severe acute asthma, when they are given intravenously in hospital. They may be helpful for troublesome nocturnal symptoms, when given as long-acting tablets.

Mild attacks. If attacks of wheezing are infrequent the occasional use of a beta-2-agonist is all that is necessary.

Moderate attacks. If the attacks of wheezing become more frequent and the inhaler is used every day a prophylactic agent should be added. The most commonly used prophylactic agent is a steroid inhaler, although sodium cromoglycate may also be used. These drugs must be administered regularly (twice a day) or the effect is soon lost. It is sensible to give the steroid after the bronchodilator as this may allow better absorbtion. Many patients are worried about the side effects of steroids. These are minimal with the usual doses of inhaled steroids.

Acute attacks may still occur which do not respond to the inhaler. High-dose beta-2 agonists can then be given via a nebulizer or spacing device. If the patient does not respond, a short course of oral steroids should be given.

Severe asthma and status asthmaticus

If the above measures are ineffective then the patient is admitted to hospital.

Treatment of status asthmaticus

Status asthmaticus is an emergency and requires constant supervision, sometimes in an intensive care unit.

1. Steroids are life saving and should be given in adequate dosage from the moment it is clear that previous remedies have been ineffective. Steroids can be given as prednisolone by mouth, 15 mg every 6 hours initially. If the patient is too ill to take drugs by mouth, hydrocortisone 100 mg can be given intravenously.

2. Regular bronchodilators are given by nebulizer.

3. Intravenous therapy may take the form of infusions of aminophylline and/or beta-2 agonists.

4. Oxygen should be given by nasal catheter. In cases where cyanosis is severe and the patient is confused or comatose, it may be necessary to pass a cuffed endotracheal tube and apply intermittent positive pressure ventilation (IPPV). The best guide in this respect is estimation of the blood gases (P_{CO_2} and P_{O_2}).

5. In no condition is good nursing care more important. Patients in status asthmaticus are frightened and exhausted and the nurse can do much to give reassurance and emotional support as well as see to the physical comforts. It is important to make sure that an adequate intake of fluid is maintained and the patient is encouraged to take a light diet.

Carcinoma of the bronchus

Lung cancer (carcinoma of the bronchus) is now the commonest form of malignant growth in Great Britain. It is commoner in men than in women and is the cause of nearly half the deaths from cancer in males. The evidence that cigarette smoking is responsible for the great increase in lung cancer is incontrovertible and indeed it has been estimated that 90% of deaths from lung cancer in men result from cigarette smoking. Cigarette smokers are much more affected than are pipe or cigar smokers. Those who give up cigarette smoking have lower death rates than those who continue to smoke, so that if the habit ceased the number of deaths caused by lung cancer would fall steeply in the course of time.

Pathology

Lung cancer can affect the body in three ways: by invasion of local tissues, by secondary deposits and by constitutional effects.

1. Local invasion. Bronchial carcinoma begins in the epithelial cells lining the bronchus. It invades the bronchial wall and spreads into the lung. This may cause ulceration and bleeding from the bronchus or it may obstruct the bronchus and lead to collapse (atelectasis) of the lung. Infection may follow, causing pneumonia or lung abscess. Spread of the malignant cells by the lymphatic system causes the glands to enlarge.

2. Malignant cells from the growth may enter the blood stream and form metastases (secondary deposits) in other organs such as the bones, the liver or the brain. These metastases may grow themselves and invade other tissues as well.

3. Constitutional symptoms are caused by the production of toxins and hormones by the tumour. These lead to general metabolic changes and to damage of the nervous system. Production of excess hormones may lead to such disorders as Cushing's syndrome.

Clinical features (local)

1. Bronchial carcinoma does not give rise to symptoms in the early stages so that the growth has normally been present for a year or more before advice is sought.

2. A cough is the commonest presenting symptom, at first ascribed to a smoker's cough. The cough becomes more persistent and purulent sputum may be produced.

3. Haemoptysis occurs eventually in most patients. Usually the sputum is blood-stained or contains small blobs of blood. Coughing up of free red blood is less common.

4. Shortness of breath is a prominent feature, usually associated with a productive cough. The dyspnoea can become severe if there is added infection or lung collapse (atelectasis).

5. Chest pain may be caused by pleurisy or by the growth invading the ribs or the intercostal nerves. Thus the pain may be worse on breathing, or it may be persistent and gnawing, depending on the cause.

6. Wheeziness may be present due to bronchial obstruction.

7. Hoarseness of the voice may be due to pressure on the recurrent laryngeal nerve which controls the vocal chords.

Clinical features (metastases)

1. Metastases in the brain may cause headaches, epileptic fits, hemiplegia or unsteadiness of gait and these may be the presenting features of a lung cancer.

2. Secondaries in the bones can lead to unexpected fractures (pathological fractures) or can be the source of unremitting pain.

3. Metastases in the liver causes enlargement of the liver and sometimes jaundice and ascites.

4. Enlargement of the lymph nodes is often painless but may lead to the diagnosis.

Clinical features (constitutional)

1. Even a small bronchial carcinoma may be associated with malaise, loss of appetite and loss of weight.

2. Clubbing of the fingers is often present and may be a clue to the diagnosis, though this occurs in other chest disorders as well, particularly bronchiectasis. The nails are curved and there is a bulbous increase in the pulp at the end of the fingers.

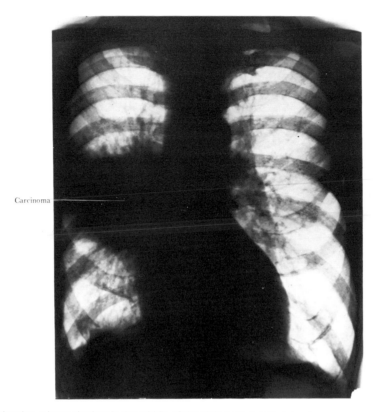

Carcinoma

Fig. 6.16 X-ray showing a large shadow in the middle of the right lung due to a carcinoma.

3. Involvement of the nervous system is common, not due to metastases but perhaps caused by a toxin from the carcinoma. It can lead to mental confusion, peripheral neuritis and unsteadiness of movement (ataxia).

4. Endocrine disorders. Sometimes excess hormones are produced by bronchial carcinoma. Excess ACTH can cause Cushing's syndrome (see p. 326) or excess parathyroid hormone (see p. 328) can lead to hyperparathyroidism.

5. Thromboses of the veins are liable to occur with bronchial carcinoma and can cause pulmonary emboli.

Diagnosis

Loss of weight and energy, particularly if associated with cough and sputum, must always arouse suspicion of lung cancer, particularly in cigarette smokers. Examination of the chest may reveal further evidence and the presence of enlarged glands or clubbing of the fingers may also lead to suspicion of the diagnosis. X-ray of the chest provides the diagnosis in most cases. A shadow in the lung associated with enlargement of the hilar glands suggests a bronchial carcinoma with lymphatic spread to the glands.

Tomography (X-rays focused on one plane) may give a clearer idea of the extent of the growth.

Examination of the sputum under the microscope may reveal the presence of malignant cells, thus confirming the diagnosis. Sometimes the aid of the physiotherapist is needed to help the patient cough up a suitable specimen.

Bronchoscopy. The bronchoscope is a lighted metal tube which can be passed into the trachea and bronchi and allows inspection of the main air passages. Snippets of tissue (biopsy) can be removed from suspicious areas and examined after suitable staining under the microscope. The fibroptic bronchoscope is of smaller bore and more flexible than the fixed tube and allows inspection of the minor bronchi.

Bronchoscopy is performed in the theatre. A tablet is sucked beforehand to anaesthetize the mouth and pharynx, and the larynx is anaesthetized by spray in the theatre. As the bronchoscope is passed, the patient's neck is extended and the head is flexed and suitably supported.

When the X-ray shadow lies in the outer part of the lung it may be inaccessible to bronchoscopy.

A needle biopsy may then be performed. The needle is inserted through the chest wall under ultrasound or CT guidance and a small tissue biopsy removed from the area involved. The biopsy is stained and examined under the microscope.

Treatment

1. Surgical resection of the tumour is the best treatment, usually pneumonectomy (removal of an entire lung) or lobectomy (removal of a lobe). Unfortunately this is seldom possible because at the time of diagnosis the tumour has already spread to the glands or has formed metastases. Surgical resection offers hope of survival and activity for a few years. Without operation, the average survival of bronchial carcinoma at diagnosis is less than a year.

2. Radiotherapy is best used for relief of symptoms such as chest pain. A short course of irradiation may relieve the pain of rib metastases or cause the regression of large glands which obstruct breathing.

3. Cytotoxic drugs. These drugs include intravenous nitrogen mustard and oral cyclophosphamide. They act by interfering with the growth processes of malignant cells without affecting healthy tissue. Unfortunately the results with lung cancer are disappointing though they sometimes cause the growth to shrink with easing of bronchial pressure.

4. In many cases, symptomatic treatment and relief of pain is all that can be achieved. A knowledge of the patient and his family background will help to decide whether he is better at home or in hospital for the terminal phase.

Prevention

Bronchial carcinoma is a distressing disorder with a poor prognosis. Since it is largely caused by cigarette smoking, nurses and doctors should do all they can to discourage this dangerous habit. All health workers should themselves set an example by not smoking and should encourage patients and their families to stop smoking. In particular, young people should be discouraged from starting the habit. Smoking advisory clinics are available to help people give up cigarettes if they are unable to do so on their own.

Atelectasis (collapse of the lung)

Collapse of the lung is not a primary disease in itself, but is caused by any disease or condition which obstructs the bronchi or interferes with the respirations. Either blockage of a bronchus or interference with the expansion of the lungs in the respiratory movement causes the affected lung or parts of the lung to collapse into a solid airless condition. This interferes with the normal respirations and causes varying degrees of distress according to the extent of the collapsed lung area.

1. Most commonly, pulmonary collapse calling for immediate treatment is seen postoperatively. Here, sedation due to the anaesthetic depresses the cough reflex and allows thick mucus to collect, which then obstructs the bronchi, causing varying degrees of collapse. Infection of the bronchi which causes excessive mucus increases this likelihood of postoperative pulmonary atelectasis.

2. Pulmonary collapse is also always a constant danger in prolonged coma and, as in postoperative collapse, calls for energetic measures in prevention and treatment.

3. Carcinoma of the bronchus commonly causes atelectasis.

4. A foreign body lodging in a bronchus.

5. Paralysis of the respiratory muscles, as seen in poliomyelitis and diphtheritic paralysis, can cause pulmonary collapse, but this form calls for specialized treatment, usually in an artificial breathing apparatus, and is discussed under the individual diseases.

6. Fluid or air accumulating in the pleural cavity can cause collapse of the lung by pressure from outside.

Symptoms and signs

Most of the diseases causing pulmonary collapse are discussed under the individual headings, so only the very common form occurring postoperatively calls for special mention here.

After operation the patient is often described as being 'chesty', with a cough, pain in the chest and difficulty in breathing. If the collapse is extensive, the dyspnoea is more severe; it causes distress to the patient and is accompanied by cyanosis. Usually a fever is present. Examination of the chest reveals the presence and extent of the atelectasis, and this is usually confirmed by an X-ray of the chest.

Treatment

Prevention is by far the most important part of the treatment. Any evidence of chest infection will naturally call for a postponement of the operation, if possible. Pre-operative breathing exercises in all patients subject to chest trouble are most valuable.

Routine encouragement of all postoperative patients to breathe deeply will reduce the incidence of atelectasis appreciably. In this connection also, early movement, frequent change of posture and getting the patient up as soon as possible are important. Analgesics may be prescribed to ease pain which otherwise might restrict mobility.

Treatment of actual collapse. Deep-breathing and coughing exercises every hour for a few minutes are very useful. Inhalation of oxygen is useful especially if dyspnoea or cyanosis is present. Postural drainage, by tipping the patient so that the collapsed area (usually the base of the lung) is uppermost, often dislodges a thick plug of mucus and expands the lung. This procedure is possible only in some cases, depending on the severity of the operation and the general condition of the patient. It is, however, a very useful and most effective measure whenever it can be applied. Chest percussion (or clapping) by a skilled physiotherapist is often combined with postural drainage.

If all the above measures fail to re-expand the affected area, then one of the several methods of aspiration of the bronchial tree will be necessary.

Passing a firm rubber catheter through the nose and into the trachea allows suction to be applied and so dislodges the thick mucus. Even if the tube cannot be passed into the bronchi, bouts of coughing occur which may be sufficient to bring up the plugs of mucus. If the above measures fail and the collapse is severe, causing acute distress and continued cyanosis, bronchoscopy will enable the obstructing mucus to be aspirated.

Pulmonary embolism

Pulmonary embolism is an important condition, especially from a nurse's point of view, as preventive measures play a large part in minimizing the frequency of the disease.

Pulmonary embolism is caused by a clot detaching itself in some part of the venous circulation, travelling in the veins, and lodging in the pulmonary artery or one of its branches. With the obstruction to the pulmonary circulation so produced, infarction of the lung or part of the lung, depending on the site of the lodgement of the embolus, occurs.

1. Venous thrombosis, especially in the large deep veins of the lower limbs and pelvis. Thrombosis in a vein occurs in several circumstances, e.g. in elderly people with slow circulation, particularly with heart failure. Prolonged rest in bed owing to a major illness or operation is also a very frequent cause.

2. Trauma to the large veins, especially in the lower abdomen during operations in this area, predisposes to thrombus formation.

3. In the puerperium a venous thrombosis is often seen 'white leg of pregnancy'.

4. The contraceptive pill, probably due to its oestrogen content, disposes to venous thrombosis.

5. In congestive heart failure a thrombus may form not only in a vein but also in the right side

of the heart. This is particularly likely in heart failure associated with atrial fibrillation.

It is from thrombosis in the deep veins, particularly the calf and pelvic veins, that embolism is most likely to arise. Thrombophlebitis of the superficial veins is much less dangerous.

Symptoms and signs

The following example is fairly typical. The patient may have recently undergone an operation and may appear to be progressing satisfactorily, or may have had a severe illness and been confined to bed for some time. In these patients there may be evidence of a venous thrombosis in a lower limb, with swelling, tenderness and slight pain in the affected leg. On the other hand there may be no such signs, or the signs may be so slight that they have escaped notice. A low-grade fever with no obvious cause is, however, often present in deep venous thrombosis and so should be viewed with great suspicion. Suddenly the patient may collapse with cyanosis and gasping respirations and die within a few minutes. Here a large embolus, sufficient to block the main pulmonary artery and so the whole pulmonary circulation, is present.

In other cases the embolus is somewhat smaller and produces severe dyspnoea, cyanosis and great distress. Pain in the chest is common, and later a cough with frank haemoptysis develops.

In some cases, multiple small emboli reach the lung and give rise to breathlessness on effort without obvious pain or haemoptysis.

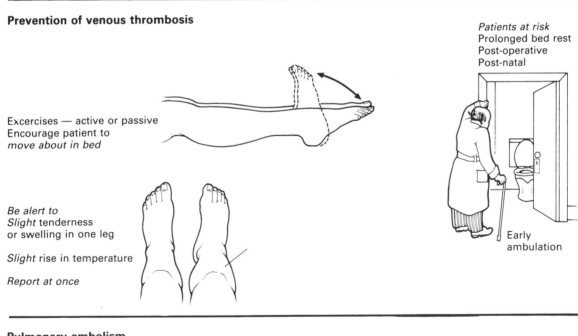

Prevention of venous thrombosis

Excercises — active or passive
Encourage patient to
move about in bed

Be alert to
Slight tenderness
or swelling in one leg

Slight rise in temperature

Report at once

Patients at risk
Prolonged bed rest
Post-operative
Post-natal

Early
ambulation

Pulmonary embolism

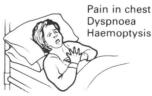

Pain in chest
Dyspnoea
Haemoptysis

Fig. 6.17 Prevention of venous thrombosis.

Treatment of pulmonary embolism

Prophylaxis. Any measures which will avoid or minimize the risk of a venous thrombosis are very valuable. Early movement of the legs in postoperative patients and early ambulation are most important. In any long standing or severe illness, especially in elderly people, passive and active movements of the legs must be undertaken early. Such exercises should form part of routine nursing care. Of course, if there is any contraindication to movement of the limb, such as a fracture or a wound, this must be taken into consideration. Heparin is frequently given subcutaneously as perioperative prophylaxis. Antiembolism stockings may also have some benefit.

If there are signs of venous thrombosis, such as pain, tenderness, or swelling of the leg, then anticoagulant therapy with heparin and warfarin is usually given. This is to prevent further spread of the thrombosis and so lessen the risk and severity of pulmonary embolism. It is important to stress that the signs of a deep venous thrombosis may be very slight, and that particular notice must therefore be taken of slight pain or tenderness in the calf, where a thrombus is especially likely to occur. This slight pain or tenderness accompanied by a low-grade fever is of particular importance, as already noted.

When embolism has occurred, a large embolus may result in sudden death. In other cases, oxygen in high concentrations to relieve the cyanosis and dyspnoea is of great value. Sedatives are usually needed for the pain and to allay the acute anxiety and shock present. Pethidine or morphine are usually given. Anticoagulant drugs, initially heparin via a continuous intravenous infusion and later tablets such as warfarin, are given to prevent further emboli.

7

Diseases of the alimentary system

DISEASES OF THE MOUTH

Stomatitis

Stomatitis is an inflammation of the mucous membrane of the mouth.

Causes

1. Viral. Herpes simplex type 1 causes an acute stomatitis and recurrent cold sores.

2. Bacterial. This is a rare form of stomatitis but may occur in malnourished patients and those with poor dentition. *Vincent's stomatitis* which is due to a number of organisms results in severe oral ulceration.

3. Fungal. The fungus *Candida albicans* can cause oral thrush. This may accompany the use of antibiotics which destroy the normal mouth bacteria and allow the fungus to grow. It is also seen in immunosuppressed patients.

4. Non-infective. Aphthous stomatitis is a recurrent painful ulceration of the mouth of unknown cause, possibly viral in origin. Mouth ulceration may also be seen in inflammatory bowel disease (see later) and can also occur as a result of adverse reactions to drugs as part of the Stevens–Johnson syndrome. Any prolonged fever or general illness particularly in the elderly or debilitated patient may predispose to stomatitis.

Symptoms and signs

The patient complains of soreness and difficulty with eating and sometimes speaking. The mucous membrane of the mouth appears red and inflamed. In aphthous stomatitis, small discrete ulcers are visible. In thrush, white plaques can be seen on the mucous membrane.

Treatment

Prevention of dehydration in the elderly or febrile patient will help prevent the development of stomatitis. In addition, regular gentle mouth toilet with sodium bicarbonate or thymol are essential. Vincent's stomatitis responds to antibiotic treatment with metronidazole and thrush may be treated with nystatin suspension given 4 times a day. Herpes simplex stomatitis is treated with acyclovir, an antiviral agent.

Glossitis

Inflammation of the tongue (glossitis) can occur with stomatitis but can also be seen in several other illnesses: (i) scarlet fever, (ii) anaemias, especially pernicious anaemia, when it is caused by vitamin B_{12} deficiency and also in association with folate deficiency.

The tongue is red and looks rather glazed. The patient complains of soreness of the tongue.

The treatment of glossitis is that of the underlying cause.

DISEASES OF THE SALIVARY GLANDS

There are three pairs of salivary glands: the parotid, the submaxillary and the sublingual glands. Their function is to secrete saliva which acts as a lubricant for the mastication of food. The constant secretion of saliva has a very essential cleansing effect. The salivary glands may be affected by various diseases. The commonest are:

Mumps (epidemic parotitis)

This is an acute infectious disease, commonest in

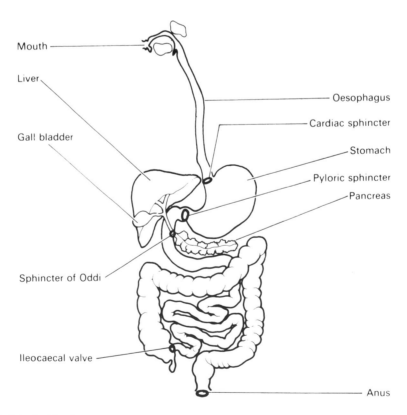

Mouth
Liver
Gall bladder
Oesophagus
Cardiac sphincter
Stomach
Pyloric sphincter
Pancreas
Sphincter of Oddi
Ileocaecal valve
Anus

Fig. 7.1 The gastrointestinal tract.

children and caused by a virus. The parotid glands become painful and swollen.

Suppurative parotitis

A suppurative bacterial inflammation of one or both parotid glands is usually the result of insufficient care of the mouth in the course of severe and debilitating illness, for example in malignant cachexia or following major surgery. Suppurative parotitis is treated by rehydration, meticulous mouth toilet, and appropriate antibiotic therapy.

Stones

Stones may form in the ducts of the submandibular and parotid glands. They cause pain and swelling of the gland, especially after eating, due to obstruction of the duct. The stone may be felt in the floor of the mouth in the case of a submandibular stone, or in the cheek in the case of a parotid stone, and can often be seen on X-ray examination. Sometimes removal of the stone alone cures the symptoms, but often secondary changes in the gland due to obstruction of the duct necessitates the removal of the whole gland (in the case of the submandibular gland) or the superficial part (in the case of the parotid gland).

Tumours of the salivary glands

Most salivary tumours occur in the parotid gland. They are slow-growing and remain well localized for many years. The commonest type is the mixed parotid tumour. Much rarer is an adenolymphoma, which is softer and sometimes bilateral. Treatment is surgical excision of the superficial part of the parotid glands containing the tumour. Sometimes temporary facial palsy occurs after this operation.

Xerostomia or dry mouth

A dry mouth may occur as a result of fever, drugs, dehydration or due to any process in which the salivary glands are destroyed.

DISEASES OF THE OESOPHAGUS

Dysphagia

Most diseases which affect the oesophagus give rise to the symptom of difficulty in swallowing or *dysphagia*. Other symptoms that may be experienced include heartburn (see later) and pain on swallowing.

Causes

1. Foreign body. Sometimes a swallowed piece of food e.g. fish bone may stick in the oesophagus and give rise to dysphagia which is often painful. The diagnosis is made on the history.

2. Carcinoma of the oesophagus. Carcinoma arising in the oesophagus is not uncommon and usually occurs in middle-aged or elderly people. It causes a progressive dysphagia, first for solid food and then for liquids. Pain may occur on swallowing but persistent pain implies local infiltration of the tumor. Weight loss and anorexia are common and anaemia and lymphadenopathy may also be present.

3. Benign stricture of the oesophagus. Benign stricture of the oesophagus occurs most often as a complication of reflux oesophagitis often in association with a hiatus hernia (see below). Reflux of gastric acid into the oesophagus causes recurrent inflammation and a stricture develops as a result of this. Frequently the patient has symptoms of heartburn but sometimes the symptoms of oesophagitis are absent and the patient presents with dysphagia alone.

Rarely, multiple strictures of the oesophagus develop following the ingestion of caustic acids and alkalis.

4. Achalasia of the cardia. Dysphagia may develop as a result of disturbance of the nervous control of the lower oesophageal sphincter (cardia). Failure of relaxation of this sphincter delays passage of food into the stomach, and the oesophagus above becomes very dilated. This condition usually occurs in women aged 30 to 40. The dysphagia takes many years to develop and may be accompanied by symptoms of reflux, regurgitation and severe retrosternal pain. In the later stages, vomiting may occur with aspiration

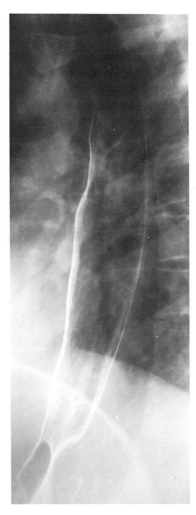

Fig. 7.2 Double-contrast barium study showing the normal oesophagus.

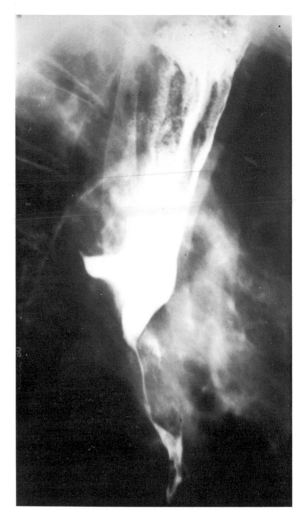

Fig. 7.3 Barium swallow showing malignant stricture at the lower end of the oesophagus.

of the contents of the oesophagus into the lungs with the development of aspiration pneumonia which is a very serious complication.

5. Extrinsic compression of the oesophagus. The conditions which most commonly cause dysphagia through extrinsic pressure on the oesophagus are:

   a. malignant growths in the mediastinum
   b. retrosternal goitres
   c. aneurysms of the arch of the aorta
   d. pharyngeal pouch.

6. Paralysis of the oesophageal muscles (bulbar paralysis). Some forms of cerebrovascular accident (stroke) and some neurological disorders, e.g. myasthenia gravis, lead to a paralysis of the oesophageal muscles with difficulty in initiating swallowing and causing dysphagia.

7. Anxiety. Acute anxiety often gives rise to a sensation of difficulty in swallowing as though there were 'a lump in the throat'. These symptoms may persist ('globus hystericus') and may become obsessional so that neither fluid nor solids will be taken.

Diagnosis

The diagnosis may be obvious from the history,

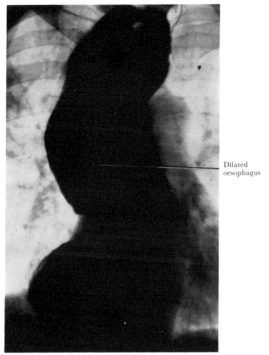

Dilated
oesophagus

Fig. 7.4   X-ray (barium swallow) showing the gross dilatation of the oesophagus in an advanced case of cardiospasm (achalasia).

e.g. swallowed fishbone. Otherwise, a barium swallow X-ray is arranged for all patients with dysphagia. In this examination, the patient is asked to swallow radio-opaque barium while X-rays are taken of the neck and chest to show the site and type of obstruction in the oesophagus. In general, irregular strictures are usually malignant, while smooth strictures are benign. Free reflux of barium from the stomach may be seen in patients with benign strictures due to reflux oesophagitis.

All patients with dysphagia should have an oesophagoscopy, usually using a flexible fibre-optic gastroscope or an oesophagoscope to confirm the diagnosis. This also enables tissue to be biopsied to identify benign or malignant disease. Computerized tomography (CT scanning) may be used to identify mediastinal masses that may be causing extrinsic compression of the oesophagus.

Treatment

1. A foreign body is removed via the oesophagoscope.

2. Carcinoma of the oesophagus may be treated by surgical removal (oesophagectomy) in the case of lower third carcinomas. Alternatively, as good results may be obtained by radiotherapy, which is the treatment of choice for tumours above the lower third. Unfortunately, these tumours have often become very advanced before presentation and therefore less than 20% of patients survive 3 years.

Alternative treatments include the dilation of the stricture caused by the tumour and more rarely nowadays the insertion of a tube to stent the blockage (e.g. Celestin tube).

3. Strictures of the oesophagus due to reflux oesophagitis need to be treated with dilatation performed at endoscopy. It is critical to treat the underlying reflux of acid so drugs such as H-2 antagonists are used to reduce acid secretion and together with antacids to protect the lower end of the oesophagus. Additionally, newer drugs are available to help maintain normal motility at the lower oesophageal sphincter. If there is a hiatus hernia present and medical therapy fails surgical repair can be undertaken.

4. Achalasia of the cardia can be treated by endoscopic dilatation of the lower end of the oesophagus and this is successful in up to 80% of patients. A few patients in whom medical therapy fails but have persistent severe symptoms surgery can be performed using Heller's procedure at which the muscle of the cardioesophageal junction is divided.

DISEASES OF THE STOMACH AND DUODENUM

Dyspepsia

The symptom of indigestion or dyspepsia means different things to different patients and may encompass a wide range of symptoms:

1. Pain. A burning pain or discomfort in the upper part of the abdomen related to eating is the classical interpretation of dyspepsia. Different patterns of pain after eating are seen in different diseases. Thus in gastric ulcer, the pain usually starts within half an hour of eating, and is made

worse by eating more food especially spicy or hot food. In duodenal ulcer, the pain usually comes on 2 or more hours after eating and is relieved by eating. Often the patient wakes at night with pain and relieves it with a glass of milk or antacid preparation.

2. Flatulence may mean either bringing up wind or passing excessive wind per rectum.

3. Heartburn. This is a burning sensation which rises from the epigastrium to the throat and is a symptom of reflux of stomach contents into the oesophagus, usually associated with a hiatus
hernia.

Other symptoms associated with diseases of the stomach and duodenum are:

1. Water-brash. This term describes the clear tasteless fluid which suddenly wells up in the mouth probably due to reflex salivation in response to duodenal ulceration.

2. Loss of appetite and weight.

3. Nausea and vomiting. Vomiting is not only a symptom of diseases of the stomach but also of disease elsewhere in the body. The actual act of vomiting consists of contraction of stomach, abdominal and diaphragmatic muscles and a relaxation of the cardiac opening of the stomach. The vomiting centre, in the medulla of the brain, which controls this complicated act. This centre is closely connected with the vagus nerve, especially with the branches from the abdominal viscera.

Vomiting can be divided into seven well-recognized groups:

1. Vomiting due to abdominal disease
   - disease of the stomach
     — acute gastritis
     — peptic ulcer
     — pyloric stenosis
     — carcinoma of the stomach
     — gastroenteritis
   - disease of other abdominal organs
     — renal and biliary colic
     — appendicitis and peritonitis
     — intestinal obstruction

2. Due to drugs. Certain drugs irritate the stomach or stimulate the vomiting centre, thus causing vomiting, and are often used for this purpose, e.g. in cases of poisoning when it is desirable to get rid of any poison in the stomach. The commonest drug used for this purpose is ipecacuanha.

3. Due to disease of the ear. The vestibular part of the ear deals with posture and equilibrium and is closely associated with the vomiting centre. Conditions affecting the vestibular apparatus often cause severe vomiting. Travel sickness and Ménière's disease are two examples of this type of vomiting.

4. Due to cerebral disease. Any disease causing raised intracranial pressure, for example cerebral tumour, abscess and meningitis, can cause vomiting by direct pressure on the vomiting centre.

5. Due to stimulation from higher cerebral centres. This class covers the vomiting resulting from emotional disorders, such as nervous tension, anxiety, fear and hysteria. This vomiting is often successfully controlled by chlorpromazine or allied drugs.

6. Metabolic diseases such as uraemia and hypercalcaemia.

7. Pregnancy.

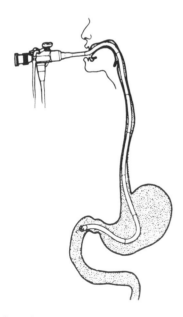

Fig. 7.5 Oesophago-gastroduodenoscope in use.

Finally it should be remembered that any severe illness can give rise to reflex vomiting.

Characteristics of vomiting in the more common diseases

Profuse vomiting is seen in patients with intestinal obstruction or pyloric stenosis. The vomiting in intestinal obstruction starts as bile-stained (green) fluid, but as the condition progresses, the vomitus begins to resemble faeces (faeculent vomiting). Acute dilation of the stomach may complicate upper abdominal operations and causes copious vomiting of brown fluid. It is prevented by the passage of a nasogastric tube following abdominal operations.

Other abdominal conditions such as appendicitis or biliary colic give rise to reflex vomiting and this is followed by retching of small quantities of fluid once the stomach is emptied. Projectile vomiting occurs in babies with pyloric stenosis and in patients with raised intracranial pressure.

Blood in the vomit may appear red if fresh. Usually the blood is degraded in the stomach and appears as dark granules well described as 'coffee grounds'. Small amounts of blood are seen in the vomitus due to carcinoma of the stomach. Vomiting of large quantities of blood is called haematemesis and is usually due to erosion of a blood vessel by a peptic ulcer or oesophageal varices.

Effects of vomiting

Vomiting is likely to have serious effects only if it is persistent and copious, as in cases of pyloric stenosis, intestinal obstruction and acute dilatation of the stomach. The main result of continued vomiting is loss of fluid and acid. The loss of fluid leads to dehydration, which causes collapse and in some cases acute renal failure. The loss of hydrochloric acid in the vomit causes the patient to develop an alkalosis which can lead to tetany (see p. 328).

Congenital hypertrophic pyloric stenosis

Congenital hypertrophic pyloric stenosis occurs in the first few weeks of life, and nearly always, for some unknown reason, in boys. The pylorus becomes thickened and hypertrophied from muscle spasm, until eventually a severe degree of stenosis is present.

Symptoms and signs

1. The infant is usually perfectly normal for the first 3 weeks or so of life, after which persistent vomiting after nearly every feed begins. The vomiting is typically described as projectile in nature, the feed being forcibly expelled for some distance.

2. The baby is hungry and greedy for his feeds.

3. Constipation is always present and stools are usually small and dark green in colour ('hunger' stools).

4. From the lack of nourishment the baby loses weight and becomes dehydrated, the skin becomes pinched and the eyes and fontanelle become sunken.

5. If the baby is examined under a good light and during a feed, peristaltic waves will be seen in the upper abdomen. These waves are due to the contractions of the stomach forcing the food against the stenosed pylorus.

6. In most cases, a firm hard contracting tumour is felt in the pyloric region. This tumour is the hypertrophied pylorus.

Treatment of congenital pyloric stenosis

Medical treatment with the use of antispasmodic drugs and intravenous fluids rarely succeeds in the case of established pyloric stenosis. A surgical operation to divide the muscle of the pylorus (*Ramstedt's operation*) is usually performed under general anaesthetic, but may be performed under local anaesthetic and is very successful at relieving the stenosis.

Gastritis

Gastritis means an inflammation of the lining mucous membrane of the stomach. It occurs in two forms, acute and chronic.

Acute gastritis

In acute gastritis there is an acute inflammation of the gastric mucosa with destruction of the superficial epithelial cells. The patient experiences epigastric pain and vomiting usually for a short period. It is not always clear what causes this but alcohol and drugs such as aspirin can be responsible. Sometimes the gastritis is severe enough to cause multiple small ulcers or acute gastric erosions which may bleed and give rise to haematemesis and melaena. Such acute ulcers may occur after severe stress such as trauma or burns.

Chronic gastritis

Chronic gastritis may follow prolonged dietary indiscretion or alcohol abuse. Recently it has been recognized that it is strongly associated with infection of the gastric mucosa by the bacterium *Helicobacter pylori* and this is probably the commonest cause of chronic gastritis. It is accompanied by atrophy of the mucosa of the stomach. Chronic gastritis is often asymptomatic but may also cause epigastric pain and anorexia.

A second form of chronic gastritis is seen in pernicious anaemia. In this disease, autoantibodies to the gastric mucosa cause chronic gastritis. In addition, the secretion of intrinsic factor required for the absorption of vitamin B_{12} by the terminal ileum is affected. The patient develops anaemia due to vitamin B_{12} deficiency.

Treatment

Acute gastritis needs no specific therapy other than removal of the underlying cause. Chronic gastritis associated with *H. pylori* requires specific treatment with antibiotics and a bismuth-containing drug to eradicate this organism. If pernicious anaemia is present this needs investigation and treatment.

Peptic ulcer

Peptic ulcer is a term used to include both gastric and duodenal ulcer. Gastric ulcers are usually single and lie on the lesser curve of the stomach. Duodenal ulcers occur in the first part of the duodenum or 'duodenal cap'.

Peptic ulcers may be acute or chronic. Acute gastric ulcers are also known as acute gastric erosions and have been described in the section on gastritis. Acute duodenal ulcers may develop as a result of severe stress, for example burns, severe injury or head injury and may bleed or perforate without prior symptoms. Chronic peptic ulcers develop from acute ulcers that fail to heal. Because of the attempt at healing at the edges of a chronic ulcer, scar tissue is formed which may lead to complications.

Cause

The exact cause or causes of peptic ulcer are unknown. Duodenal ulcers are commoner than gastric ulcers. *H. pylori* infection is a common cause.

Gastric ulcer

Most patients with gastric ulcers have normal or low acid outputs and so other factors are involved in ulcer production including chronic gastritis and alterations in mucous production.

Duodenal ulcer

Patients with duodenal ulcers secrete excess acid. It has recently been recognized that infection with *H. pylori* may increase gastric acid production and thus cause duodenal ulcers.

Other factors

Peptic ulcers are commoner in men, elderly patients, and in patients with a family history. Weaker associations are with smoking (for duodenal ulcers), with diet and psychological factors such as stress.

Symptoms

Pain. Epigastric pain or discomfort are the major features of peptic ulcer disease. It may be possible to distinguish the pain of gastric and duodenal ulcers. Pain from gastric ulcer often occurs soon after eating and is aggravated by eating. Pain

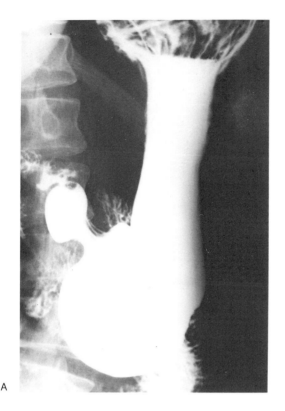

A

from duodenal ulcer is sometimes described as a 'hunger pain' and is relieved by eating. The patient with a duodenal ulcer often wakes at night with pain and relieves it by eating.

Other symptoms

Vomiting may occur, especially if the pain is severe, and often relieves the pain of gastric ulcer. Severe vomiting suggests a complication such as perforation. Patients may vomit blood in small quantities. In cases of severe bleeding from the upper gastrointestinal tract, the motions can become black and 'tarry' from the large amount of altered blood present. Black tarry motions from upper gastrointestinal haemorrhage are known as *melaena*. In contrast, blood in the motion in lower intestinal bleeding is red or plum-coloured and is usually on the outside of the specimen, e.g. in carcinoma of the lower colon, haemorrhoids and colitis. Heartburn and flatulence may also occur. Appetite is usually good in patients with duodenal ulcer but patients with gastric ulcer are sometimes afraid to eat, and lose weight. Peptic ulcer symptoms are often periodic with exacerbation in the spring and autumn.

Diagnosis

The suspicion of peptic ulcer disease can only be confirmed by barium meal X-ray or more usually by endoscopy.

Barium meal X-ray

A specialized X-ray examination, known as a *barium meal*, will show up the stomach and duodenum and usually any ulcer that may be present. After suitable preparation the patient is examined under an X-ray screen immediately after drinking barium sulphate (the patient must have nothing to eat or drink for 6 hours before the X-ray; in addition, all medicines should have been stopped). Barium is opaque to X-rays and it therefore outlines the whole stomach and duodenum. In this way, an ulcer crater may be seen. Occasionally, however, even though an ulcer is present, the X-ray may not reveal it.

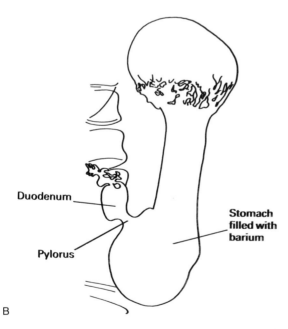

Duodenum

Pylorus

Stomach filled with barium

B

Fig. 7.6 A, B. Barium meal showing stomach, pylorus and first part of duodenum.

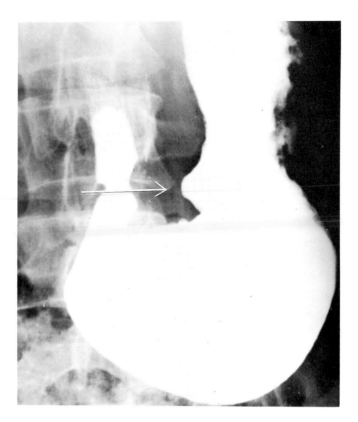

Fig. 7.7   X-ray (barium meal) showing an ulcer on the lesser curvature of the stomach.

Endoscopy (gastroscopy)

The interior of the stomach can be inspected with a gastroscope. This is a flexible fibre-optic instrument which when passed into the stomach allows a good view of the stomach and the duodenum. A biopsy of the edge of the ulcer may be taken using biopsy forceps which may be passed through the gastroscope. Endoscopic biopsy also allows examination for the presence of the bacterium *H. pylori*.

Treatment

General advice Meals should be taken at regular intervals and frequent small meals of bland food is the usual recommendation. Spicy, fried or vinegary foods should be avoided, as should alcohol.

Smoking delays the healing of ulcers and patients should be advised not to smoke. Drug treatments for other conditions, e.g. arthritis, should be reviewed and drugs known to cause irritation to the stomach discontinued, e.g. aspirin, anti-inflammatory drugs.

Anxiety and depression should be treated. Stress should be minimised as far as possible as stress causes an exacerbation of symptoms. Complete bed rest in hospital will allow gastric ulcers to heal but is very expensive treatment!

Drug treatment for pain relief, antacid drugs such as magnesium trisilicate or aluminium hydroxide may be used to treat mild episodes of discomfort and indigestion.

Duodenal ulcer

The treatment of duodenal ulcers in the last few years has changed with introduction of H2 antagonists. These agents can heal most cases of duodenal ulcer but need to be taken for 4–6 weeks. Unfortunately, the ulcer and symptoms are liable to return after a time so that further courses of these drugs may be needed. With the recognition that *H. pylori* infection is a factor in recurrent duodenal ulceration a combination of acid inhibition and antibiotics can be used to eradicate this organism, and this results in a very low ulcer recurrence rate. More powerful acid inhibitory drugs, such as omeprazole, also have a role in treating ulcer disease which is resistant to first-line H2 antagonist therapy.

Gastric ulcer

H2 antagonists are the mainstay of treatment, but the other agents mentioned previously for duodenal ulcers are used if indicated. Additionally, it is essential to ensure that the ulcer has healed so follow up X-rays or endoscopy with biopsy are needed. This is because of the risk that such an unhealed ulcer may be malignant.

Surgical treatment of peptic ulceration

Duodenal ulcer Surgery is indicated in patients who have had severe symptoms in whom medical treatment has failed. The commonest operation is a highly selective vagotomy (proximal gastric vagotomy) which reduces the secretion of acid by the stomach by ablating the vagal innervation to the acid secreting area. Truncal vagotomy, where the entire vagus nerves are divided as they enter the abdomen around the oesophagus, will have the same effect but must be

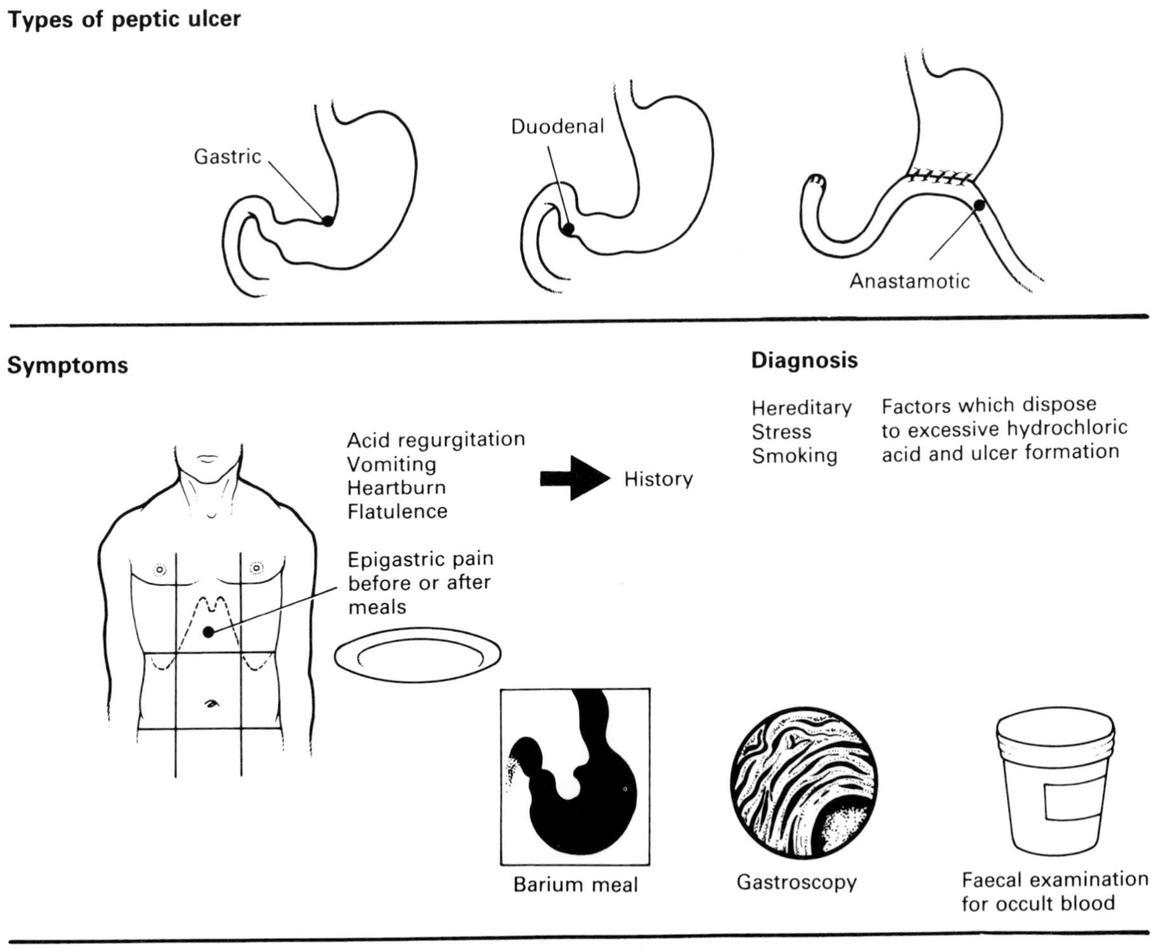

Types of peptic ulcer

Gastric

Duodenal

Anastamotic

Symptoms

Diagnosis

Acid regurgitation
Vomiting
Heartburn
Flatulence

History

Epigastric pain
before or after
meals

Hereditary
Stress
Smoking

Factors which dispose
to excessive hydrochloric
acid and ulcer formation

Barium meal

Gastroscopy

Faecal examination
for occult blood

Fig. 7.8 Peptic ulcer.

combined with a pyloroplasty as the normal innervation of the pylorus is also destroyed and the stomach will not otherwise empty. Partial gastrectomy is also effective in reducing acid secretion and may be undertaken in severe ulceration.

Gastric ulcer Partial gastrectomy to remove the ulcer is the treatment of choice if medical therapy fails to heal the ulcer or if it is uncertain if the ulcer is malignant.

For both gastric and duodenal ulceration, surgery is mandatory in the presence of complications, in perforation, severe haemorrhage and pyloric stenosis.

Complications of peptic ulcer

1. Haemorrhage
2. Perforation
3. Pyloric stenosis
4. Malignant change.

Haemorrhage

Peptic ulcers may erode a blood vessel and cause bleeding. Both duodenal and gastric ulcers may

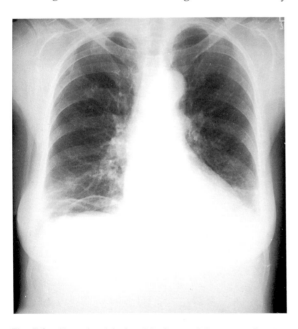

Fig. 7.9 Air under right hemidiaphragm following perforation of peptic ulcer.

cause haematemesis, but this is more common with gastric ulcers. However, melaena may be the only symptom. If the haemorrhage is severe, signs of shock are present:

the skin becomes cold and clammy
the pulse becomes very rapid
the patient is usually very restless
there is a fall in blood pressure.

Important factors affecting the management of haematemesis are the age of the patient, the amount of blood lost, whether there is continued bleeding and the presence of other medical conditions.

Treatment General measures. If the haemorrhage is severe, the patient is shocked and measures to overcome this must be taken at once (see below). The patient is kept at absolute rest, and raising the foot of the bed helps to maintain blood pressure. Adequate warmth is necessary, but care must be taken to avoid overheating, which only makes the condition worse. A half-hourly or one-hourly pulse and blood pressure chart is kept to monitor the patient's progress. A falling blood pressure and a rising pulse are an indication of continued haemorrhage.

Transfusions In patients with copious haemorrhage and severe shock, as revealed by a persistently rapid pulse of over 100, a systolic blood pressure below 100 mmHg and restlessness, restoration of the blood volume is required immediately. This is achieved initially with plasma expanders but transfusion should be started with packed red cells and fresh frozen plasma as soon as these have been cross-matched. A strict watch must be kept for transfusion reactions. Critically ill and elderly patients will require central venous cannulation to ensure venous access together with monitoring of central venous pressure and urine output.

With patients who do not immediately require a transfusion, close observation of the pulse rate and blood pressure, as already mentioned, is essential, as if the haemorrhage continues a blood transfusion may become necessary.

If the abdomen becomes distended, as may happen with a large haemorrhage, a small enema may be ordered. To keep the stools soft and

Surgery essential

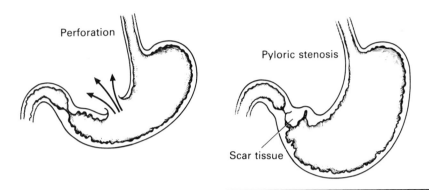

Surgery advisable

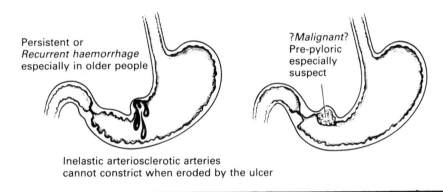

Inelastic arteriosclerotic arteries
cannot constrict when eroded by the ulcer

Fig. 7.10 Indications for surgical treatment of peptic ulcer.

prevent straining, one or two ounces of liquid paraffin daily are useful. The patient must be warned against straining at stool as this may restart bleeding.

Diet Whether or not the patient is given food by mouth depends on the doctor in charge. In the acute stages the patient should be nil by mouth as they will need an endoscopy and may need an operation. In the convalescent period the usual practice is to allow food by mouth as for patients with an acute ulcer, that is, small frequent feeds of a bland non-irritating variety. Some patients feel like eating more than others, and in the first few days it is wise to accede to the patient's wishes within the limits of the diet mentioned.

Drugs Cimetidine or ranitidine tablets have a powerful effect in blocking the production of acid in the stomach but have not been shown to affect the mortality rate of severe upper gastrointestinal haemorrhage. However, since acid can exacerbate bleeding from the ulcer, these drugs may be useful.

Endoscopy This should be arranged as soon as the patient has been resuscitated or within 12–24 hours of admission in less severe bleeding as this will enable the diagnosis to be confirmed. In some cases if the ulcer is seen direct therapy may be applied to the ulcer to prevent bleeding from it recurring.

Surgical intervention In most patients the haemorrhage subsides with the above treatment, but it does persist in a minority of cases, usually in elderly patients with large chronic ulcers. The arteries in elderly people are more likely to be arteriosclerotic and therefore do not contract down so readily in order to control the bleeding. In these elderly patients with persistent haemorrhage, surgery may be advised after the shock has been overcome with adequate transfusions of blood. For gastric ulcer, partial gastrectomy is the operation of choice. For duodenal ulcers, the bleeding is usually controlled by under running the blood vessel in the ulcer and a vagotomy and pyloroplasty performed to allow the ulcer to heal.

Other causes of haematemesis and melaena Before leaving the discussion of haemorrhage as a complication of peptic ulcer, it is convenient here to mention the other causes of haematemesis and melaena. It should be remembered, however, that in 90% of cases the cause is peptic ulcer.

1. gastric erosions
2. carcinoma of the stomach
3. cirrhosis of the liver causing portal hypertension and bleeding from oesophageal varices
4. blood diseases (purpura, leukaemia, vitamin K deficiency)
5. swallowed blood e.g. from epistaxis or following operations on nose and throat.

Perforation

A peptic ulcer may perforate through into the peritoneal cavity and is one of the common causes of an 'acute abdomen'. There is shock with severe and generalized abdominal pain. When the patient is examined the abdomen is found to be held absolutely rigid. These are the signs of peritonitis which is due to the release of gastric contents into the peritoneal cavity. This requires urgent surgical intervention to over-sew the perforated ulcer and to allow drainage of the abdominal cavity.

Pyloric stenosis

A chronic ulcer, when it heals, produces scar tissue. If the ulcer is situated near the pylorus the scar tissue may obstruct the pyloric opening, thus causing a pyloric stenosis. In severe cases, very

little food may pass through into the duodenum. Usually, there are the following symptoms and signs:

1. Vomiting is frequent and copious, a history of vomiting of food eaten on a previous day being most characteristic of this condition.
2. The loss of weight varies with the degree of the stenosis, but it is very marked in the severe cases.
3. Constipation is usually present.
4. On passage of a nasogastric tube, the gastric juice content is found to be as much as 500 to 700 ml.
5. Barium meal examination will show that the stomach is very dilated and there is great delay in emptying.

Malignant change

Some gastric ulcers may undergo malignant change. Duodenal ulcers rarely become malignant.

Carcinoma of the stomach

Carcinoma of the stomach is one of the commonest cancers and occurs in middle-aged or elderly people.

Symptoms and signs

The symptoms of carcinoma of the stomach are often very similar to peptic ulcer:

1. Epigastric pain may mimic the dyspepsia of peptic ulcer but often the pain is more persistent and less periodic.
2. Loss of appetite is early and fairly constant.
3. There is progressive weight loss. This is not usually a feature of uncomplicated peptic ulcer.
4. Anaemia is often present.
5. Jaundice may develop in the late stages owing to the spread of the tumour to the liver.

Because the symptoms of carcinoma of the stomach in the early stages are very similar to peptic ulcer, the diagnosis may be missed until the diseases is advanced.

Diagnosis

The diagnosis is usually suspected on the above

symptoms. The development, for the first time, of indigestion in middle-aged or elderly people is significant. Confirmation of the diagnosis is obtained by barium meal examination and endoscopy, which allows biopsy and histological confirmation. It is nearly always possible to distinguish a malignant from a benign gastric ulcer by gastroscopy and biopsy.

Treatment

In 95% of patients, the disease cannot be cured and treatment is usually palliative. If the growth has not progressed too far, either partial or total gastrectomy will relieve the symptoms and offers the only chance for cure. If the tumour is not resectable, a bypass operation such as gastrojejunostomy may relieve some of the symptoms, e.g. due to pyloric stenosis. In a few selected cases, particularly in younger patients, palliative chemotherapy is now a treatment option but the outcome is still poor.

Hiatus hernia

This is a common disorder and may occur in any age group and in either sex but the typical patients are overweight middle-aged women. Part of the stomach protrudes through the oesophageal opening (hiatus) of the diaphragm into the thorax. The hernia is not necessarily permanent but can slide into the thorax, especially when the patient bends forward after a heavy meal. Reflux of gastric acid into the oesophagus occurs giving rise to a burning discomfort in the upper abdomen and behind the sternum in the chest (*heartburn*). The inflammation in the oesophageal mucosa hernia can give rise to bleeding and anaemia. The diagnosis of hiatus hernia can be confirmed by a barium meal X-ray with the patient tilted downwards on the X-ray table to demonstrate the hernia above the diaphragm.

To avoid symptoms the patient should:

1. reduce weight and abstain from heavy meals
2. avoid tight clothes around the abdomen

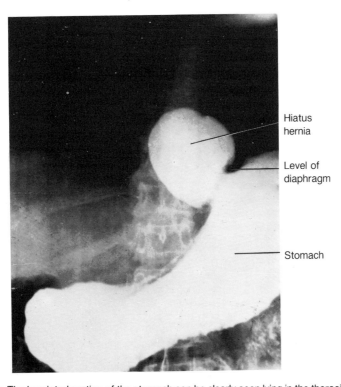

Hiatus hernia

Level of diaphragm

Stomach

Fig. 7.11   Hiatus hernia. The herniated portion of the stomach can be clearly seen lying in the thoracic cavity above the diaphragm.

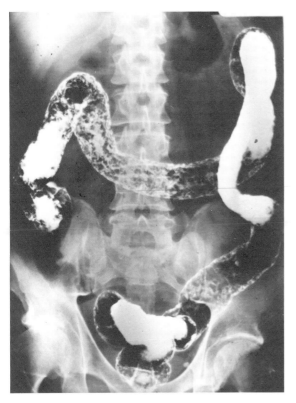

Fig. 7.12 X-ray (barium enema) showing the appearance of the normal colon.

3. avoid lying or sitting in a hunched-up position, especially after meals
4. raise the head of the bed at night.

Antacids are helpful in relieving discomfort, and particularly antacid preparations combined with a viscous alginate (gaviscon) which coats the lower end of the oesophagus.

H2 antagonists or omeprazole are used to treat the oesophagitis as for reflux and usually succeed in bringing about symptom relief. Rarely an operation to repair the opening in the diaphragm is necessary in patients with severe symptoms who do not respond to medical measures or who develop complications (stricture of the oesophagus).

DISEASES OF THE INTESTINES

Disorders of the intestine may give rise to vomiting, abdominal pain, constipation and diarrhoea.

Vomiting

This has been described on page 154.

Abdominal pain

Abdominal pain may be of two varieties:

1. Colicky pain, which comes and goes every 5–15 minutes and is felt in the mid-line. This pain makes the patient uncomfortable and restless.
2. Peritoneal pain, which is due to inflammation of the peritoneum. This pain is constant and sometimes severe. It makes the patient lie still as any movement aggravates the pain.

Constipation

Constipation means delay in evacuation of the bowels. It is important to remember that normal bowel habit varies considerably from person to person.

Causes

1. Habit. If the normal desire to have the bowels open (call to stool) is ignored for social reasons then the normal defecatory reflex, evoked by the presence of faeces in the rectum, is gradually lost. The stool becomes hard and dry due to water absorption. This type of constipation is a particular problem in the elderly. Chronic constipation results in loss of muscle tone in the rectum and causes difficult or incomplete evacuation of the bowels which aggravates the condition.
2. Diets low in fibre cause slow intestinal transit and the formation of small hard stools.

Local causes

1. Anal conditions. Painful anal conditions such as anal fissure or strangulated haemorrhoids will result in constipation. It is difficult to know whether haemorrhoids cause or are caused by constipation.
2. Any disease causing obstruction to the

bowel, especially the large bowel, will cause constipation.

   3. Megacolon (see p. 175)

Treatment

The treatment of constipation is that of the cause. Usually, habit constipation responds to phosphate or soap and water enemas. In milder cases purgatives, either as suppository or by mouth, may suffice. However, if purgatives such as senokot or milpar are tried, their use should be discontinued as soon as possible as purgative abuse may cause constipation in the long term. Once constipation has been relieved, the institution of a high fibre diet, possibly with the addition of a dietary bulking agent such as normacol or fibogel, will help to prevent recurrence. In the elderly or demented patients, chronic constipation may be a very difficult problem.

Diarrhoea

When unformed stools are passed, diarrhoea is said to be present. Diarrhoea is a common and important symptom of intestinal disease, its severity and nature varying according to the disease. It is impossible here to give all the causes of diarrhoea, but a classification of the main causes is useful.

Causes of acute diarrhoea

1. Acute gastroenteritis
   (a) infective gastroenteritis
   (b) food poisoning
   (c) chemical poisoning
2. Appendicitis (some patients)
3. Enteric fever
4. Dysenteries
5. Anxiety.

Causes of chronic diarrhoea

1. Inflammatory diseases
   (a) ulcerative colitis
   (b) regional ileitis (Crohn's disease)
   (c) diverticulitis
   (d) tuberculosis
2. Carcinoma of the colon
3. Coeliac disease and tropical sprue
4. Vitamin B deficiency (pellagra)
5. Thyrotoxicosis
6. Irritable bowel syndrome.

For the purpose of diagnosing the cause of diarrhoea, and also of assessing the effects of treatment, monitoring of the character of the stools is of great importance.

Acute gastroenteritis

Acute enteric infections are common in infants and children and have a significant mortality. Predisposing factors are poor nutrition, prematurity in infants and immunodeficiency. Breast-fed babies are virtually immune to gastroenteritis. The cause is either bacterial (*Salmonella*, *Shigella* and some strains of *E. coli*), or viral (Rota virus).

Symptoms and signs

   1. The disease usually occurs in children under 2 and is very serious in infants under 1 year.

   2. The onset may be very abrupt, the infant being well one moment and in a matter of hours seriously ill. The severity of the attack varies from a mild rapidly cured condition to a fulminating fatal disease.

   3. The infant vomits his feeds and this vomiting is persistent. Diarrhoea sets in quickly and the stools are characteristically frequent, watery and green in colour. In severe cases the stools may be a bright orange colour and extremely frequent.

   4. The infant is very lethargic and signs of dehydration rapidly appear in any severe case, i.e. the eyes become sunken, the fontanelle depressed and the skin, when pinched, remains in a fold. The whole aspect of the child is one of severe toxicity and lethargy. Fever may also be present.

   5. Bronchopneumonia is a common complication.

Treatment

Acute infective gastroenteritis must be treated as

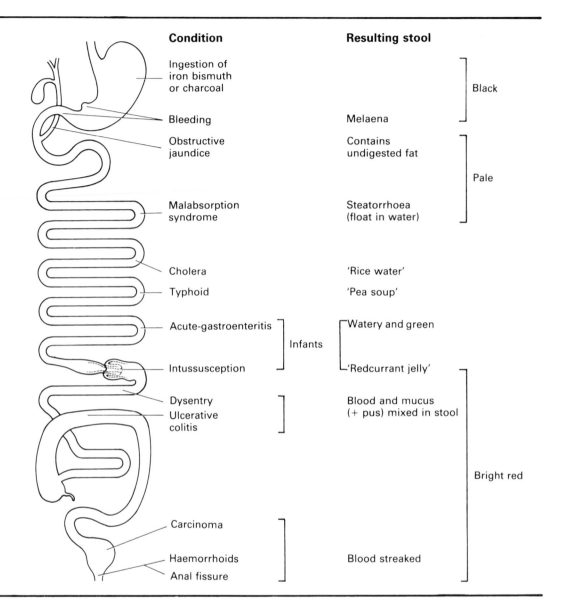

Condition | **Resulting stool**

Ingestion of iron bismuth or charcoal ⎤ Black

Bleeding — Melaena ⎦ Black

Obstructive jaundice — Contains undigested fat ⎤ Pale

Malabsorption syndrome — Steatorrhoea (float in water) ⎦ Pale

Cholera — 'Rice water'

Typhoid — 'Pea soup'

Acute-gastroenteritis ⎤ Infants ⎡ Watery and green

Intussusception ⎦ ⎣ 'Redcurrant jelly'

Dysentry / Ulcerative colitis ⎤ Blood and mucus (+ pus) mixed in stool

Carcinoma — ⎤

Haemorrhoids / Anal fissure ⎦ Blood streaked

Bright red

Fig. 7.13 Characteristics of the stools in various ailments.

a medical emergency for two reasons:

1. To prevent spread to other children the strictest isolation precautions should be taken at the outset.

2. To prevent the disease becoming worse with a possible fatal outcome.

   a. Warmth. The infant must be nursed in a warm well-ventilated room. Adequate warmth is essential.

b. Initial period of starvation. This is necessary in all cases, and during this time only, boiled water, glucose water or a glucose/electrolyte solution is given by mouth. The total amount of liquid required in the 24 hours should be calculated on the basis of 165 ml of fluid per kg body-weight, plus an additional amount of 150 to 450 ml to overcome any existing dehydration. These feeds must be given in small frequent amounts to prevent recurrence of the vomiting and also to avoid tiring the infant. To carry out these measures will call for all the skill and attention that the nurse can give.

c. Treatment of dehydration. Infants with severe dehydration i.e. with marked lethargy, sunken eyes, depressed fontanelle and pinched skin, must be given fluid by the intravenous route as soon as possible. Delay in giving intravenous fluid in these cases can be fatal. Intravenous therapy is also necessary when boiled water is not tolerated by mouth. Half-strength saline, dextrose-saline and Hartmann's solution are the usual types of fluid given.

d. Feeding. After the preliminary period of starvation, which usually varies from 12 to 36 hours according to the persistence of vomiting and the frequency of stools, milk feeds are started. At first one part of the milk diluted in three or four parts of water is given, as the infant will not tolerate stronger feeds. If the infant keeps down the feeds, then the concentration of milk in each feed is gradually increased until finally the infant is taking full strength milk mixtures appropriate to his age. It usually takes approximately 2–3 days to re-establish normal feeds.

Breast milk is the ideal milk for an infant, but when an infant who is artificially fed is recovering from an attack of gastroenteritis it is best to keep him on a half-cream milk for a short period as too much fat is not well tolerated.

e. Drugs. Antibiotics have been shown to encourage the growth of pathogenic bacteria in the intestine and should not be given unless the infection spreads outside the intestine.

Intestinal obstruction

Intestinal obstruction falls into two categories:

1. Acute. This is due to obstruction of the small bowel, usually due to adhesions from a previous abdominal operation or due to a strangulated inguinal or femoral hernia.

2. Chronic. This is due to obstruction of the large bowel from a carcinoma of the colon, diverticular disease, Crohn's disease or chronic severe constipation in the elderly.

Symptoms and signs

1. Vomiting. This is usually severe and occurs early in acute obstruction, but is a late symptom in chronic obstruction. In the later stages, vomit may become thick and brown and is described as faeculent.

2. Pain. Colicky, abdominal pain occurs early and is more severe in acute obstruction.

3. Abdominal distension. This is usually the major symptom of chronic obstruction.

4. Constipation. In chronic obstruction, constipation is an early symptom. In acute obstruction, residual motion in the lower bowel may continue to be passed for some hours after onset of the obstruction.

Diagnosis

The diagnosis is usually made on the symptoms and signs. It is very important to look for a cause of the obstruction, i.e. strangulated hernia, previous operation scar, faecal impaction. In addition, abdominal X-rays taken supine will show distended loops of bowel and on erect X-rays, fluid levels will be visible.

Treatment

The initial treatment is to correct severe dehydration with intravenous fluids. Normal saline, often supplemented with potassium, is usually used. In addition, it is essential to pass a nasogastric tube to empty the stomach and relieve discomfort. The patient's fluid balance must be carefully monitored. Thereafter, the treatment of obstruction is of the cause. Faecal impaction may be relieved by a manual evacuation and enemas. Otherwise, a surgical operation is usually needed to deal with a strangulated hernia or abdominal adhesions. In the case of large bowel obstruction due to carcinoma or diverticular disease, a hemicolectomy may be performed or in cases of left colon disease, a transverse colostomy is usually the first treatment to relieve the obstruction. The disease can then be dealt with later by a left hemicolectomy after the bowel has returned to normal size.

Acute appendicitis

This is a common surgical emergency which can occur at any age, but often affects young people. The cause is either obstruction of the appendix by a faecolith (hard inspissated faecal pellet) or by infection of the lymphoid tissue under the mucosa.

Symptoms and signs

The patient complains of abdominal pain which starts centrally and is colicky and then moves to the right iliac fossa and becomes more constant. Vomiting, nausea and loss of appetite are associated with the pain. Constipation is usually present but occasionally there may be diarrhoea. On examination, the tongue is usually furred and there are signs of mild dehydration. There is tenderness in the right iliac fossa. In late cases, a mass may be felt.

Diagnosis

This is made on the symptoms and signs. X-rays and laboratory investigations are unhelpful except the patient may have a raised white count.

Treatment

The treatment of appendicitis is appendicectomy, usually as soon as possible after the diagnosis has been made. However, if a mass is present, conservative treatment may be commenced. The patient is forbidden anything by mouth. An intravenous infusion is instituted to replace lost fluid and antibiotics are given. If the patient responds and the mass reduces in size, oral fluid may be introduced over the next few days. The patient is discharged home once the mass has disappeared and appendicectomy is arranged in 2–3 months' time. This is necessary to prevent recurrence.

Complications of appendicitis

1. Perforation of the appendix may lead to:

(a) generalized peritonitis due to spread of infection throughout the abdomen

(b) formation of an abscess around the appendix
The greater omentum helps to limit the spread of infection by adhering around the site of infection. This is an appendix mass. It may resolve spontaneously with conservative treatment, or burst to cause generalized peritonitis.

(c) pelvic abscess. Infection may track down into the pelvis and cause an abscess which may eventually discharge into the rectum.

2. Wound infection. This commonly follows appendicectomy for appendicitis, though the incidence has been reduced considerably with prophylactic antibiotics. Should pus exude from the wound, it is essential to open the wound fully by traction and sinus forceps to allow the wound to drain. After cleaning with chlorhexidine solution in water, the wound is packed with ribbon gauze soaked in eusol (sodium hypochlorite solution) and liquid paraffin. The dressing is changed daily. The wound is allowed to heal from the bottom upwards. Usually the scar is no worse than if healing had occurred normally.

3. Portal pyaemia. This complication of spread of infection via the portal blood stream to cause multiple abscesses in the liver is nowadays rarely seen due to the routine use of prophylactic antibiotics prior to appendicectomy.

Diverticular disease

Small outpouchings of the lining (mucosa) of the large bowel may form, probably due to spasm of the bowel causing increased intraluminal pressure. This is associated with a western (low residue) diet. These diverticulae occur usually in the sigmoid colon. Diverticular disease occurs in 50% of people over the age of fifty. It is completely asymptomatic in 90% of cases but some people may suffer from intermittent constipation and diarrhoea and left iliac fossa pain. However, if infection develops, an abscess may form in the wall of the colon causing acute diverticulitis.

Symptoms and signs

The patient is usually middle-aged or elderly. Pain in the left iliac fossa associated with nausea and vomiting are the presenting symptoms. The patient is usually constipated. On examination there is tenderness in the left iliac fossa. The temperature is usually raised and signs of dehydration may be present.

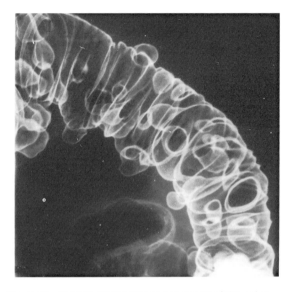

Fig. 7.14 Multiple diverticulae in a segment of the colon.

Diagnosis and treatment

The diagnosis is made on clinical symptoms and signs. The treatment is to rest the bowel. The patient is given nothing by mouth, and if vomiting occurs, a nasogastric tube is passed. An intravenous infusion is instituted to replace lost fluid and antibiotics are usually given. On this regime, the condition usually settles spontaneously. Once resolved it is important to arrange a barium enema examination and sigmoidoscopy to exclude a carcinoma of the colon which may co-exist.

Complications

These may be acute or chronic.
Acute complications are as follows:

1. Peri-colic abscess. The infection may spread outside the wall of the bowel to form an abscess around the colon. The patient is usually ill with a swinging fever. Otherwise the symptoms and signs are the same as for acute diverticulitis. The abscess usually resolves by rupturing into the colon. The abscess cavity may be seen on barium enema X-ray taken 3 weeks after the symptoms have resolved.

2. Perforation. Occasionally an inflamed diverticulum may rupture, causing generalized peritonitis either due to infection or due to the escape of faeces into the peritoneal cavity (faecal peritonitis). The patient complains of sudden onset of pain in the left iliac fossa becoming severe and generalized. On examination, the patient is very ill and the abdomen is rigid. It may be impossible to distinguish this from a perforated peptic ulcer. The treatment is surgical. The area of colon affected is resected (sigmoid colectomy) and the two ends are either brought out as a colostomy

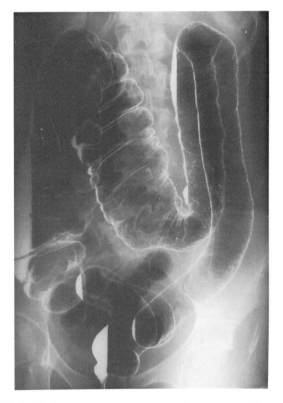

Fig. 7.15 Barium enema from a case of ulcerative colitis showing a section of colon which is narrowed and has lost its normal haustral pattern.

and rectal fistula, or an anastomosis to join the two ends may be performed. The mortality for this condition is very high.

3. Haemorrhage. Rarely, acute diverticulitis may result in massive haemorrhage from the large bowel.

Chronic complications Chronic diverticulitis or diverticular disease results from repeated attacks of acute diverticulitis. Repeated episodes of inflammation lead to different complications.

1. Stricture. The symptoms are similar to carcinoma of the colon (see later) with increasing constipation causing the passage of small 'rabbit-like' stools. The stricture may become severe enough to cause intestinal obstruction.

2. Fistula. Occasionally, an abscess caused by diverticulitis may rupture into the vagina or bladder causing a fistula. This can only be treated by surgery to remove the affected bowel and repair the fistula.

Ulcerative colitis

Ulcerative colitis is a chronic inflammatory disease of the large bowel. It causes ulceration of the mucosal membrane of the rectum and can involve the whole colon. The cause is not known.

Symptoms and signs

1. The disease is most common in young and middle-aged people. It is a chronic relapsing condition which may temporarily clear up spontaneously or under treatment, only to recur.

2. Chronic diarrhoea, with watery stools containing blood and mucus, is the main complaint. In severe cases, the stools may be as frequent as ten to twenty a day and may consist entirely of blood and pus with no faecal matter.

3. Abdominal colic sometimes accompanies the diarrhoea and the abdomen may be very tender to the touch.

4. General features include malaise, lethargy and anorexia.

5. In a severe case, the patient is toxic, wasted and anaemic with features of an acute abdomen.

Diagnosis

The diagnosis is usually made on the characteristic symptoms and confirmed on sigmoidoscopy. A sigmoidoscope is a rigid tube with a light and lens attached. It is passed per rectum and through it the mucous membrane of the rectum and sigmoid colon may be seen. In ulcerative colitis, the mucous membrane will appear grossly inflamed and ulcerated and will bleed easily on contact. A sigmoidoscopy is also an important means of excluding other causes of chronic diarrhoea with the passage of blood in the stools, especially carcinoma of the lower colon. A rectal biopsy can be taken, and the small fragment removed can be examined under the microscope.

The colonoscope is a flexible fibre-optic instrument which allows visualization of the whole colon. It is valuable because it allows biopsies to be taken from the entire colon and so is useful in assessing the activity and extent of the colitis. A barium enema X-ray will also show the extent and degree to which the colon is affected. The colon looks narrowed and does not contract normally. Ulceration may be demonstrated throughout the colon. The stool must be examined in the laboratory to exclude disorders such as amoebic dysentery. The haemoglobin must also be checked to reveal the extent to which the patient is anaemic and the serum albumin may be low.

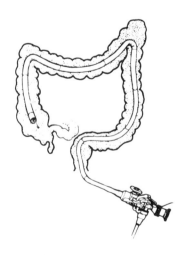

Fig. 7.16 Colonoscopy.

Complications

1. Haemorrhage. Moderate bleeding from the bowel is common in ulcerative colitis but occasionally a massive and life-threatening haemorrhage can occur.

2. Perforation. In acute cases, the bowel becomes distended (toxic dilatation) and erosion of the mucosa may lead to perforation and peritonitis.

3. Carcinoma. After many years, chronic ulcerative colitis may give rise to carcinoma of the colon.

Treatment of ulcerative colitis

Ulcerative colitis can be a chronic disorder and even when apparently cured for many years is liable to relapse. However many patients never have further trouble after the initial attack so there is every reason to adopt an optimistic attitude. Some patients with ulcerative colitis have underlying anxiety as to the nature of their illness and as to their future. The nurse should discuss fears expressed by the patient. Records must be kept of the nature and number of stools passed and whether the stools contain blood or mucus. In acute cases, the fluid intake and output should also be monitored and in severe attacks treatment should be in hospital.

Rest. In an acute phase, particularly when the temperature is raised and the diarrhoea is severe, the patient should be nursed in bed, usually in hospital. The period of bed rest will be determined by progress and in a severe case several weeks may be necessary.

Diet. In the acute phase, the diet is likely to be determined by what the patient can manage so that heavy meals should be avoided. In the long term, a diet containing sufficient protein and high in roughage is more likely to be beneficial than the low-residue diet previously recommended. The patient soon learns that some types of food give rise to diarrhoea in their case and so will avoid them.

Fluids

In severe acute colitis the patient may be unable to eat or drink so they are kept nil by mouth. These patients require intravenous fluid replacement and occasionally parenteral nutrition.

Drugs

1. Prednisolone and other steroid preparations are the most effective remedy in the acute phase. Prednisolone given by mouth in adequate doses reduces the inflammation of the colonic mucous membrane with relief of constitutional symptoms and control of the diarrhoea. Unfortunately, the long-term use of steroids can cause dangerous complications and is therefore avoided if possible. If a patient is particularly unwell and unable to tolerate oral medication steroids can be given intravenously. When the rectum is particularly involved, prednisolone can be administered in the form of suppository or as an enema. The enemata are supplied in plastic containers with nozzle attached. The patient can be taught to insert the lubricated nozzle attached into the rectum, best done while lying on the left side, and the solution then squeezed in. The nozzle and bag are then discarded and the patient lies on his front for about half an hour.

2. Sulphasalazine (salazopyrin) or other drugs containing 5-amino salicylate are effective as long-term treatment for preventing relapse of ulcerative colitis.

3. Codeine and related drugs may help to control diarrhoea, while antispasmodic agents such as mebeverine are useful for relieving the abdominal colic.

4. Iron is given for the anaemia.

5. Vitamins. The diet should contain all the necessary vitamins, but some patients need supplements of vitamins. Vitamins B and K are particularly likely to be deficient.

Blood transfusions may be necessary to correct anaemia which delays healing.

General measures. Owing to the chronic and relapsing nature of the illness and the anxiety factor which is usually present, patients with ulcerative colitis demand all the understanding and continual reassurance which the doctor and the nurse can give.

Surgical intervention is needed:

1. Where medical treatment after adequate trial has failed and the patient suffers chronic ill-health.

2. In long-standing cases where carcinoma is suspected.

3. In cases of intestinal obstruction due to strictures formed by healing of the ulcers. The surgical treatment usually carried out is removal of the whole colon (colectomy), leaving the patient with a permanent ileostomy. The patient wears an appliance over the opening and the bag is emptied two or three times a day. The patient can lead a normal and active life and can take a full diet.

Crohn's disease

Crohn's disease is difficult to distinguish from ulcerative colitis in many cases because the symptoms are often similar. It affects mainly the terminal ileum but also the colon and indeed any part of the gastrointestinal tract may be involved. Inflammation occurs through the whole thickness of the bowel wall and leads to areas of thickening and rigidity. Strictures and adhesions are common so that loops of bowel become matted together to form palpable masses which obstruct the bowel. Perforations may occur as can the development of fistulae between the bowel and the skin or other intra-abdominal organs.

Symptoms and signs

As with ulcerative colitis, chronic diarrhoea and abdominal colic are common symptoms. In addition, however, intestinal obstruction may occur with severe pain and vomiting. These symptoms may be associated with fever and considerable loss of weight. Bleeding from the rectum is not uncommon, sometimes associated with abscess formation in the rectum or anal region.

Diagnosis

Small-bowel barium studies may show areas of ulceration and narrowing in the ileum and a barium enema is necessary to demonstrate colonic involvement. Colonoscopy and sigmoidoscopy will allow further assessment of the bowel

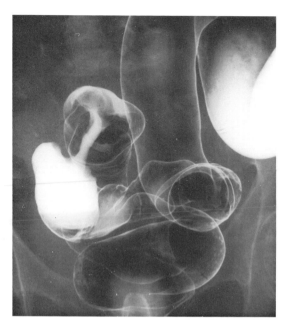

Fig. 7.17 Barium enema showing classical 'apple-core' appearance of a malignant stricture of the sigmoid colon.

and enable biopsies to be taken to determine the diagnosis. Again, a full blood count and stool cultures should be performed.

Diet. In some patients the diarrhoea may respond to dietary changes but in general the diet is as for ulcerative colitis.

Drugs. Codeine (60 mg three times daily) may help the diarrhoea. Steroids such as prednisolone can be used to tide the patient over a severe attack, and sulphalazine can be used for patients with colonic disease. Antibiotics such as metronidazole can be given when there are abscesses in the peri-anal region.

Surgery. Surgery may become obligatory when intestinal obstruction or abscess formation occurs and, indeed, the majority of patients with Crohn's disease require surgery at some stage. The obstructed area of bowel is resected but unfortunately in some patients the condition recurs after a time in some other part of the bowel.

Irritable bowel syndrome

This term is applied to many patients, commonly young women, who complain of frequent attacks of diarrhoea, abdominal discomfort, flatulence and a sense of distension in the abdomen. Investigations, including examination of the stools, sigmoidoscopy and barium enema, do not reveal any organic disease and the disorder is regarded as functional with psychological factors being important.

Reassurance and explanation are often helpful, and a discussion as to possible social or domestic stresses may give a lead as to the nature of the disorder. Antispasmodic drugs may give some symptom relief.

Carcinoma of the colon

Carcinoma of the colon and rectum is the second commonest cancer in the United Kingdom. It usually occurs in middle-aged or elderly people but can arise in young people. Two-thirds of the cases occur in the rectosigmoid region of the large bowel.

Symptoms and signs

1. Change in bowel habit. Mechanical obstruction of the colon or constipation often alternating with bouts of diarrhoea are the main symptoms. This is usually progressive.

2. Bleeding per rectum is another common symptom. Patients often consider the passage of blood per rectum to be due to 'piles'. Unfortunately, if a carcinoma of the colon or rectum is present the diagnosis may be delayed because of this misapprehension until the disease is advanced.

3. Acute intestinal obstruction. In some patients the first sign of carcinoma of the colon may be intestinal obstruction.

4. In advanced cases anaemia wasting and hepatomegaly due to metastases are present.

Diagnosis

This is usually made on the symptoms of alternating constipation and diarrhoea, abdominal colic, and in many cases the presence of visible or occult blood in the faeces. If the carcinoma is in the rectum a digital examination will reveal a

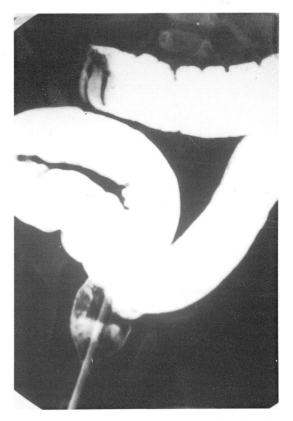

Fig. 7.18 Barium enema showing invaginated section of bowel and failure of barium to travel beyond this.

palpable hard mass. A sigmoidoscopy will detect a growth situated in the rectum or sigmoid colon and allow it to be biopsied. An X-ray examination (barium enema) is most useful in confirming the diagnosis. The tumour may show as a filling defect, ulcer or stricture. Colonoscopy is useful for the confirmation of doubtful lesions as biopsies can be taken.

The treatment of carcinoma of the colon is surgical wherever possible. Usually the tumour can be removed by hemicolectomy. The prognosis of this tumour is better than most. About half of the patients are alive 5 years after presentation and if the tumour is confined to the mucosa at removal the 5 year survival is over 95%.

Malabsorption syndrome

This condition is due to failure of the small intestine to absorb the products of digestion. Fat appears prominently in the stools so that the condition is often called *steatorrhoea*, but this is only one aspect of malabsorption since glucose, vitamins, minerals and other foodstuffs are also poorly absorbed. Three clinical states are included under this heading:

1. Coeliac disease occurs mainly in children but also in adults. This has been shown to be due to an intolerance of gluten a protein in wheat and certain other cereals. As a result of this idiosyncrasy the small intestine mucosa atrophies and thus fails to function properly when gluten is present in the diet.

2. Idiopathic steatorrhoea in adults. Here the cause of the malabsorption is usually unknown though damage to the small intestine by such diseases as tuberculosis or malignant infiltration may be found later.

3. Tropical sprue, occurring especially in India and China, is also of unknown origin.

Symptoms and signs

1. The patients are undernourished, wasted and easily fatigued. Loss of appetite is a marked feature. Children with coeliac disease show abdominal distension and fail to grow and thrive.

2. The characteristic features are chronic diarrhoea with very large, bulky, pale, offensive stools. The appearance of the stools is due to the large excess of fat which they contain.

3. Many complications may arise which are best described according to their cause:

a. deficient absorption of the following vitamins:
   (i)   folic acid and vitamin B_{12} resulting in a pernicious (macrocytic) type of anaemia
   (ii) vitamin D causing rickets in children and osteomalacia in adults; the vitamin D deficiency is also responsible, in conjunction with a deficient absorption of calcium, for the tetany seen in sprue
   (iii) vitamin B complex causing a sore tongue (glossitis) and peripheral neuritis
   (iv) vitamin K resulting in prothrombin deficiency and haemorrhagic manifestations

b. deficient absorption of minerals:
   (i)   iron, causing a hypochromic anaemia:
   (ii) calcium, causing tetany and softening of the bones (osteomalacia)

c. the combination of the deficient absorption of fats, carbohydrates, minerals and vitamins causes the lack of growth and infantilism seen in children with coeliac disease.

Treatment

During the active stages of the disease, bed rest is essential to a rapid recovery. Diet is of the utmost importance in all causes of malabsorption. In coeliac disease the main essential is to exclude the wheat protein, gluten. This is achieved by cutting out all foods made with wheat flour and by using corn flour or soya bean flour. When gluten is excluded from the diet, children with coeliac disease are able to tolerate fat in the diet to a much greater degree. In sprue, it has not yet been proved that a gluten-free diet is as beneficial as in coeliac disease.

The diet in idiopathic steatorrhoea and coeliac disease should contain a high-protein, low-starch and low-fat content as well as excluding gluten. All the missing vitamins must be given, especially A, D, B complex and K. Calcium should also be added to the diet. Food is best given in small amounts at frequent intervals, the amount being gradually increased as the condition improves.

Folic acid (and in some cases vitamin B_{12}) is given when a macrocytic anaemia is present. If a hypochromic anaemia is present this denotes a deficiency of iron, and ferrous succinate or ferrous gluconate should be given.

Acute intussusception

Acute intussusception usually occurs in infants about the time of weaning. It may be mistaken for acute gastroenteritis. In intussusception, part of the intestine becomes invaginated into the intestine immediately below it. The invaginated part of the intestine can then travel onwards for a considerable distance in the gut. The result of intussusception is to produce an acute intestinal obstruction. An intussusception usually starts at the lower end of the ileum near the ileocecal valve.

Symptoms and signs

1. Breast-fed infants under 1 year are usually affected.
2. The onset is sudden with abdominal colic. The infant has attacks of screaming and draws up its legs.
3. Vomiting starts early and is severe and repeated.
4. After the first motion the infant passes only pure blood and mucus from the bowel the 'red-current jelly' stool.
5. A typical sausage-shaped tumour is usually palpable in the abdomen. This tumour is the invaginated portion of the intestine. On rectal examination the lower end of the invaginated bowel may be felt in some cases. The finger when withdrawn will be covered in blood.

Diagnosis and treatment

Intussusception must be distinguished from the other acute illnesses in infants in which blood and mucus are passed in the stools. Acute bacillary dysentery (usually due to the Sonnei bacillus) is the condition which is most likely to be confused with acute intussusception. In the dysentery cases, the vomiting and the screaming attacks of colic are slight or absent and an abdominal tumour is not felt. The treatment of intussusception is immediate operation to relieve the obstruction. The invaginated portion of intestine is 'milked back', great care being needed to prevent the bowel tearing. If, as happens in some cases, the bowel is gangrenous, then resection of the gangrenous part is necessary.

Megacolon

Megacolon is the term used to describe a number of congenital and acquired conditions in which the colon is dilated. In many instances it is secondary to chronic constipation but in children

Hirschsprung's disease needs to be excluded. This latter condition occurs due to a disturbance in the nerve supply to the lower part of the colon in the rectosigmoid region. This region becomes narrowed and thickened with the result that the bowel above the contracted segment becomes enormously dilated.

The cardinal signs of megacolon are extreme constipation and abdominal distension. In children, the symptoms date from soon after birth, and in severe cases the abdomen becomes enormously distended with coils of bowel visible through the abdominal wall. Evacuation of the bowel may take place only at intervals of weeks, and in these severe cases death can ensue from toxaemia and intestinal obstruction. X-ray examination (barium enema) reveals the grossly distended large bowel.

Treatment of megacolon consists of resection of the narrowed segment of the colon (rectosigmoidectomy).

Intestinal worms (helminths)

Worms often inhabit the intestinal tract. Those most commonly found in western countries are:

1. threadworms
2. roundworms
3. tapeworms.

In tropical countries there are many other types of worm as well which cause serious ill-health, with severe anaemia as a particular feature.

Threadworms

Threadworm infection is extremely common, especially in children, the tiny white worms being seen in the faeces or around the anus. Marked peri-anal itching is present. The child becomes infected by swallowing the eggs (ova). Continuous re-infection takes place through the child scratching the anus and thereby infecting the hands.

Treatment

As most of the children and even adults in the

family are usually infected with threadworms at the same time, it is most important for all members of the family to be examined and for those infected to be treated together; failing this, re-infection will take place.

1. Eradication of the worms. A suitable anthelmintic (drug which kills worms) is given after the bowels have been well opened by a mild purgative. Piperazine or mebendazole are the drugs of choice.

2. Prevention of re-infection. This is most important. The anal region must be properly cleansed after each motion. The hands must be washed after visiting the toilet. The underclothes, night attire and linen should be boiled after all infected members of the family have been treated.

Roundworms (Ascaris lumbricoides)

Roundworm infection results from eating or drinking contaminated food (particularly raw vegetables and salads) or water. The worms mainly inhabit the intestines but occasionally invade the bile ducts, liver or trachea. In adults, the main symptoms are abdominal pain, diarrhoea or constipation, while in infants, enuresis (bed-wetting) and convulsions are common. With many patients the first sign is the presence of the worms in the motions. Piperazine usually eradicates the infection.

Tapeworms

Tapeworm infection occurs in both adults and children. There are two common types: *Taenia saginata*, derived from infected cattle, and *Taenia solium* from infected pigs. Man becomes infected through eating infected beef or pork which has been insufficiently cooked. Adequate cooking of beef and pork destroys the worms.

Tapeworms grow to a length of many feet. The worm, which has a flat white appearance, is made up of a head and individual small segments which usually drop off in turn and are passed in the faeces. The symptoms of tapeworm infection are slight, usually consisting of excessive appetite, mild abdominal colic and perhaps some loss of weight. There are several effective anthelmintics used for the treatment of tapeworms, niclosamide being the commonest.

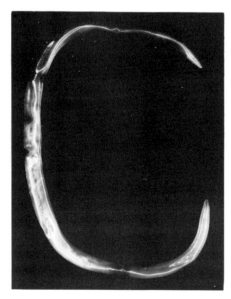

Fig. 7.19 Roundworm.

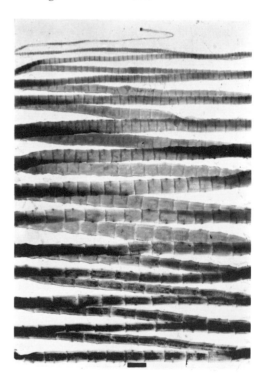

Fig. 7.20 Tapeworm.

Hydatid cysts

Hydatid disease is rare in this country but is seen in visitors from abroad, particularly Australia and the Middle East. The worm, *Taenia echinococcus*, is small (about 0.5 cm long) and lives in the intestine of the dog. The eggs, which it passes in the faeces, contaminate food ingested by man, sheep and rabbits, who are the intermediate hosts. The ova transform into a larval state in the intestine. The larvae penetrate the intestinal wall and enter various organs, especially the liver, where cysts are formed. Dogs eat the infected viscera of sheep and rabbits, the worms develop in the dog (primary host) and so the cycle continues.

Clinical features Cysts in the liver may grow to a great size leading to abdominal swelling and discomfort; sometimes pressure on the bile ducts causes jaundice.

The diagnosis should be suspected in a patient from abroad with a large liver. Surgical treatment is sometimes needed to remove the cyst.

DISEASES OF THE PERITONEUM

Inflammation of the peritoneum (*peritonitis*) is often seen as the result of a spread of infection from the intestinal tract or pelvic organs. Most cases of acute peritonitis are caused by such surgical conditions as acute appendicitis, perforated peptic ulcer or acute salpingitis (inflammation of the Fallopian tubes). Rarer types of acute peritonitis are those due to perforation of a typhoid ulcer in the intestines and the primary pneumococcal peritonitis, usually resulting from a generalized infection. Apart from the above forms of acute peritonitis there remains tuberculous peritonitis.

Tuberculous peritonitis

This is usually due to reactivation of a tuberculous focus in the peritoneum with concurrent pulmonary, gastrointestinal or genital TB. The infection is due to bovine tubercle bacilli.

Symptoms and signs The onset is slow and gradual. Vague abdominal pain with fever, loss of weight and appetite are the main symptoms. In later stages, the abdomen is distended by ascites (fluid in the peritoneal cavity). Treatment is a prolonged course of antituberculous chemotherapy (see page 134).

Ascites

Ascites is the presence of fluid in the peritoneal cavity, and may be caused by many different types of disease bearing little relation to each

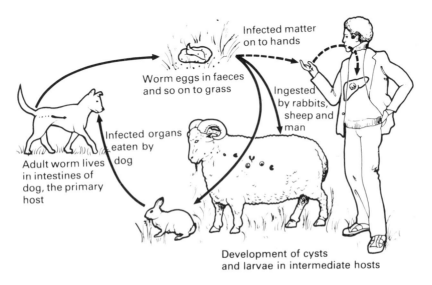

Infected matter on to hands

Worm eggs in faeces and so on to grass

Ingested by rabbits, sheep and man

Infected organs eaten by dog

Adult worm lives in intestines of dog, the primary host

Development of cysts and larvae in intermediate hosts

Fig. 7.21 Hydatid cysts.

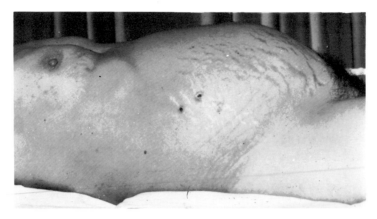

Fig. 7.22 Ascites. The abdomen is grossly distended. The two puncture marks from the paracentesis can be clearly seen.

other. It is convenient, therefore, to summarize the main types of ascites according to the causative diseases:

Causes of ascites

Congestive heart failure This is the commonest cause of ascites and the fluid is present as part of a generalized oedematous state.

Diseases of the peritoneum (a) Secondary carcinoma of the peritoneum caused by spread (metastases) from other organs, particularly the ovaries, stomach and colon causes marked ascites that may need frequent tapping. The general condition of the patient is poor, severe wasting and anaemia being present. Treatment is directed towards the patient's comfort but in some cases cytotoxic drugs (such as nitrogen mustard) or radioactive gold can be injected into the peritoneum in the hope of killing the malignant cells. (b) Tuberculous peritonitis. The ascites is accompanied by a general wasting, fever and diarrhoea. The fluid seldom needs tapping.

Diseases of the liver (a) Carcinoma of the liver, usually secondary spread from other organs such as the lungs, stomach or intestines, may result in ascites. (b) Cirrhosis of the liver. Ascites is present in the late stages of most cases of cirrhosis. It is caused by pressure on the portal vein from the fibrous tissue in the liver. Enlarged veins are often present in the abdominal wall (caput medusae).

Glomerulonephritis Ascites, as part of a general oedema, is sometimes present in cases of glomerulonephritis, and always in the nephrotic syndrome.

Adhesions

Adhesions may form in the peritoneal cavity as a result of infection. Here, the adhesions play a useful role in limiting the spread of infection. In the very young and elderly, the ability of the peritoneum and greater omentum to form adhesions, is not as good as in the adult. This means that diseases such as appendicitis and diverticulitis more often lead to generalized peritonitis in the young and elderly.

In addition to this protective effect, adhesions may cause disease by forming bands that obstruct the bowel and cause intestinal obstruction. These adhesions usually follow abdominal surgery. Multiple adhesions causing recurrent intestinal obstruction may be due to the talc on surgeons' (and scrub nurses') gloves, and it is very important to wash the talc off with sterile water before commencing an operation.

8

Diseases of the liver, biliary tract and pancreas

ANATOMY OF THE LIVER

The liver is the largest organ in the body, weighing about 1.5 kg. It is situated beneath the right half of the diaphragm. The upper border lies between the fifth and sixth ribs and the lower border is sometimes felt below the right lower rib margin on inspiration. There are two main lobes of the liver, the right and the left, and two smaller lobes, the caudate and quadrate. The normal liver consists of masses of hepatocytes (liver cells) supported by a framework of fibres (reticulin). The liver cells are grouped into lobules with a hepatic vein at the centre and portal tracts at the periphery. Portal tracts contain a branch of the portal vein, a branch of the hepatic artery and small bile ducts. Running between the masses of liver cells are tiny bile channels which drain into the bile duct within the portal tract; these in turn join to make up the common hepatic duct. The hepatic duct then joins the cystic duct from the gall-bladder to form the common bile duct which opens into the duodenum.

There is a second type of cell (the Kupffer cell) within the liver; Kupffer cells are phagocytic and they belong to the reticulo-endothelial system. They will be discussed further in the next section.

FUNCTIONS OF THE LIVER

The liver plays an important role in many metabolic processes. It receives blood from the portal vein and so all nutrients absorbed from the gut, with the exception of fats which are transported via the lymphatic system, pass through the liver before entering the systemic circulation.

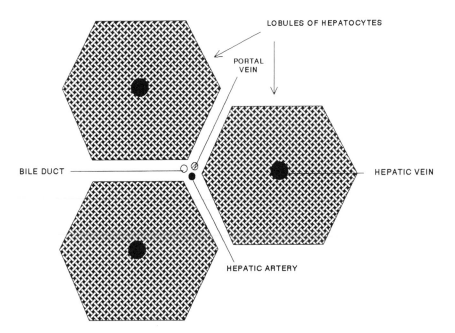

Fig. 8.1 Normal liver architecture.

Carbohydrate metabolism

The liver stores glucose, an important energy source, in the form of glycogen. Glycogen can be broken down to glucose to maintain blood glucose levels during periods of fasting.

Protein synthesis

The liver synthesises many of the plasma proteins including albumin, carrier proteins, such as transferrin (iron) and caeruloplasmin (copper) and most of the proteins involved in blood coagulation. During this process, urea is formed from ammonia in the Krebs cycle (see below) and is excreted as a waste product by the kidneys.

Fat metabolism

Fats, including VLDL (very low density lipoprotein) and HDL (high-density lipoprotein) cholesterol, and triglycerides, are synthesized by the liver cells. Cholesterol is also broken down to bile salts and these are excreted in the bile (see below).

Storage functions

Many vitamins and other substances, including vitamins D and B_{12}, iron and folate are stored in the liver.

Excretion and detoxication

Bile salts and cholesterol are excreted in the bile. Bile salts are important in aiding the proper digestion and absorption of fats and fat-soluble vitamins, such as vitamin K, from the gut. Ammonia, which is formed during protein metabolism, is converted to urea which is less toxic and is excreted by the kidneys. Many drugs are detoxicated by the liver. Fat-soluble drugs may be converted to water-soluble compounds allowing excretion in the bile. Steroid hormones are inactivated in the liver. Bile pigments are derived from the breakdown of old red blood cells. The cells release haemoglobin which is split into a protein part (globin) and haem which contains iron. After removal of the iron, the haem molecule is converted to bilirubin in cells of the reticulo-endothelial system in the liver and spleen. Bilirubin is then transported in the blood

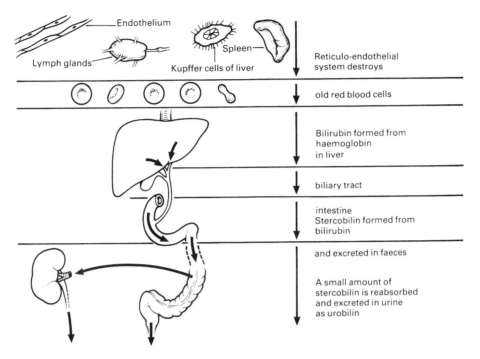

Fig. 8.2 Normal bile pigment formation and circulation.

stream (as unconjugated bilirubin) to liver cells. Bilirubin is combined with an acid molecule in the liver cells (conjugated bilirubin) and then excreted into the biliary tract and eventually emptied into the duodenum. In the intestine the bilirubin is broken down by bacteria to stercobilinogen, a pigment that gives the faeces their normal dark brown colour. In the absence of stercobilinogen the faeces are pale. In addition to being excreted in the faeces, a small amount of stercobilinogen is reabsorbed back into the blood stream, to be partially excreted in the urine. This small amount of pigment which is excreted in the urine is given the name urobilinogen, although it is identical with stercobilinogen.

INVESTIGATIONS IN LIVER DISEASE

Blood tests

Various blood tests are available which help to assess the functional state of the liver. These include serum bilirubin, serum albumin and the prothrombin time, a coagulation test which is very sensitive to acute liver damage. The liver cell enzymes, serum aspartate aminotransferase (AST) and serum alanine aminotransferase (ALT), leak out into the blood when liver cells are damaged – as in viral hepatitis. Alkaline phosphatase tends to be high in biliary obstruction. In alcoholics the red blood cells may be enlarged (macrocytosis) on a full blood count and levels of the enzyme gamma glutamyl transferase (GGT) may be raised.

Urine tests

Bilirubin in the urine is always abnormal and indicative of liver disease (see under jaundice).

Liver biopsy

A liver biopsy is a relatively simple procedure, which may be performed under local anaesthetic, and involves only an overnight stay in hospital. A needle (e.g. Menghini or Trucut) is inserted into the liver and a fragment of liver tissue withdrawn to be examined under the microscope. It is important for assessing the severity of disease (e.g. in alcoholism) and may sometimes help with the diagnosis of unexplained abnormalities of liver function, liver enlargement, drug-related liver disease and liver tumours. Patients must be able to lie flat and hold their breath. Biopsy can be dangerous, especially if biliary obstruction is present (when bile leaks may occur) or the patient has a bleeding tendency. The risk of the procedure can be reduced by performing it under ultrasound or CT guidance (see below). Following a biopsy the patient must remain in bed for 24 hours. Pulse and blood pressure must be measured quarter-hourly for the first hour and half-hourly for the next five hours because of the risk of haemorrhage.

Liver scans and radiological investigations

Three methods are available for looking at the general structure of the liver (the biliary system will be dealt with separately):

1. *Ultrasound scanning*. Sound waves can be bounced off the liver and its size and the presence of tumours or abscesses can be seen. Distortion of the sound wave pattern can be seen when the liver tissue is damaged, for example by cirrhosis. Ultrasound is difficult when the patient is obese.

2. *CT (computer tomography) scanning*. This involves a computer producing a picture of a slice through the patient from a series of X-ray beams. Slices through the liver can show the presence of cysts, abscesses or tumour.

3. *Radio-isotope scans*. These involve injecting a radio-isotope into the blood system, which is then taken up by liver cells. Liver tumours can often be well demonstrated. Decreased uptake of isotope indicates disease of liver tissue, especially alcoholic liver disease.

Jaundice

Jaundice is the term given to the yellow discolouration of the skin and conjunctiva caused by an excess of bile pigment, bilirubin, in the blood-stream (Plate 6). Jaundice is very common and frequently the predominating sign in many diseases of the liver and biliary tract. There are two main types, depending on how the excess bilirubin builds up in the blood stream:

1. *Haemolytic jaundice*. This is due to an increased load of bilirubin arriving at the liver cell as a result of increased red blood cell breakdown, as in haemolysis. Newborn babies and infants are more susceptible to haemolytic jaundice and their livers are less able to cope with an excess of bile pigments. The causes of haemolysis of the red blood cells which may give rise to haemolytic jaundice are discussed under haemolytic anaemias.

2. *Liver cell destruction and cholestasis*. Cholestasis is the failure of bile flow from the liver cell to the duodenum. It used to be called obstructive jaundice. Liver cell damage and cholestasis cause jaundice because bilirubin cannot be excreted by the liver cells into the bile passages so that the forward flow of bile along the bile passages does not occur. The bile is re-absorbed into the blood stream, thereby causing jaundice.

Causes of liver cell damage

1. Acute hepatitis, commonly of viral origin
2. Liver toxins, e.g. carbon tetrachloride, paracetamol
3. Chronic hepatitis – this may follow acute hepatitis
4. Liver cell damage may occur secondarily to long-standing biliary obstruction
5. Hypoxia
6. Idiopathic (i.e. unknown) – not all the causes of liver cell disease are known.

Causes of cholestasis within the liver (intrahepatic cholestasis)

Intrahepatic cholestasis is often associated with liver cell damage caused by:

1. viral hepatitis
2. drugs, e.g. chlorpromazine
3. cirrhosis (some cases)

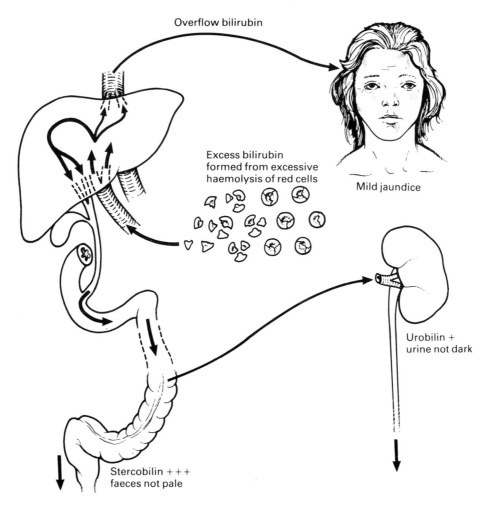

Overflow bilirubin

Excess bilirubin
formed from excessive
haemolysis of red cells

Mild jaundice

Urobilin +
urine not dark

Stercobilin +++
faeces not pale

Fig. 8.3 The mechanism of haemolytic jaundice.

4. cholangitis (inflammation of the bile ducts)
5. infiltration of the liver, e.g. by carcinoma
6. rare disorders, e.g. biliary cirrhosis.

Causes of cholestasis outside the liver (extrahepatic cholestasis)

1. Gall-stones in the common bile duct
2. Carcinoma of the head of the pancreas, ampulla of Vater (where the common bile duct joins the duodenum), or, rarely, bile duct
3. Fibrosis and stricture of the bile duct
4. Obstruction and pressure on the ducts from outside by tumours or enlarged lymph glands.

Signs and symptoms associated with jaundice

Cholestatic jaundice causes a deep greeny-yellow colour of the skin, the faeces are pale as bile pigments fail to reach the intestine, and the urine is dark brown owing to the presence of bilirubin. Bile salts accumulate in the blood causing severe itching of the skin. The lack of bile salts reaching the bowel means that fat soluble vitamins cannot be absorbed. Failure to absorb vitamin K leads to prothrombin deficiency and a prolonged blood clotting time. Cholesterol is also retained because it is usually converted into bile acids and excreted in the bile. In some cases, particularly patients with primary biliary cirrhosis, this may cause

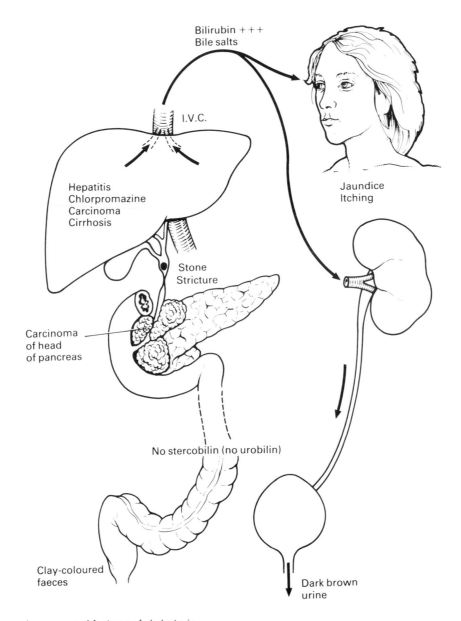

Fig. 8.4 The main causes and features of cholestasis.

xanthomatosis – yellow nodular accumulations of cholesterol on the exterior surfaces, pressure areas, scars and around the eyes.

In haemolytic jaundice the jaundice is usually mild and bile pigments (stercobilinogen) can reach the gut, so the faeces are a normal colour. In fact, excess bile pigments reach the gut so more sterco-bilinogen (urobilinogen) is absorbed and excreted in the urine, and the urine contains excess urobili-nogen but not bilirubin. Bile salts do not accumu-late in the blood stream so itching does not occur.

Other signs and symptoms of liver disease

These will be discussed in more detail under the

different diseases. It is important to note the age and sex of the patient as acute hepatitis is commonest in young people, gall-stones and alcoholic liver disease are more usual in middle age, and carcinoma, especially of the head of the pancreas, mainly occurs in elderly patients. Alcoholic liver disease is more common in males and primary biliary cirrhosis is usually a disease of women.

INDIVIDUAL DISEASES OF THE LIVER

Viral hepatitis

Viral hepatitis refers to infections of the liver caused by the hepatitis viruses (A–E). Other viruses can cause hepatitis, particularly cytomegalovirus (CMV) and Epstein–Barr virus (EBV), which causes glandular fever.

Hepatitis A

Hepatitis A is spread by the faeco-oral route with an incubation period of 2–6 weeks. It is the commonest cause of viral hepatitis and occurs more frequently in areas of poor sanitation. It is usually a mild infection in children which goes unnoticed. In young adults it usually causes symptoms with fever, loss of appetite, nausea and pain under the right rib margin. After a few days or weeks, jaundice and dark urine develop. The faeces may be clay-coloured if cholestasis occurs. Examination of these patients usually reveals jaundice and a swollen tender liver. Blood tests of liver function and a look for antibodies to hepatitis A may help to establish the diagnosis. Patients can be looked after at home but may be admitted to hospital for social reasons, if the disease is severe with features such as bruising, fluid retention or confusion, or the diagnosis is in doubt. In hospital, patients should be barrier nursed and care is taken with disposal of faeces, as the virus is excreted in the stool. There is no specific treatment and no special diet is necessary. The illness usually resolves over 3–4 weeks. Very occasionally patients relapse. A vaccine to hepatitis A is being developed, but at present protection to travellers to endemic areas can be given by intramuscular injection of pooled human immunoglobulin.

Hepatitis B

Hepatitis B is a very widespread infection with an incubation period of 2–6 months. It is transmitted by blood and blood products, including inoculation by contaminated syringes used in surgical and dental procedures and tattooing. Hepatitis B can also be transmitted by sexual intercourse, especially among male homosexuals, and possibly by kissing. Infection can be passed by mothers to their babies, either across the placenta or during breast feeding.

Acute hepatitis B usually causes a prodromal illness (non-specific viral illness preceding the hepatitis), similar to that with hepatitis A infection, before jaundice appears. Some patients with hepatitis B have skin rashes or joint pains. The diagnosis can be confirmed by liver function tests and by finding hepatitis B surface antigen in the blood, the so-called Australia antigen, as it was first discovered in an Australian aborigine. As with hepatitis A, there is no specific treatment and patients are nursed along the same lines. Great care should be taken when handling blood, syringes and needles. Blood should be transported in special labelled containers.

Relapses of hepatitis B can occur but, in addition, hepatitis B can cause chronic liver disease (chronic hepatitis and cirrhosis) as the virus is not completely cleared from the liver cells. Chronic infection affects about 5% of the world population and is associated with a high incidence of liver cell carcinoma in certain areas. Patients who continue to have the hepatitis E antigen in the blood remain highly infectious. Chronic hepatitis B infection can respond to the antiviral agent, α interferon, with eradication of the virus in 40% of cases.

Hepatitis B infection was a major problem in haemodialysis units and as a complication of blood transfusion. In the United Kingdom, infection in dialysis units has been controlled by preventing infected patients and staff from entering the unit. Screening potential blood donors for Australian antigen has also greatly helped to reduce post-transfusion hepatitis. Hepatitis B immunoglobulin can be given to people who have come into contact with hepatitis B-infected material. Prevention of infection relies on risk avoidance and immunization for high-risk groups. A vaccine derived from human plasma has been available for some years and now a genetically engineered vaccine is widely available. It is being offered to particular patients, hospital staff or other groups who are at increased risk of acquiring the infection.

Hepatitis C

Hepatitis C is the major cause of the infection previously called *non-A non-B* hepatitis. This virus has similar epidemiological and clinical features to hepatitis B. It is now the cause of almost all post-transfusion hepatitis. At present there are no confirmatory tests in routine use but they may shortly be introduced for screening blood for transfusion. The acute illness is usually mild but may be fulminant. Chronic hepatitis C infection may respond to α interferon. There is a high incidence of liver cell carcinoma in association with chronic hepatitis C infection in certain parts of the world.

Hepatitis D

Hepatitis D (delta virus infection) is transmitted with hepatitis B in certain cases and leads to worsening of the hepatitis B related disease.

Hepatitis E

Hepatitis E behaves like hepatitis A, being spread by the faeco-oral routes. Major epidemics of hepatitis E occur in the Indian subcontinent and other parts of the tropics. It attacks adults more commonly than children, in contrast to hepatitis A, and is particularly serious when it affects pregnant women, with a death rate of over 20% in this group. The clinical features are the same as for hepatitis A and treatment is symptomatic. There is no associated chronic infection.

Other hepatitis viruses may exist, since not all the cases of blood-borne hepatitis are hepatitis B or C positive.

Alcoholic liver disease

The daily consumption of alcohol needed to produce liver disease varies between individuals but women are much more susceptible to alcoholic liver damage than men. The upper safe limit for men is about 60 g, and is 30–40 g for women; one alcoholic drink contains about 8 g (one unit). Alcohol is metabolized by enzymes in the liver. Excess alcohol leads to the formation of acetaldehyde and severe upset in fat metabolism. As a result, the serum triglyceride levels rise and alcohol-induced fatty liver develops. A fatty liver has no symptoms and is reversible when drinking is stopped. The next, and more serious effect of alcohol, is alcoholic hepatitis, when injured liver cells die and the liver becomes acutely inflamed. A patient with alcoholic hepatitis who continues to drink may go on to develop cirrhosis, where the whole structure of the liver becomes disorganized and nodules develop. Ultimately, liver cell carcinoma (hepatoma) develops in 10–15% of cirrhotics.

Patients with alcoholic liver disease may have only mild symptoms such as anorexia, morning retching and diarrhoea, accompanied by a large liver. If acute alcoholic hepatitis develops often following a binge, they can quickly become very ill with fever, jaundice, abdominal pain and a large tender liver. They may also have signs of hepatic encephalopathy (see below). The blood film of such patients typically shows large red blood cells, plentiful neutrophils and a shortage of platelets. Liver function tests are abnormal with a high bilirubin and high enzyme levels. Patients with alcoholic cirrhosis may slowly develop signs of portal hypertension (see below) but at any time they can become very ill, especially if acute alcoholic hepatitis or a hepatoma develops on top of the cirrhosis. The damaged liver can no longer cope with the additional burdens and the term 'decompensation' is used to describe this.

The only treatment likely to benefit an alcoholic is complete abstinence – the 5-year survival rate for patients with cirrhosis who continue to drink is only 30%. Family and medical support is essential to achieve this. Patients with acute alcoholic hepatitis or decompensated cirrhosis should be admitted to hospital. Treatment includes a low salt, low protein diet, folic acid, vitamin B complex, prompt treatment of any infections, diuretics for ascites and treatment of hepatic encephalopathy if this is present (see below). Some patients with acute alcoholic hepatitis are given steroids but there is no good evidence that steroids are beneficial.

Chronic hepatitis and cirrhosis

There are two types of chronic hepatitis:

1. Chronic persistent hepatitis may follow viral hepatitis or some drugs. It is not serious and does not progress to cirrhosis. Patients have mild liver enlargement. No treatment is required except the avoidance of alcohol or the incriminating drug.

2. Chronic active hepatitis is more serious because it may progress to cirrhosis. The liver becomes inflamed, fibrous septa develop and liver cells die. Causes of chronic active hepatitis include viral hepatitis, alcohol, various drugs such as sulphonamides and methyldopa, and autoimmune ('lupoid') liver damage, which may be associated with systemic lupus erythematosus (SLE) or inflammatory bowel disease. Patients with autoimmune disease may improve on steroids, but otherwise there is no specific treatment.

Hepatic cirrhosis follows whenever masses of liver cells die. The architecture of the liver is upset and any re-growth of liver cells causes fibrosis and nodules to develop. Cirrhosis often follows on from chronic active hepatitis and so the causes are similar: the commonest are viral hepatitis and alcoholism, and others include drugs and autoimmune disease (primary biliary cirrhosis) but often the exact cause is unknown (cryptogenic). Cirrhosis leads to liver failure and obstruction to the flow of blood from the portal vein (portal hypertension).

Liver transplantation has recently become more widely available and is particularly used for the patients with chronic active hepatitis and cirrhosis. Patients with autoimmune disease are most likely to benefit from transplantation, although it is not yet clear if the condition returns in the new liver. Alcoholics can do very well with liver transplants if they abstain from alcohol, and they must do this for at least 6 months prior to the operation. Liver transplants have also been given to people with liver tumours and acute liver failure as a result of viral or drug-induced damage, especially due to paracetamol overdose, but the outcome is much less successful in this group of patients, as a result of tumour in other sites or tumour recurrence in the case of the former, and the systemic consequences of the decompensated hepatic failure in the latter case.

Portal hypertension

The portal vein drains blood from the stomach, intestines, spleen and pancreas and takes it to the liver. The blood is usually under low pressure (5–10 mmHg) but any obstruction to blood flow may cause the pressure to rise – *portal hypertension*. Obstruction to the flow of portal venous blood can occur within the portal vein itself, within the liver or as blood leaves the liver through the hepatic vein. Cirrhosis is a major cause of portal hypertension as it affects the small branches of the portal vein within the liver.

The clinical effects of portal hypertension are as follows:

1. Large blood vessels (collateral channels) develop wherever there is a communication between the portal and systemic (general) circulation, so helping to reduce the portal pressure by allowing blood to escape into the systemic venous system. These blood vessels develop between the oesophagus and stomach (*oesophageal varices*), in the retroperitoneal tissues, in the rectum (*causing haemorrhoids*) and around the umbilicus. Sometimes these blood vessels burst and cause torrential bleeding – usually from oesophageal varices.

2. The size of the spleen increases. This may result in anaemia, leucopenia (a low white blood cell count) and thrombocytopenia (low platelets).

3. Ascites – collection of fluid in the peritoneal cavity.

Bleeding from oesophageal varices

This causes a high mortality and is a medical emergency. The patient must first be resuscitated and peripheral and central venous lines are often

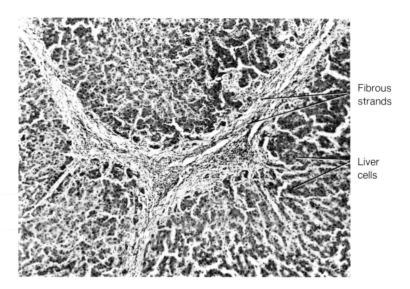

Fibrous
strands

Liver
cells

Fig. 8.5 Cirrhosis of the liver. Section of the liver to show the dense strands of fibrous tissue present. The liver cells are beginning to degenerate.

required so that plasma expanders and whole blood can be given quickly. Blood should be taken for cross-matching (at least 6 units), haemoglobin, urea (elevated due to release from digested blood) and electrolytes, clotting studies and liver function tests.

All vital signs and fluid balance need to be carefully monitored. Following resuscitation an endoscopy is usually performed so that the exact site of bleeding can be confirmed. Bleeding from varices may be controlled either by drugs or by direct pressure. Infusion of vasopressin acts by constricting blood vessels which supply the portal circulation but re-bleeding is common when the infusion is stopped. The Sengstaken–Blakemore tube is very effective but has to be carefully inserted as the oesophagus can be ruptured. Aspiration of nasopharyngeal secretions may also occur. Once initial resuscitation has been performed bleeding can be controlled by endoscopic sclerotherapy. A sclerosant is injected into the varices through the endoscope and the resulting inflammatory reaction obliterates the varices.

Long-term treatment of portal hypertension

Many different types of treatment – medical and surgical – have been tried to reduce the risk of bleeding from oesophageal varices. Beta-blockers slow the pulse rate and hence reduce portal pressure and may be beneficial. A more commonly used approach is regular endoscopic sclerotherapy. There are also several operations available, aimed at draining blood away from the portal circulation into the systemic circulation, for example, by joining the portal vein to the inferior vena cava or by joining the splenic vein to the left renal vein. A major problem with these operations is the high incidence of hepatic encephalopathy afterwards, due to decompensation of liver function as a result of the anaesthetic and surgical stress. Recently it has been possible to join the portal and systemic circulations using a metal stent inserted by a radiologist during angiography, and this comparatively safe procedure may produce better results.

Liver failure

This means that the liver is no longer able to carry out its various metabolic functions. Liver failure may result from chronic liver disease (cirrhosis, chronic active hepatitis, alcoholic liver disease or extensive tumours) or from fulminant hepatic failure (usually secondary to viral hepa-

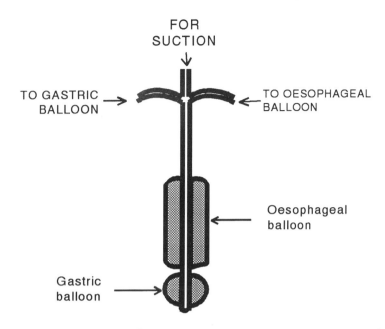

Fig. 8.6   Sengstaken–Blakemore tube.

titis or paracetamol over-dose). The effects of liver failure are as follows:

1. Jaundice
2. Hepatic encephalopathy; this term refers to the psychiatric manifestations of liver failure, extending from mild confusion to deep coma
3. Bleeding tendency, giving rise to haemorrhage
4. Ascites
5. Osteomalacia and osteoporosis, causing bone pains and fractures
6. Sensitivity to many drugs – especially sedatives and analgesics which may precipitate hepatic encephalopathy.

Severely ill patients should be nursed in an intensive care unit. Patients with fulminant hepatic failure (whose livers were functioning normally prior to their illness) have the potential for full recovery, although only about 30% of those in deep coma will recover. Each complication has to be treated individually as there is no specific treatment for liver failure and machines are not available to take over the function of the liver in the same way as kidney machines do in renal failure. Hepatic encephalopathy can be precipitated by a protein load, either from the diet or

following gastrointestinal bleeding, constipation, which increases ammonia absorption, infection, particularly of the ascitic fluid, diuretics, which may cause a low potassium (hypokalaemia), and drugs, especially narcotics. Patients with hepatic encephalopathy should be treated with a protein-free diet, sedatives are contraindicated and the bowel should be cleared with lactulose, given both orally and by enema, to reduce ammonia absorption. Oral neomycin should be prescribed to reduce the number of bacteria in the gut. Bowel bacteria produce toxic substances which are absorbed and, since they cannot be detoxicated by the liver, make the encephalopathy worse. Diuretics should be avoided, electrolyte imbalances should be corrected and infection should be looked for and treated.

Liver tumour

The most common liver tumours are metastases from carcinoma elsewhere in the body. The liver usually enlarges and may become tender. Metastases rarely upset the function of the liver but their presence is usually associated with a poor prognosis. Primary liver cell carcinoma (hepatoma) is one of the commonest tumours in the world, although it is seen infrequently in the United Kingdom. Carcinoma may be the end result of chronic hepatitis B infection. In Africa, the tumour is associated with aflatoxin which is produced by the fungus, aspergillus flavus. Aflatoxin contaminates stored grain. Liver carcinoma causes weight loss, abdominal pain, fever and, later, abdominal swelling due to ascites and a large liver. A blood test can help in the diagnosis of hepatomas as the alpha-fetoprotein is usually very high. The prognosis is poor although some patients do well following surgical resection of the tumour.

Other diseases affecting the liver

The liver may be involved in many diseases in addition to the ones described above. Some of these are common – such as the large tender liver seen in patients with right-sided heart failure, or the large fatty liver which develops in some diabetics. Many tropical infections affect the liver including malaria, amoebic liver abscess, schistosomiasis and lassa fever. Children are not exempt from liver disease. Those with cystic fibrosis may have mild liver disease which can progress to cirrhosis in those that survive to adolescence. Several inherited disorders also affect the liver and they include defective metabolism of iron and copper so that huge amounts of these minerals build up in the liver, and various disorders of glycogen and fat metabolism.

DISEASES OF THE BILIARY TRACT

Gallstones

The biliary tract comprises the hepatic duct which drains bile from the liver, the cystic duct which joins the hepatic duct to the gall bladder where bile is stored, and the common bile duct which drains bile from the hepatic and cystic ducts into the duodenum. Stones may develop in the gall bladder due to an excess of one or more of the normal constituents of bile, cholesterol or bilirubin. Normally, these constituents are held in

solution by the detergent action of the bile salts. Gall stones usually develop in the gall bladder as this is where bile is concentrated by the reabsorption of water.

Gall stones may remain asymptomatic for years. However, they may also give rise to a variety of different illnesses:

1. *Flatulent dyspepsia.* Chronic indigestion with flatulence is associated with gall stones. It is generally aggravated by eating fatty foods which cause the gall bladder to contract.

2. *Biliary colic.* In this condition, a stone temporarily becomes stuck in the biliary tract. This usually occurs in the neck of the gall bladder causing abdominal pain with vomiting, which can be severe. An attack may last up to 12 hours after which the stone becomes dislodged, relieving the pain. Stones may also become stuck in the common bile duct, causing biliary colic and jaundice.

3. *Acute cholecystitis.* If a stone which has become stuck in the neck of the gall bladder or cystic duct does not become dislodged then the gall bladder becomes distended and inflamed.

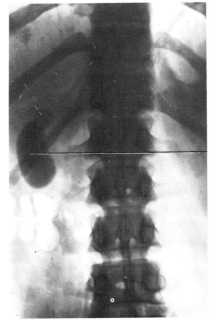

Gall-
bladder

Fig. 8.7 X-ray (cholecystogram) of the normal gall bladder.

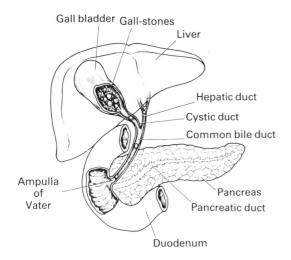

Fig. 8.8 Diagram of organs in upper abdomen showing where gall stones may be found.

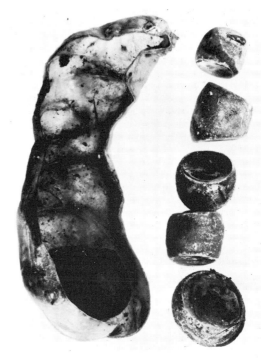

Fig. 8.9 A large distended chronically inflamed gall bladder filled with gall stones.

This is usually sterile but secondary bacterial infection may occur. This condition is characterized by epigastric and right-sided abdominal pain with fever and usually lasts 2 to 4 days. Treatment is to rest the gall bladder by making patients nil by mouth. Intravenous fluids are given to prevent dehydration and antibiotics may be prescribed. The condition usually responds to these measures. Once the acute attack has settled removal of the gall bladder, cholecystectomy, is usually performed within a few days.

4. *Empyema of the gall bladder.* If acute cholecystitis fails to resolve and infection supervenes, the gall bladder may fill with pus. This is known as an empyema of the gall bladder. It may respond to the same measures as acute cholecystitis or may rupture causing peritonitis in which case an emergency operation is necessary.

5. *Mucocoele of the gall bladder.* This is a rare condition which develops when a stone blocks the outlet of the gall bladder which then transiently fills with mucous.

Occasionally, a stone may pass from the gall bladder into the common bile duct where it may give rise to three different conditions:

1. *Cholestatic jaundice.* Blockage of the common bile duct due to a gall stone produces a triad of pain, fever and jaundice. The blockage is often intermittent and so the patient experiences intermittent abdominal pain. These features may distinguish this cause of cholestatic jaundice from the other main cause – carcinoma of the pancreas.

2. *Ascending cholangitis.* The presence of a stone in the common bile duct may lead to infection which results in a high fever, rigors and jaundice.

3. *Acute pancreatitis.* This will be considered later.

Diagnosis

Gall stones may be suspected on the clinical history of flatulent dyspepsia or a previous attack of biliary colic or cholecystitis. In the latter cases, it is usual to allow the symptoms to settle before performing any investigations. As gallstones can only be seen on plain X-ray in 10% of patients, other investigations are usually needed to show them. Most gallstones can be seen by looking at the biliary tract with ultrasound. The stones block the echo waves causing shadows. If ultrasound

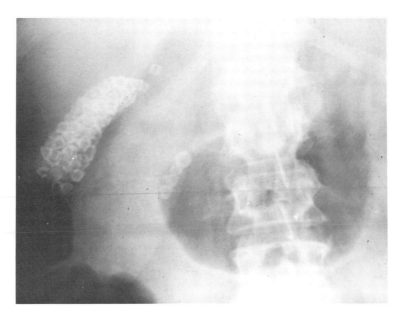

A

does not show a stone then an oral cholecysto-gram can be performed. On the evening before the examination, the patient swallows a radio-opaque dye in the form of tablets. This dye is absorbed and excreted in the bile and becomes concentrated in the gall bladder. Stones are shown as filling defects in the gall bladder, although often the gall bladder is not seen due to inflammation or a blocked cystic duct. This investigation should not be performed in patients with jaundice as the bile will not pass into the biliary tract.

Treatment

Patients with gall stones are usually offered surgical removal of the gall bladder (*cholecystectomy*) as once gall stones have given trouble, further attacks usually occur. During cholecystectomy, a further X-ray of the common bile duct is taken (*per-operative cholangiogram*) to exclude the presence of gall stones in the common bile duct. If these are found, they are removed. Following exploration of the common bile duct a T-tube is left in place for bile drainage to allow the biliary tract to heal. Another cholangiogram is performed through the T-tube before it is removed to confirm that no stones have been left. If stones are found at this stage they can be extracted

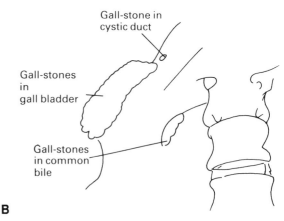

B

Fig. 8.10 A, B. Multiple gall stones.

through the T-tube by a Dormier basket.

Drugs, such as ursodeoxycholic acid, can be used to dissolve gall stones in patients who are not fit for surgery, but they take a long time to work (6 months to 2 years), are often not effective, and may cause diarrhoea.

ANATOMY AND FUNCTIONS OF THE PANCREAS

The pancreas lies retroperitoneally, its head encircled by the duodenum and its tail lying in contact with the spleen. The exocrine pancreas secretes into the duodenum enzymes to digest proteins, fats and carbohydrates, and bicarbonate to neutralize the acid entering the duodenum from the stomach. The endocrine pancreas contains nests of hormone producing cells (Islets of Langerhans), the main hormones being insulin and glucagon (See chapter 13).

DISEASES OF THE PANCREAS

Tumours

Carcinoma of the pancreas is fairly common. The main symptoms are upper abdominal pain radiating through to the back due to erosion of local nerves, and, for tumours involving the pancreatic head, cholestatic jaundice due to obstruction of the common bile duct which runs through this region. Other symptoms include weight loss, anorexia, thrombophlebitis and anaemia.

Investigations

It may be difficult to distinguish between cholestatic jaundice due to carcinoma of the pancreas and gall stones. Usually, the jaundice is progressive in cases of carcinoma. A variety of investigations may help in the diagnosis:

1. *Ultrasound.* This may show a tumour in the pancreas and often shows dilatation of the bile ducts. Gall stones may also be demonstrated.
2. *ERCP (endoscopic retrograde cholangiopancreatography).* This is performed by inserting a cannula into the lower end of the biliary and pancreatic ducts via an endoscope in the duodenum. Radio-opaque dye is injected which shows any obstruction in the duct. ERCP can be used in treating carcinoma of the pancreas by inserting a *stent* (hollow tube) through the obstruction in the bile duct to relieve the jaundice. It can also be used therapeutically to remove gall stones in the common bile duct.
3. *CT scan.* This X-ray investigation allows the visualization of a mass in the pancreas.

Treatment

The treatment of carcinoma of the pancreas is usually palliative as the disease is often advanced before symptoms develop, and most patients are dead within 9 months. The tumour rarely responds to chemotherapy or radiotherapy. Occasionally, the tumour can be removed at operation. An operation may be performed to relieve the jaundice by joining the gall bladder to the small bowel, but this is usually done by inserting a stent endoscopically.

Acute pancreatitis

In this condition, pancreatic necrosis occurs, probably because enzymes of the pancreas become activated while still in the pancreas and cause autodigestion of the organ. The two main causes are gall stones and excessive alcohol ingestion.

Symptoms and signs

The patient complains of sudden onset of severe abdominal pain radiating to the back. Usually the patient is shocked and this may be severe. In addition, nausea and vomiting are present. The patient is restless, the pulse is rapid and the blood pressure is usually low. The abdomen is tender even to light touch. Occasionally bruising occurs around the umbilicus or in the flanks. The diagnosis is made by finding a high serum level of the pancreatic enzyme amylase.

Treatment

Acute pancreatitis presents as an emergency. Diamorphine or pethidine may be necessary to relieve pain. The patient should be kept nil by mouth and a nasogastric tube should be passed for regular aspiration of stomach contents. Fluid should be given by intravenous drip while the patient is still vomiting or in shock. Records must be kept of the fluid intake and output, the pulse, the blood pressure and the temperature which may be subnormal in the early stages. Oxygen should be given via a face mask since patients usually have a lack of circulating oxygen (hypoxia). In most cases, the condition subsides over a few days or a week, but in severe cases patients may need to be nil by mouth for weeks and intravenous nutrition may be required. In some cases cysts or abscesses may develop needing drainage. The mortality from acute pancreatitis is less than 1% for mild cases, but is over 50% in severe cases.

Chronic pancreatitis

Chronic pancreatitis is characterized by intermittent bouts of severe abdominal pain and marked weight loss secondary to anorexia. Vomiting may occur. Loose stools containing a high fat content-(*steatorrhoea*) result from the failure to absorb fat due to pancreatic enzyme loss (*pancreatic insufficiency*). Damage of the islet cells may lead to diabetes. The serum amylase may be raised during an acute attack. The diagnosis can be made by showing pancreatic calcification on an abdominal X-ray or CT scan, or a dilated, dis-

torted pancreatic duct on ERCP. Stools should be collected for three days for a faecal fat estimation to confirm steatorrhoea, and levels are usually very high.

Treatment

The most important treatment is for the pain. Patients usually require very strong pain-killers, such as pethidine or morphine, and may become analgesic addicts. The fat content of the diet should be restricted and alcohol avoided. Diabetes may require insulin. Tablets containing pancreatic enzymes are given to aid digestion of food. They should be taken with each main meal. Part or all the pancreas may be removed surgically if pain is intractable but this is usually effective only if patients abstain from alcohol and even then results are variable.

9

Diseases of the nervous system

This chapter is divided into three sections:

1. Anatomy and physiology
2. Symptoms and signs of neurological diseases
3. Diseases of the nervous system

ANATOMY AND PHYSIOLOGY

Knowledge of the anatomy and physiology of the nervous system is particularly important in understanding its diseases. As only a simplified account can be provided here, the nurse studying this chapter is encouraged to supplement her reading of the structure and function of the nervous system.

The nerve cell (neuron) is the basic unit of the nervous system. It has a cell body, where the nerve impulse or signal starts, a long projecting fibre (axon) along which the nerve impulse travels, and a terminal containing a chemical (neurotransmitter) which the impulse releases outside the cell. This released chemical then activates the cell body of the next neuron and the impulse or signal travels on. The nervous system comprises such chains of neurons, some in pathways with a known purpose (e.g. motor or sensory).

The nerve cells in the brain and spinal cord form part of the 'central' nervous system, and those lying outside them the 'peripheral' nervous system. The nerve cells are supported by 'glial' cells. In peripheral nerves, glial cells form a jacket called a 'myelin sheath' around the larger nerve fibres. In the central nervous system, glial cells are of two types, astrocytes and oligodendrocytes.

Nerve cells receive essential nutrition (e.g.

glucose) and oxygen via the blood supply.

Motor system

The motor system can be divided into two parts: the 'pyramidal' system, which is responsible for voluntary movement, and the 'extrapyramidal' system, which controls posture and co-ordination. The main pathway of the pyramidal system is illustrated in Figure 9.1. The starting point of this pathway are the brain cells located in a part of the cortex responsible for movement, therefore called the motor cortex. Fibres from these cells project to the spinal cord, forming a bundle or tract as they pass downwards through different structures. An important feature to note is that the pyramidal tract from the right motor cortex crosses to the left side of the spinal cord in the region of the medulla; hence the right motor cortex controls movement in the left side of the body. Similarly, the pyramidal tract arising from the left motor cortex crosses in the medulla to the

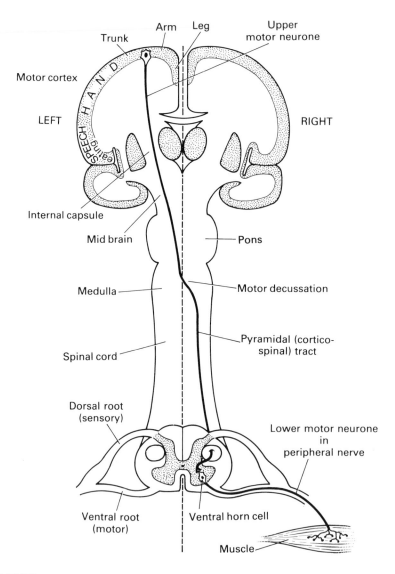

Fig. 9.1 The motor system.

right side. Because the motor fibres cross over in this way a disease in the right motor cortex, or right pyramidal tract above the point of crossing, will produce its effects on the left side of the body.

The terminals of the pyramidal tract activate nerve cells (motor neurones) lying in the ventral spinal cord. Motor neurones project directly to muscles, forming a 'neuromuscular junction'. Impulses along motor neurones make the muscles they supply contract.

The nerve cells in the motor cortex and its fibres are collectively referred to as the 'upper motor neurone' and the motor neurones as the 'lower motor neurone'; we shall see later that this division of the motor system is very important in locating the site of disease in the nervous system, as a disease affecting the upper motor neuron produces a different set of signs from those produced by a disease affecting the lower motor neuron.

Sensory system

There are various forms of sensation such as touch, vibration, hot and cold, joint position sense and pain: the nerve pathways that carry the impulses that lead to these sensations form the 'somatosensory' system. In addition, there are the special senses of sight, hearing, smell and taste, which have specialized receptor organs and their separate pathways. The nerve terminals in the peripheral organs (e.g. skin, bladder, joints) form the starting point of impulses that lead to sensation. There are two relay points in the somatosensory system. The sensory fibres enter the dorsal spinal cord, where they first relay with spinal cord cells. These project to the thalamus to form the second relay with cells which in turn project to the sensory cortex. As is the case with the main motor system, the main sensory system which leads to the sensation of touch crosses over to the opposite side of the body in the medulla; hence, a disease of the left sensory cortex will lead to abnormal sensation in the right side of the body.

The reflex

A simple functional unit of the nervous system is

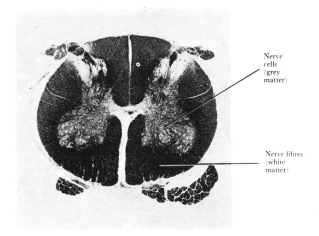

Fig. 9.2 Section of normal spinal cord. The central mass of grey matter (nerve cells) can be clearly distinguished from the surrounding white matter.

the 'reflex', which may be elicited without the conscious effort of the subject. It consists of two arcs: the sensory, and the motor. Reflexes are divided into superficial (e.g. abdominal) or deep (e.g. tendon). To explain the deep tendon reflex action we shall consider the knee jerk. When the tendon of quadriceps muscle is tapped over the knee, the sudden stretch of the muscle sends signals in the sensory nerves up to the spinal cord. This signal activates motor cells in the spinal cord, which lead to activation and contraction of the quadriceps muscle. The typical jerk of the knee results. Note that in this reflex the impulses go only via the lower motor neuron and all parts have to work at full speed and in unison for a jerk to be seen. It is only in diseases affecting the lower motor neuron and local sensory system that this deep tendon reflex is lost.

Autonomic system

This comprises the nerves which regulate the various bodily functions that do not require voluntary control (e.g. digestion), and help maintain a constant internal environment (e.g. a steady blood pressure).

The peripheral autonomic nervous system is divided into two parts: the 'sympathetic' and 'para-sympathetic' nervous systems. The sympathetic nervous system originates from the thoracic and upper lumbar spinal cord, and, with the exception of fibres supplying sweat glands (which have acetylcholine as the neurotransmitter), the neurotransmitters it secretes are noradrenalin and adrenalin (in USA epinephrine). The sympathetic system prepares the body for emergencies – there is an increase in heart rate, blood is diverted from the skin to the muscles, the airways dilate, and the sweat rate increases. Parasympathetic nerves leave the central nervous system in some cranial nerves (e.g. the vagus) and the sacral spinal cord, and use acetylcholine as their neurotransmitter. In contrast to the sympathetic system, the parasympathetic system activates functions appropriate to rest, such as digestion and urogenital function. It slows the heart rate, and diverts blood to the gut.

Recently, a group of substances known as neuropeptides have been discovered in the auto-nomic nerves, and they also serve as neurotransmitters.

Higher functions

These include consciousness, language and memory. In the great majority of adults, the organization of language is located in the left cerebral hemisphere. This fact is often used to diagnose the site of cerebral disease. Memory is divided into short-term and long-term; it is the short-term memory that is disrupted by a number of disease processes, and, indeed, by old age.

SYMPTOMS AND SIGNS IN NEUROLOGICAL DISEASES

These are used to locate the site of a disease, diagnose its nature, and monitor its progress in relation to treatment.

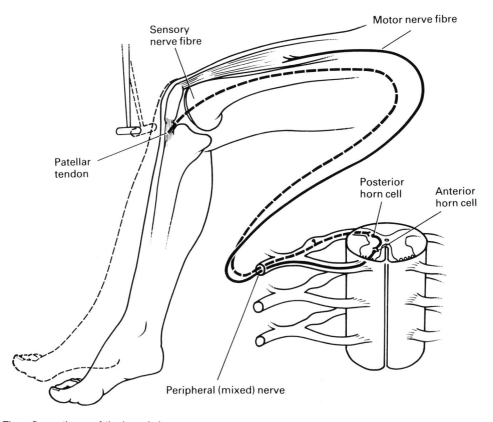

Fig. 9.3 The reflex pathway of the knee jerk.

Motor

The main symptoms are weakness, uncoordinated or 'extra' movements, and stiffness or floppiness. Weakness may result from an abnormality in the motor pathway (upper or lower motor neurone), the neuromuscular junction, or the muscle itself. The weakness may be mild ('paresis') or severe ('plegia'). Common forms of paralysis include: hemiplegia, paralysis of one side of the body; paraplegia, paralysis of both lower limbs; and monoplegia, paralysis of one limb. Further symptoms and signs help distinguish between upper and lower motor neurone disorders (see Table 9.l). In upper motor neurone disorders, the weakness is accompanied by stiffness ('spasticity'), increased deep tendon reflexes and an abnormal plantar reflex (i.e. the toe moves upwards on stroking the sole of the foot). Lower motor neurone disorders are associated with floppy ('flaccid') muscles, wasting of muscles, decreased reflex responses, and a normal plantar reflex (i.e. toe moves towards the sole). Double vision ('diplopia') may result from weakness of muscles that move the eyeballs. 'Tremors' are rhythmical rapid movements, and may occur either as exaggerations of the physiological tremor or as marked abnormal writhing or jerking movements (athetosis, chorea, hemiballismus) in disorders of the extra-pyramidal system. 'Nystagmus' is a term which describes a jerking movement disorder of the eyeballs. 'Ataxia' refers to incoordination of movement, and may be often best seen when the patient is asked to walk. The manner of walking ('gait') is characteristic in a number of diseases. For example, in Parkinson's disease, there is a shuffling, short-step gait. In hemiplegia, the patient drags the paralysed leg, and the paralysed arm is held close to the side.

Sensory

Disturbances of sensation include:

Anaesthesia: loss of sensation of touch
Analgesia: loss of sensation of pain
Hyperalgesia: increased pain sensation
Paraesthesia: sensation of pins and needles, 'tingling'.

Each of the various sensations – touch, pain, heat and cold, joint position, vibration – may be tested. Peripheral nerve lesions usually cause a loss of sensations from the region supplied by the nerve.

The special senses include sight, hearing, smell and taste. Visual loss may present as loss of ability to read at a distance (loss of acuity), or loss of part of the normal view (loss in the visual field), or double vision (diplopia). Hearing disturbance may present as deafness or 'tinnitus' (a persistent whistling or buzzing sound). Tuning fork tests may distinguish between neural and other causes of deafness such as an ear blocked with wax.

DISEASES OF THE NERVOUS SYSTEM

Infections

Meningitis

The meninges consist of three sheaths covering the brain and spinal cord: the pia, arachnoid and dura mater. Meningitis (inflammation of the meninges) is the most common and important disease affecting the meninges. The infection may be blood borne or from local spread.

Table 9.1

Changes in the affected limbs	In upper motor neurone disease	In lower motor neurone disease
1. Paralysis (loss of power)	Present, often not complete. Tends to affect *whole* limbs	Present, usually complete. Affects *groups of muscles* in a limb or limbs
2. Tones of muscles	Stiff and rigid (spastic)	Limp (flaccid)
3. Wasting of muscles	Usually slight	Usually marked
4. Tendon reflex	Present (usually exaggerated)	Absent
5. Abdominal reflexes	Absent	Present
6. Plantar reflex	Extensor response (Babinski's sign present)	Normal flexor response
7. Sensation	Usually only slightly disturbed	Sensory disturbances more evident

Symptoms and signs The commonest features are headache, neck stiffness and clouding of consciousness.

1. *Onset.* This is in most cases quick (hours or days) with the exception of the tuberculous type. The patient is severely ill, with fever.

2. *Headache.* This is constant and persistent. It comes on early and is associated with vomiting.

3. *Altered consciousness.* The patient is drowsy and irritable, and often delirious. He resents being touched or disturbed.

4. *Neck rigidity.* There is a marked stiffness of the neck. The patient lies turned away from the light, as photophobia (dislike of light) is present.

5. *Convulsions or fits.* These are common, especially in infants.

6. *Kernig's sign.* This is the resistance met with on attempting to straighten the flexed (bended) knee, as this movement stretches the inflamed meninges, causing pain.

Types of meningitis

1. *Pyogenic meningitis.* Meningococcal meningitis is by far the most common form in the adult, and often occurs in epidemics. *Haemophilus influenza* and *E. coli* are sometimes responsible in childhood; the onset and course may be particularly rapid in children. In streptococcal and staphylococcal meningitis there may be evidence of infection in the ear (otitis media), mastoid or other sinuses (sinusitis); the meningitis may develop as a result of local spread of infection to the meninges.

2. *Tuberculous meningitis.* Here the onset may be gradual (over weeks) before the characteristic picture of meningitis occurs. The accumulation of purulent exudate over the base of the brain may affect the emerging cranial nerves.

3. *Viral meningitis.* This is usually less severe, and may occur in epidemics.

Diagnosis of meningitis It is important to exclude a cerebral abscess and a CT scan will normally be carried out before a lumbar puncture to confirm the diagnosis. A needle with a stilette in it is inserted, under the strictest aseptic technique, between the third and fourth or fourth and fifth lumbar vertebrae, passing through the dura mater and into the subarachnoid space. On withdrawing the stilette the cerebrospinal fluid (CSF) flows through the needle. Normal CSF comes out drop by drop at a certain pressure (which can be measured by a special manometer) and, most importantly, is always crystal clear.

In meningitis, the CSF is cloudy and spurts out under high pressure, and in pyogenic meningitis it may be frankly purulent. By examining the fluid in the laboratory and culturing the organism, the exact type of meningitis can be ascertained; this procedure is particularly important for diagnosing an early case of tuberculous meningitis.

Nursing Patients with meningitis are severely ill, so that they require the most skilled nursing. They may resent all disturbance, so that great patience on the part of the nurse is needed to make sure that the patient gets sufficient fluids; an intravenous infusion may be necessary. The patient is best nursed in a subdued light because of the photophobia. Quietness is essential as noise is badly tolerated. Barrier nursing is necessary to prevent the spread of infection. Careful neurological observation is essential, to detect any signs of deterioration. General treatment includes bed rest, and analgesia in the form of paracetamol and codeine may be given for headache.

Special treatment

Pyogenic meningitis. The introduction of antibiotic drugs has completely changed the outlook in pyogenic meningitis. Before these drugs were used, the majority of cases of meningitis died. Now the vast majority recover. Depending on the severity and type of infection, it is usual to give sulphonamides and penicillin (up to 2 million units every 2 to 4 hours). Chloramphenicol may be given in addition, especially in children. Penicillin (10 000 to 20 000 units) is sometimes given by the intrathecal route, i.e. by a lumbar puncture. The antibodies must be given intravenously, and should be started on suspicion of meningitis, often by the GP, before any investigations are performed. Early antibiotic treatment can be life-saving.

Tuberculous meningitis. Chemotherapy has also changed the course of this disease. Streptomycin,

Anatomy

Pia mater closely invests brain, spinal cord and issuing nerves

Arachnoid mater

Dura mater is tough and inelastic

Subarachnoid space contains cerebrospinal fluid. CSF is increased in quantity and therefore pressure in *meningitis*

Brain

Pia

Arachnoid

Dura

Spinal cord

Lumbar cistern containing CSF, cauda equina and filum terminale

Signs and symptoms

High fever-pulse relatively slow
Neck rigidity
Photophobia
Withdrawn and irritable
Vomiting
Headache

Lumbar puncture

Lower end of spinal cord

L1
L2
L3
L4
L5
S1

Arachnoid + Dura (spinal flexed)

CSF cloudy and under pressure

Treatment

Fluids ++
Quietness
Dim light
Patience

Appropriate chemotherapy

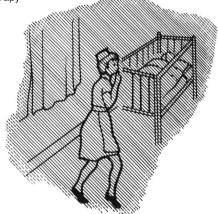

Fig. 9.4 Meningitis.

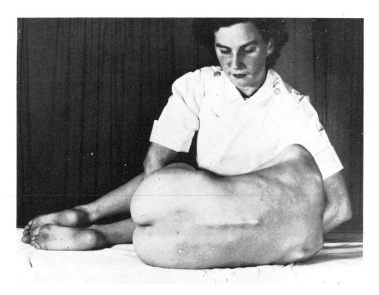

Fig. 9.5 The position of the patient for lumbar puncture. The spine must be fully flexed.

para-aminosalicylic acid (PAS) and isoniazid are given until the sensitivity of the organism is known, after which the two most effective agents are continued for at least 6 months. In serious cases, drugs may be given intrathecally. Pyridoxine is given to prevent the neurotoxic effects of isoniazid, and anticonvulsants may be necessary, especially in children.

Encephalitis

Encephalitis is an inflammation or infection of the cells in the brain and may arise from several causes, e.g. different viruses, or as an immune complication of vaccination.

Epidemic viral encephalitis occurs in many parts of the world. The patient usually complains of headache and drowsiness, which may be followed by fits and coma. Herpes simplex encephalitis is a common and grave condition which is treated with intravenous infusion of the anti-herpes viral drug acyclovir at the onset of infection.

Cerebral abscess

A cerebral abscess is usually caused by spread of infection from septic disease in the ears, mastoid cells or nasal sinuses. A cerebral abscess can also result from a septic embolus lodging in the brain, particularly in cases of bronchiectasis.

Symptoms and signs These are essentially the same as for cerebral tumours (see below), with the addition of fever. There will be the signs of increased pressure and also the localizing signs according to the site of the abscess in the brain. Signs of infection, like fever and raised white cell count help to distinguish abscess from tumour. Evidence of septic ear disease or bronchiectasis also helps in the diagnosis.

Treatment Antibiotics are of great value, but, in addition, operation to evacuate the abscess may be necessary. Penicillin and streptomycin may be injected locally into the abscess cavity after evacuation of the abscess. The primary focus of infection (ear, mastoid, etc.) must also be dealt with by the appropriate measures.

Poliomyelitis (infantile paralysis)

Poliomyelitis is caused by a virus which specifically attacks the anterior horn (motor neurone) cells in the spinal cord. It may also affect the brain, especially the midbrain, producing encephalitis. The encephalitis caused by the poliomyelitis virus is known as polioencephalitis.

Poliomyelitis tends to occur in epidemics in the autumn.

Spread of infection The virus grows in the intestinal tract and is excreted in the faeces. It is more likely to spread where sanitation is neglected and where hygiene is poor. Transmission is by contamination of food and also by droplet infection.

Symptoms and signs

1. Children and young adults are most commonly affected, but the disease varies in different epidemics; in recent years, older patients have been affected. The onset is sudden, with fever, headache and the general feeling of malaise.

2. Stiffness of the neck with pain in the back are common in early symptoms. In some patients, the disease may progress no further than this stage, which is known as the preparalytic stage. These abortive attacks are often suspected and diagnosed during an epidemic.

3. Other cases go on to the stage of paralysis. Here, one or more limbs or the trunk muscles may become paralysed. The areas most commonly affected are the legs, shoulder girdle muscles (especially the deltoid), intercostal muscles or diaphragm. Any part of the body may, however, be affected. The paralysed part is limp and the deep tendon reflexes are lost. Wasting of the muscle is an early and prominent feature. This is a typical example of a lower motor neuron paralysis.

4. Pain in the affected muscles is usually present and in some cases may be very pronounced. The muscles are usually tender to touch in the acute stage.

5. In cases where the brain cells are affected (polioencephalitis), paralysis of some of the cranial nerves, such as the seventh (facial) nerve with a resulting weakness of one side of the face, occurs. More important, however, is the paralysis of the vital centres (bulbar paralysis) which may develop. Paralysis of the respiratory centre, with marked dyspnoea and cyanosis, is a common form of bulbar paralysis. Respiratory failure in poliomyelitis may also be caused by paralysis of the intercostal muscles and diaphragm.

Pharyngeal paralysis is another important result of bulbar paralysis. Pharyngeal paralysis causes difficulty in swallowing with consequential accumulation of secretions in the throat which may lead to choking and asphyxia.

Diagnosis and course The sudden onset after a few days of fever, during an epidemic, of a flaccid paralysis of a limb or part of a limb allows the diagnosis to be readily made. The diagnosis may be confirmed by examination of the cerebrospinal fluid, which will show an increase in the number of the white cells.

The paralysis usually reaches its maximum in the first few days, after which it remains stationary.

Paralysis is particularly likely to occur where strenuous physical exercise had been undertaken in the preceding few days. Slow gradual improvement usually takes place over the next few months, but it may take as long as a year before the maximum recovery had been effected. In some cases complete recovery may take place, but in others residual paralysis with severe wasting of the muscles remains.

Treatment of poliomyelitis

Active immunization. After years of research, an active and safe vaccine has been produced which offers good protection against paralytic poliomyelitis. This vaccine has already done much to eradicate the dreaded effects of a disease so long known as infantile paralysis. Today, the vaccine most widely used throughout the world is an attenuated or weakened form of live virus. This vaccine is usually taken orally. The first dose can be given when the child is 2 months old and two further doses within the first 6 months. A booster dose can be given at the age of 18. This virus, too weak to lead to any ill effects, nevertheless causes the formation of sufficient antibodies to provide immunity for several years. All susceptible members of the family should be immunized at the same time. Parents and carers of young children undergoing vaccination should also have a booster as they excrete the polio virus in their nappies.

Curative. The patient is nursed at complete rest and barrier nursing is carried out. Masks, gowns and gloves should be worn and the faeces must be handled with care and disposed with promptly. It is essential to wash the hands carefully after toileting.

The affected limbs must be placed in a position of optimum rest. It is most important that paralysed muscles not be stretched as permanent damage may result. (See page 209 for the proper care of paralysed limbs and the prevention of pressure sores.)

Passive movements are started from the onset, and it is for this reason that any splints used should be capable of easy removal. Prolonged rigid fixation of a limb in heavy splints must at all costs be avoided. As soon as the pains and the acute tenderness of the muscles subside active exercises are started, preferably under the supervision of a skilled physiotherapist. Baths are very useful in that active exercises of the muscles are carried out with greater ease in water. Physiotherapy may have to be continued for months or even years to ensure the maximum degree of recovery possible.

Special orthopaedic appliances, such as walking callipers, may be necessary, and in some cases operations may be performed to aid movement in the paralysed parts.

If the respiratory muscles (intercostals and diaphragm) are affected, respiratory failure may develop, and for these cases special apparatus known as a respirator (iron lung) is available to help the patient over the acute phase. Several different types of respirator are used and all require the utmost skill in management. Patients who have to be placed in a respirator are naturally very apprehensive and often terrified. Constant reassurance and explanation of the benefits to be gained are needed to allay this anxiety.

In the bulbar form of poliomyelitis, pharyngeal paralysis may be present, causing an inability to swallow which can lead to choking and asphyxia as a result of the accumulation of secretions in the throat. A suction apparatus must, therefore, always be available at the bedside to remove the mouth secretions. Postural drainage helps to prevent the accumulation of secretions in the throat and so these patients are best nursed in the prone or semiprone position with the foot of the bed elevated. See Figure 9.6.

The bulbar form of poliomyelitis, with its pha-

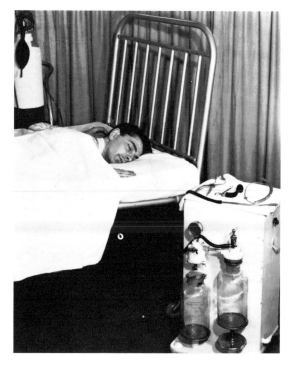

Fig. 9.6 The various instruments, suction apparatus and oxygen necessary for nursing a patient with pharyngeal paralysis. They must always be available at the bedside.

ryngeal paralysis and also paralysis of the respiratory centre, calls for the greatest care and constant attention to ensure that a clear airway is at all times maintained. Tracheostomy is often needed in poliomyelitis to maintain a clear airway. Patients with acute respiratory and bulbar paralysis must never be left unattended. Finally, it should be realised how apprehensive patients suffering from poliomyelitis are. As progress may be very slow and may take many months or years, the need for continued sympathy, understanding and encouragement for these patients must be stressed.

Herpes zoster

Herpes zoster is a common disease caused by reactivation of the virus responsible for an earlier (childhood) attack of chickenpox. It is often known as shingles and involves the posterior nerve roots. Any nerve can be affected.

Symptoms and signs At first there is a pain along the affected nerve, which is followed soon

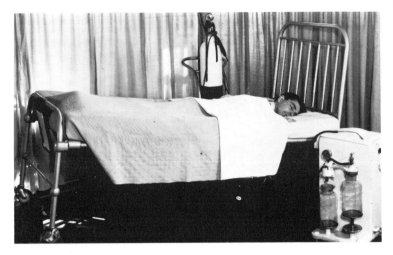

Fig. 9.7 The correct position for nursing a patient with laryngeal paralysis. The prone (or semiprone) position with the head on one side and elevation of the foot of the bed allow the maximum drainage of the mouth secretions. The patient should be turned frequently from side to side.

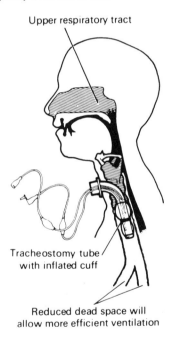

Fig. 9.8 Tracheostomy tube in situ.

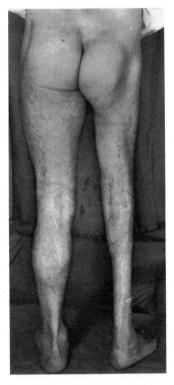

Fig. 9.9 Poliomyelitis, late stage of the disease, showing permanent wasting of the muscles of the right leg.

after by the characteristic eruption. This takes the form of small blebs, or vesicles, scattered along the line of nerve so that they map out the path of the affected nerve. The vesicles dry up to form crusts.

The pain, particularly in elderly patients, may be most severe and persistent, lasting perhaps for many weeks or months after all signs of the eruption has gone. The pain may be so severe as to lead to marked mental depression.

Two nerves are commonly the site of herpes zoster infections:

1. The ophthalmic division of the fifth cranial nerve with resultant pain and eruption above the affected eye. The cornea of the eye may also be affected, leading to corneal ulceration.

2. The intercostal nerves, when pain and the typical eruption occur in a girdle fashion around one side of the chest.

In severe cases with a lot of pain, the patient is treated in bed. A light dusting powder, such as zinc oxide, is used for the eruption. The anti-viral drug acyclovir may be prescribed. Sedatives and analgesics are usually needed to relieve the pain. Carbamazepine or amitriptiline may be required in severe cases.

In cases affecting the eye, particular attention must be paid to prevent or minimize corneal ulceration. Hyoscine or atropine drops are instilled into the eye to dilate the pupil; hot bathing may also be useful.

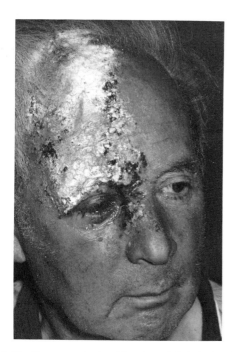

Fig. 9.10 Herpes zoster involving the ophthalmic division of the trigeminal nerve.

Syphilis of the nervous system

Syphilitic disease of the central nervous system, often known as neurosyphilis, is now an uncommon disorder. There are three main types: meningovascular, tabes dorsalis and general paralysis of the insane (GPI).

Meningovascular syphilis

Particularly in the second stage of syphilis, changes can occur in the meninges and the vessels of the brain. A rare cause of meningitis not previously mentioned is syphilis. The symptoms and signs of syphilis meningitis are exactly the same as those in other acute forms.

Tabes dorsalis

Pathology The form of neurosyphilis known as tabes dorsalis occurs in the tertiary stage of syphilitic infection from 5 to 15 years after the primary stage. The main lesions are in the posterior columns of the spinal cord, and as these carry sensory impulses the early predominating symptoms tend to be sensory.

Symptoms and signs Men are more commonly affected, usually in middle life. A juvenile form of tabes, however, is seen in congenital syphilis.

1. The earliest symptoms are the characteristic 'lightning pains', so called because they last for a few brief seconds, shooting up and down or through the legs. They are often likened to the effect of pins being stuck into the limb.

2. Disturbances of bladder function occur early, usually consisting of difficulty in holding the urine or, in other cases, retention of urine.

3. The ataxic gait is often so predominant that the other name for tabes dorsalis is locomotor ataxia. The patient tends to fall about, especially when the eyes are closed or in a dark room. The patient characteristically walks with the feet wide apart and with marked stamping of the feet.

4. The loss of the sensation of pain, causing unfelt damage to the joints, can lead to gross swelling, marked destruction and deformity. Extreme abnormal mobility without pain is the typical result of these changes. Similar trophic

joint changes, which are commonly known as Charcot's joints, can and do occur in any neurological disease where the sensation of pain in a joint is lost. The absence of the sensation of pain allows repeated trivial injuries to effect the destructive changes in the joints.

5. Sudden acute severe abdominal pain with vomiting may occur, which may give the appearance of an acute abdomen. This attack is known as a gastric crisis of tabes. Similar crises may affect other parts, e.g. the larynx, causing difficulty in breathing.
6. The pupils of the eyes become narrowed and irregular.
7. The deep tendon reflexes, especially in the ankle and knee jerks, are absent from an early age.

Diagnosis The lightning pains and the marked ataxic gait form the clinical basis of the diagnosis. A lumbar puncture is, however, usually done, when changes such as an increase in cells and in the protein in the cerebrospinal fluid are found to be present. Serological tests are performed to confirm the diagnosis.

General paralysis of the insane (GPI)

General paralysis of the insane, like tabes, arises in the tertiary stage of syphilis. It affects the higher centres of the brain and also the pyramidal motor tracts. The name is descriptive, emphasizing the predominant changes, i.e. a paralysis associated with insanity.

Symptoms and signs

1. *Mental changes.* The earliest symptoms are usually a deterioration of intellect and abnormal behaviour on the part of the patient, particularly as regards personal appearance and moral conduct. Eventually, complete dementia sets in.
2. *Paralysis.* This mainly affects the legs, causing a paraplegia (paralysis of both lower limbs). The paralysis may progress so that the patient becomes immobile and incontinent.
3. Convulsions or fits are frequent.

Diagnosis The mental changes combined with paralysis and often with fits suggest the diagnosis. Other tests are performed as previously described.

Treatment of neurosyphilis

1. The specific treatment for neurosyphilis, as for all types of syphilitic infection, is large doses of penicillin. At least 10 million units are given over a period of approximately 14 days. A second course may be necessary.
2. *Tabes dorsalis.* Re-educational exercises to improve the walking are extremely useful and may enable a patient to get about who otherwise would be bedridden.

AIDS

AIDS, or the acquired immunodeficiency syndrome, is associated with a variety of neurological syndromes. These include peripheral neuropathy, myelopathy, dementia, opportunistic infections in the brain (such as toxoplasmosis and tuberculosis), as well as lymphoma of the brain.

Vascular diseases of the brain
Strokes (Fig. 9.11)

Causes A stroke is a common disease and may be caused by three different kinds of lesion in the cerebral arteries, all of which may produce a similar clinical picture:

1. *Cerebral thrombosis.* Particularly in elderly people, the cerebral arteries are affected by arteriosclerosis, in which the lining of the arteries becomes thickened and roughened. The flow of blood may be obstructed and 'clotting' occurs. This clot (thrombus) blocks the artery and deprives part of the brain of its blood supply.
2. *Cerebral haemorrhage.* Rupture of a blood vessel produces haemorrhage into the brain. This event is more common in cases of hypertension.
3. *Cerebral embolism.* An embolus, or detached clot, may lodge in one of the cerebral arteries and produce a stroke. This variety of stroke is seen in diseases where a clot forms on the carotid arteries in the neck or the left side of the heart, and is carried up in the blood stream to lodge in one of the cerebral vessels. The diseases which most frequently cause a clot in the left side of the heart are: (a) mitral stenosis with atrial fibrillation, (b) myocardial infarction and (c) subacute bacterial endocarditis.

Causes

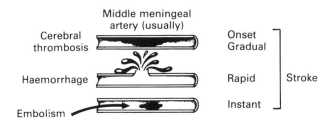

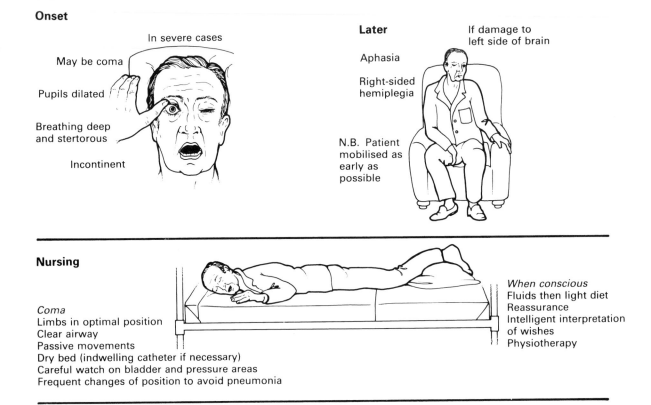

Onset

In severe cases

May be coma

Pupils dilated

Breathing deep
and stertorous

Incontinent

Later

If damage to
left side of brain

Aphasia

Right-sided
hemiplegia

N.B. Patient
mobilised as
early as
possible

Nursing

Coma
Limbs in optimal position
Clear airway
Passive movements
Dry bed (indwelling catheter if necessary)
Careful watch on bladder and pressure areas
Frequent changes of position to avoid pneumonia

When conscious
Fluids then light diet
Reassurance
Intelligent interpretation
of wishes
Physiotherapy

Fig. 9.11 Strokes.

Symptoms and signs

1. The symptoms and signs of cerebral thrombosis, haemorrhage and embolism may be the same, except for the onset. In thrombosis it may take hours or even days, while in embolism the onset is very sudden. In haemorrhage the onset is fairly sudden.

2. In many cases, the patient becomes drowsy and lapses into unconsciousness (coma), or may become comatose suddenly. The breathing may become deep and noisy, and the pupils dilated. Incontinence of urine and faeces is present. In mild cases, which are usually due to cerebral thrombosis, the first sign of a stroke may be paralysis without unconsciousness.

3. The patient in severe cases may die without regaining consciousness. In other cases, when the patient regains consciousness the various signs

and symptoms resulting from the lesion may become more apparent. Paralysis and loss of sensation on the opposite side of the body may be present (as previously mentioned, sensory and motor tracts from the brain cross-over to the opposite side of the body in the brain stem). If the lesion is on the left side of the brain, the language area may also be affected, leading to a loss of language ability (aphasia) in addition to a right hemiplegia.

4. The course of the disease may vary considerably. The patient often regains some power of movement, and this may be gradual over some weeks.

Assessment of 'level of consciousness' The nurse has to monitor the progress of the unconscious patient, and alert the medical staff in the event of deterioration. A neurological observation chart is usually kept by the bedside of the seriously ill patient. One important assessment is the 'level of consciousness', changes of which help monitor progress. The following description of observations may be used to communicate the level of consciousness:

1. Alert and orientated. Patient knows his name, where he is, what time of day it is.
2. Obeys commands. Patient moves limbs, shuts eyes, or performs some act when asked to do so.
3. Responds to painful stimuli. Patient moves limbs, grimaces, when pinched or stimulated in other ways.
4. Unresponsive.

Other important signs, too, are useful in assessing deterioration, and may be associated with increased pressure inside the skull (which is in effect a 'closed box') following stroke and other diseases or head injury:

1. Decreased pulse rate.
2. Increased blood pressure.
3. One or both pupils dilated, and later unresponsive to light; this is an important sign.
4. Change in rate or pattern of breathing.

Treatment of strokes
Nursing. During the stage of coma the nursing

of the patient is of the utmost importance. As in any case of coma with paralysis, certain dangerous problems are very prone to arise which, if possible, must at all costs be prevented.

1. A clear airway must be maintained so that the patient does not become asphyxiated through the tongue falling back in the mouth. The patient's head is best put on the side, and if necessary an airway should be inserted. If there is any difficulty over drainage of the mouth secretions, the patient is best nursed in the prone or semiprone position. Suction should always be available.

2. Pressure sores (Fig. 9.12) are very liable to develop in any prolonged coma, especially in elderly people, and particularly if paralysis is also present. In the case of strokes, the vast majority of the patients are elderly and, as paralysis is often present, pressure sores are very liable to occur unless carefully nursed. For this reason preventive measures, such as attention to the skin over the pressure areas and frequent changes of the patient's position (every 2 hours), are particularly important. Draw sheets and incontinence aids should be used to keep the patient clean and dry.

3. Frequent changing of the patient's position and physiotherapy will also help to avert another prevalent danger – pneumonia. If pneumonia should develop, antibiotics may be given.

4. Careful watch on bladder function is necessary. As has already been stated, either incontinence of urine (which is more usual) or, in some cases, retention of urine with a distended bladder, may occur. In cases of retention, when the bladder becomes grossly distended, an overflow dribbling of urine can occur. A large distended bladder is felt as a tense rounded mass in the middle of the abdomen above the pelvis. In either case, an indwelling catheter in the bladder with closed drainage bag attached may be necessary.

5. Nutrition and fluids may be given intravenously or via a nasogastric tube. Later, when the patient has recovered consciousness, fluids and a light diet may be given by mouth.

Treatment of the paralysed limbs It is essential to put the paralysed limbs through a full range of

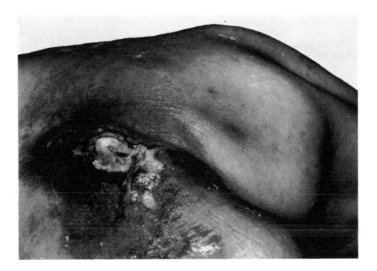

Fig. 9.12 Pressure sore.

passive movements several times a day from the very start of the illness. Passive movements help to prevent arthritis and fixation of the joints.

All weight must be taken off the paralysed limbs. The paralysed limbs must be put in the best position for the prevention or minimization of deformities. The affected leg should be prevented from rotating outwards by the proper use of sandbags or firm pillows. The leg should be in a position of extension with the knee slightly flexed to relax the muscles. A small pad or pillow placed under or just below the knee helps to maintain this position. To prevent pressure on the heels a small flat pillow should be placed under the ankles. On no account must heel rings be used to prevent pressure sores, as they themselves cause pressure. A foot-board or pillow at the end of the bed will help to prevent foot-drop. A small pillow should be placed in the axilla on the affected side to prevent adduction of the arm and to relax the muscles. The whole stress of treatment of hemiplegia is to mobilise the patient as early as possible. The patient must not be kept in bed if he is able to sit in a chair, and active movements and exercise must be organized, usually by the physiotherapist. Walking needs a conscious effort of will by the patient, and the experience is often a distressing one, needing constant reassurance and encouragement. With the aid of a Zimmer walking frame or a four-legged stick, the patient can be educated to balance himself and to gain confidence.

If the hemiplegia is on the right side, language disturbance is likely to be present. A patient so affected is greatly upset to find that he cannot understand others or express himself, and nurse will take care to offer reassurance and try to anticipate his needs. A speech therapist will be able to help the patient to articulate his words and improve speech.

Occupational therapy has the major role to play in rehabilitation. The occupational therapist can prepare the patient for the various day-to-day tasks needed on returning home. Climbing the stairs, using the bath and the lavatory, eating and preparing of meals, all these functions, previously accepted without thought, now become matters of effort and re-learning. A visit to the home by the therapist will reveal any unexpected difficulties that need to be provided for. Discussion with the family by the nurse, the doctor and the social worker may help to restore confidence. In doubtful cases, a trial visit home for a day or a weekend before discharge from hospital should be arranged. In many areas, rehabilitation centres provide special facilities for the further education of the hemiplegic patient.

Medical treatment

1. Hypertension is the most important predisposing cause of a stroke, and if high blood

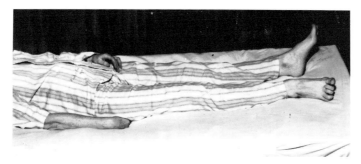

Fig. 9.13 Right hemiplegia. The leg is externally rotated and the foot is dropped. The paralysed arm is adducted and the hand curled under the body.

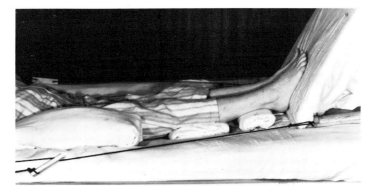

Fig. 9.14 The correct positioning of the lower limb in hemiplegia. The large firm pillow against the thigh prevents external rotation of the whole leg. The pillow just below the knee slightly flexes the knee and relaxes the muscles. The small pillow under the ankles prevents pressure on the heels and the foot-board overcomes the foot-drop.

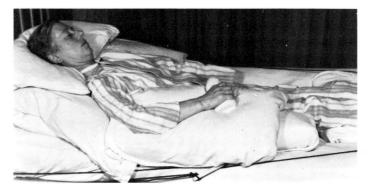

Fig. 9.15 The correct positioning of the upper limb in hemiplegia. The pillow prevents adduction of the arm and the hand-roll keeps the fingers and thumb opposed to each other.

pressure is found, treatment is indicated by drugs (see p. 86). Too great a reduction in blood pressure is not advised, since this might diminish the cerebral blood flow.

2. If the stroke has been caused by an embolus from atrial fibrillation, anticoagulant therapy (p. 93) can be used to prevent further clot formation, and digoxin can be used to slow the heart rate.

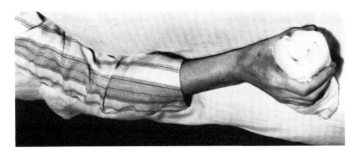

Fig. 9.16 Close-up view of the hand with the hand-roll in place to show the proper positioning of the fingers, thumb and wrist.

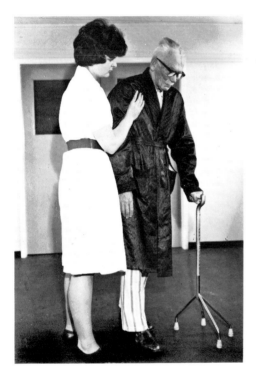

Fig. 9.17 Right hemiplegia. Mobilizing the patient.

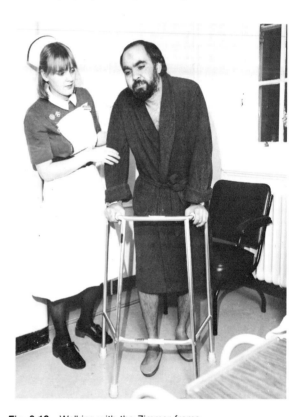

Fig. 9.18 Walking with the Zimmer frame.

Subarachnoid haemorrhage

A haemorrhage into the subarachnoid space may occur spontaneously, and in these cases, rupture of an unsuspected cerebral aneurysm or arterio-venous malformation is usually the cause. Small aneurysms of the cerebral arteries (berry aneurysms) are not uncommon, and are a result of congenital weakening of the arterial wall. These aneurysms usually do not give rise to symptoms unless they rupture. In older people, subarachnoid haemorrhage is relatively more likely to be associated with a severe hypertensive haemorrhage than to a congenital aneurysm. Head injury, especially with a fracture of the skull, may also cause subarachnoid haemorrhage.

Symptoms and signs

1. The onset is usually sudden with intense headache and vomiting. If the haemorrhage is large, the patient may be comatose and convulsions may occur.

2. The pulse is slow. Neck rigidity is a charac-

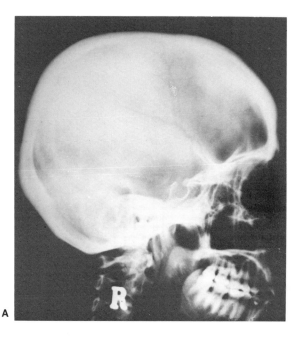

A

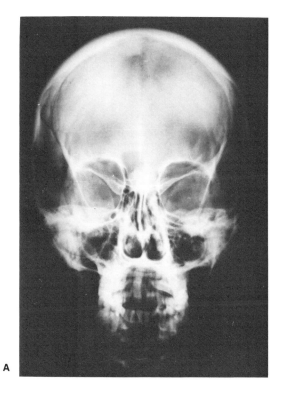

A

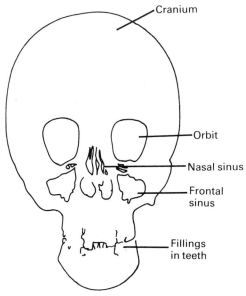

B

Fig. 9.19 A, B. X-ray showing frontal view of skull, and diagram indicating particular features.

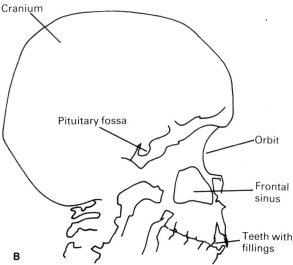

B

Fig. 9.20 A, B. X-ray showing side-view of skull, and diagram indicating particular features.

teristic feature. Photophobia may occur.

3. The urine may contain albumin and sugar.

4. In some cases paralysis of the cranial nerves and limbs develops.

Diagnosis The picture of intense headache, vomiting, neck rigidity and slow pulse resembles that of meningitis. A lumbar puncture, however, will establish the diagnosis, as in subarachnoid haemorrhage the cerebrospinal fluid is heavily bloodstained and not purulent as in meningitis. Angiography is also very helpful in the diagnosis and is done before any operative procedure. A radio-opaque dye is injected into the carotid artery and an X-ray of the skull then taken. The dye outlines the blood vessels and may show up the aneurysm.

Treatment The neck of the aneurysm is clipped surgically if it is accessible, or the body of the aneurysm may be wrapped. Patients treated medically must be nursed at complete rest, everything being done for them to eliminate the least possible strain. The patient remains in bed for about 6 weeks. Recurrence of rupture of the aneurysm is not uncommon and often occurs within a week after the initial attack. Some patients get a severe secondary spasm of cerebral vessels in the days after the haemorrhage, which may result in death.

Headache

1. Headache is often a feature of any general illness and many common infections are ushered in by a headache.

2. Tension headaches occur in nervous subjects when under stress. The headache is often described as 'like a tight band round the head'; it is sometimes at the back of the head. There is no aura and it is not associated with vomiting. It usually responds to simple analgesics.

3. Despite a popular misconception, hypertension does not usually cause headaches. However, if the blood pressure is very high, headaches and vomiting may occur.

4. Cerebral tumours may present with headaches and the physician always has this possibility in mind when confronted with a patient who has begun to get episodes of headache. Investigation may be necessary to make sure of the diagnosis.

5. Temporal arteritis (see p. 343). This inflammation of the temporal arteries is commonest in the elderly and the headache is associated with malaise, pyrexia and sometimes mental confusion. As involvement of the central artery of the retina may cause blindness, early diagnosis, followed by treatment with corticosteroids, is necessary.

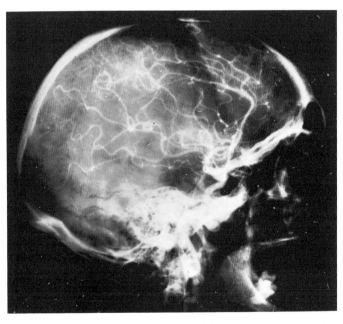

Fig. 9.21 Cerebral angiogram in a normal person. The opaque dye is injected into the carotid artery so that the carotid artery and cerebral blood vessels are clearly outlined.

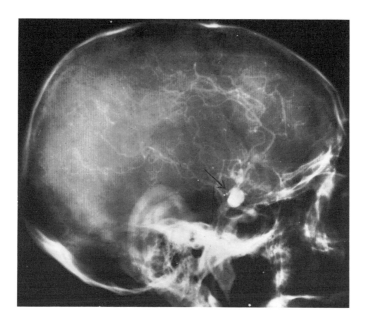

Fig. 9.22 Cerebral angiogram showing a large aneurysm.

Migraine

Migraine is a form of paroxysmal 'vascular' headache, often occurring in more than one member of a family. Migraine has various characteristics, but not every migraine sufferer has all these symptoms:

1. The headache is often preceded by an 'aura'. This usually consists of a visual disturbance with flashes of light, zigzags of varying colours or even partial loss of vision, or the aura may be a sense of numbness and tingling on one side of the face or body. The aura may last for up to half an hour and is followed by the headache.

2. The headache is often throbbing in character, worse on one side of the head, and frequently associated with anorexia, nausea or vomiting. The headache may last many hours or, rarely, for several days.

3. Attacks of migraine may occur at times of relaxation after spells of intense activity or stress, particularly at the weekends.

4. Attacks of migraine can be precipitated in different subjects by different trigger factors. Certain foods (e.g. chocolate, cheese, alcohol), certain drugs (e.g. contraceptive pill), strong light, excessive exercise, emotional upsets or premenstruation may dispose to a migraine attack.

Pathology

Migraine is thought to be due to changes in the cerebral blood vessels. In the aura stage, the vessels become constricted while the throbbing headaches are associated with a subsequent fullness and dilatation of the vessels.

Migraine subjects should learn what trigger factors are liable to precipitate an attack and how to avoid them.

Sometimes, when migraine becomes very frequent and due to stress, a course of sedation may help to reduce the frequency of the attacks.

Propranolol, pizotifen and clonidine are sometimes successful in preventing attacks, if taken regularly.

If given at the first intimation of an attack, ergotamine or sumatriptan can be effective in preventing the attack from developing.

Convulsions (fits)

Convulsions or fits are commonly seen in a wide

variety of diseases and tend to occur more frequently in infants and children than in adults; a fit or convulsion in an infant often takes the place of a rigor in an adult. On the other hand, epilepsy is a disorder characterized by repeated fits for which, in many cases, no cause may be found.

Symptomatic fits

Symptomatic fits are those in which there is some underlying discoverable cause. In contrast to symptomatic fits, idiopathic fits (or epilepsy) are those recurring fits without any obvious cause which are frequently seen in children and adults. Symptomatic fits are much more frequent than idiopathic epilepsy, so they will be described first. Again, for the sake of convenience, we can divide symptomatic fits into (1) those in infants and children, and (2) those in adults.

Common causes of fits in infants and children Fits or convulsions are very commonly seen in infants. Any severe general illness or fever in an infant may start with a convulsion. Whooping cough, measles, pneumonia and otitis media commonly cause convulsions in infants.

Gastrointestinal disturbances are another frequent cause of fits, especially in the first year of life; gastroenteritis and intestinal worms may be associated with convulsions. Simple digestive upsets, especially in the teething stage, may also cause fits.

Diseases of the central nervous system (such as meningitis, cerebral tumours, hydrocephalus and the various forms of paralysis due to maldevelopment or injury which are so often seen in infants) are especially liable to cause repeated fits.

Common causes of fits in adults The following is a brief list of the more common conditions in adults in which convulsions occur:

(a) Following severe head injury
(b) Uraemia (renal failure)
(c) Severe hypertension (hypertensive encephalopathy)
(d) Toxaemia of pregnancy (eclampsia)
(e) Cerebral tumours
(f) Neurosyphilis
(g) Hypoglycaemia

(h) Hysteria.

Idiopathic epilepsy

This is the term given to the frequently seen recurring fits without obvious underlying cause. Epilepsy usually begins in childhood, rarely occurring for the first time in adult life. Fits which do start for the first time in adult life, therefore, usually have some definite underlying cause and so come into the category of symptomatic fits.

There are two main forms of epilepsy, major epilepsy (grand mal) and petit mal.

Grand mal (major epilepsy)

In this form, fits occur with loss of consciousness and usually in well-defined stages:

1. *The warning.* This takes different forms in different people, e.g. a peculiar sensation, an odd taste or smell, a sense of nausea etc. The aura may not occur in some cases.

2. *Tonic stage.* In this stage the patient falls unconscious, often with an epileptic cry. All the muscles go rigid, the breathing ceases and the patient goes blue in the face. The tongue is frequently bitten.

3. *Clonic stage.* Spasms of the muscles occur, resulting in violent movements of the limbs. Frothing at the mouth and incontinence of urine and faeces are also usually present.

4. *Stage of coma.* After the clonic spasms, the patient remains in a coma, which, however, quickly passes into a deep ordinary sleep if the patient is not awakened. The duration of the fit is hardly ever more than two minutes and may be much less. In severe cases, fit may succeed fit, causing the condition of status epilepticus. This may go on for hours and, if the fits are not controlled, death from exhaustion can occur.

Petit mal or absence attacks

Minor fits are more common than major fits, and may occur separately or in a patient also suffering from major fits. The attacks are much briefer and often more numerous. The fit may last only for a second or two and is sometimes known as an

Symptomatic fits: common causes

Children

Tumours
Meningitis
Hydrocephalus
Maldevelopment
Injury

Fever

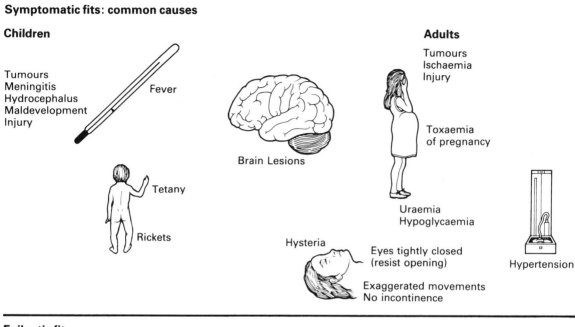

Tetany

Rickets

Brain Lesions

Adults

Tumours
Ischaemia
Injury

Toxaemia
of pregnancy

Uraemia
Hypoglycaemia

Hysteria

Eyes tightly closed
(resist opening)

Exaggerated movements
No incontinence

Hypertension

Epileptic fits

Begin in childhood

Warning
Loss of consciousness with tonic
and clonic stages
Incontinent

Tongue often bitten
Brief coma
Can lead to
status epilepticus
(continued convulsions)

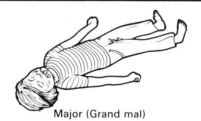

Major (Grand mal)

Minor (Petit mal)
Transient loss of consciousness
No convulsions

Fig. 9.23 Some common causes of convulsions.

'absence'. This loss of consciousness may be so brief that the patient only feels 'dazed' and onlookers may not notice anything wrong. No convulsions occur, the patient merely staying still with a vacant expression and ceasing any action he may be carrying out.

Partial seizures and post-epileptic automatism

Post-epileptic automatism occasionally follows an epileptic fit. In this state, which may last for several hours, the patient may carry out actions and procedures of which he is unaware and has no recollection afterwards of what has been done. The importance of this state is that the patients may perform actions which can have serious legal consequences. The term 'psychomotor epilepsy' is used to describe disorders of behaviour often associated with loss of memory (amnesia) where this is due to epilepsy. As such seizures often originate in the temporal lobe.

Course and diagnosis The diagnosis of a single attack of loss of consciousness is often difficult if no reliable witness has observed the episode.

A fainting attack (syncope) is a common occurrence, especially in young people, and has to be differentiated from epilepsy. Syncope is due to a temporary deprivation of the blood supply to the brain and is associated with a slow pulse and a fall in blood pressure. It is liable to occur on standing too long in a warm room or, in some susceptible people, at the sight of blood or even the mention of a medical matter. It is usually preceded by a swimmy feeling and sweating so that there is some warning that something is wrong. The face is pale, the pulse is slow and weak and the skin is moist. Convulsive movements rarely occur and are not sustained. Although the subject may sink to the floor, recovery soon takes place and there is no prolonged confusional state on recovery.

In an epileptic attack there is usually no discernible precipitating factor. The convulsive movements may be strong and persistent and may be followed by a confusional state. The pulse is full and rapid and there is no sweating. The electroencephalogram (EEG) may be of help in confirming this diagnosis. This is a recording of the electrical activity of the brain and it may reveal abnormalities when epilepsy is present. Where either is available, computerized axial tomography (using the CT scanner) or magnetic resonance imaging (MRI) provide a composite series of pictures of the brain and reveal the presence of any abnormal areas (Fig. 9.24).

Treatment of epilepsy

Management of the fit. A major fit is often very alarming to the uninitiated onlooker and the nurse should remain calm and prevent others from acting rashly. It is usually not necessary to do anything more than to ensure that the person having the fit is out of harm's way, for example from traffic or from an electric fire. Obstruction to the patient's movements should be removed and something soft, such as a folded jacket, placed under the head. Tight clothing around the neck can be carefully loosened if this is not likely to

frighten a semi-conscious patient. When the convulsions have ceased, the patient can be turned onto the side in a semi-prone position to aid breathing and comfort. The patient is often confused for a time after a major fit and the nurse can offer reassurance and sympathy during this phase.

It is never wise to restrain convulsive movements or to try to put anything between the teeth. Especially in undiagnosed cases, the nurse may be a vital witness of the seizure and her observations may allow a firm diagnosis to be reached. A record should be made of onset of the attack, the nature of the convulsions, the recovery stage and the pulse rate. In 'status epilepticus', consciousness does not recover between attacks. Here, urgent measures to stop the recurring fits are necessary. Injections of diazepam, intravenous or intramuscular, are valuable. If this is not successful intravenous infusion of an appropriate anticonvulsant is tried.

Prevention of the fits. Apart from advising the patient to avoid any triggers of attacks, a number of drugs are prescribed in the treatment of epilepsy, either alone or in combination. These include carbamazepine, phenytoin, clonazepam, sodium valproate, phenobarbitone, and primidone.

Ethosuximide and sodium valproate are particularly successful in the treatment of petit mal, and carbamazepine in partial seizures. Newer anticonvulsants such as clobazam, vigabatrin and lamotrigine may be added in combination to one or two of the above in severe cases.

Regular supervision of patients taking antiepileptic drugs is necessary, since side-effects may occur. The level of drug should be measured in the blood so that the dose can be monitored according to response.

Later management In some children the attacks are so frequent despite all treatment that admission to special schools is necessary. Adults liable to epilepsy must find employment which would not involve danger if a fit occurred; they should not drive vehicles unless they have been free of convulsions for a legally accepted period, and should not work at heights or near machinery.

Operative measures may be carried out in

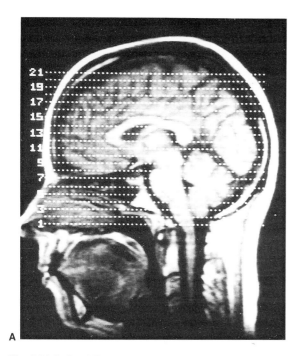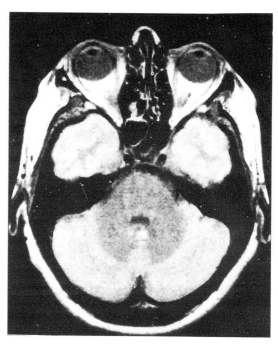

Fig. 9.24 A, B. MRI scan: sagittal (**A**) and axial (**B**) images of a normal magnetic resonance scan (MRI). This provides better detail of structures within the brain substance than a CT scan.

some cases of severe epilepsy to remove a focal abnormality in the brain. Removal of part of the temporal lobe, in what is called temporal lobe epilepsy, is the most common operative treatment at present.

Many cases of epilepsy tend to lessen in severity when adult life is reached, and in some patients the fits may cease completely. Some severe cases may, however, be associated with mental deterioration, and these patients are best treated in special homes.

Coma

Apart from epilepsy, a number of different conditions may cause unconsciousness or coma. Common causes of coma:

1. Drug overdose. This is a common cause of coma in young people today. It should be realised that tranquillisers and antidepressants are prescribed for those who are anxious or depressed, and such patients are most likely to attempt suicide. Not all cases of deliberate overdose really mean to commit suicide. Often the taking of too many tablets is a gesture to demonstrate to others the depth of misery or despair that is being experienced. The tablets most commonly used are aspirin, paracetamol, sedatives and antidepressants.

2. Injury, especially head injury. In most severe cases there is a fracture of the skull and laceration of the brain (contusion). The term concussion is often used to describe a transitory loss of consciousness due to a head injury.

3. Cerebrovascular accident. This includes cerebral haemorrhage, thrombosis or embolism.

4. Diabetic coma (see p. 311). The onset is gradual, usually ushered in by vomiting. There is a deep sighing respiration with breath smelling of acetone and the urine containing sugar and acetone.

5. Hypoglycaemia (see p. 307). Liable to occur in any diabetic taking insulin.

6. Alcoholic coma. The breath smells strongly of alcohol. Alcohol can induce hypoglycaemia even with moderate intake.

7. Hepatic coma. The end stage of severe liver destruction.

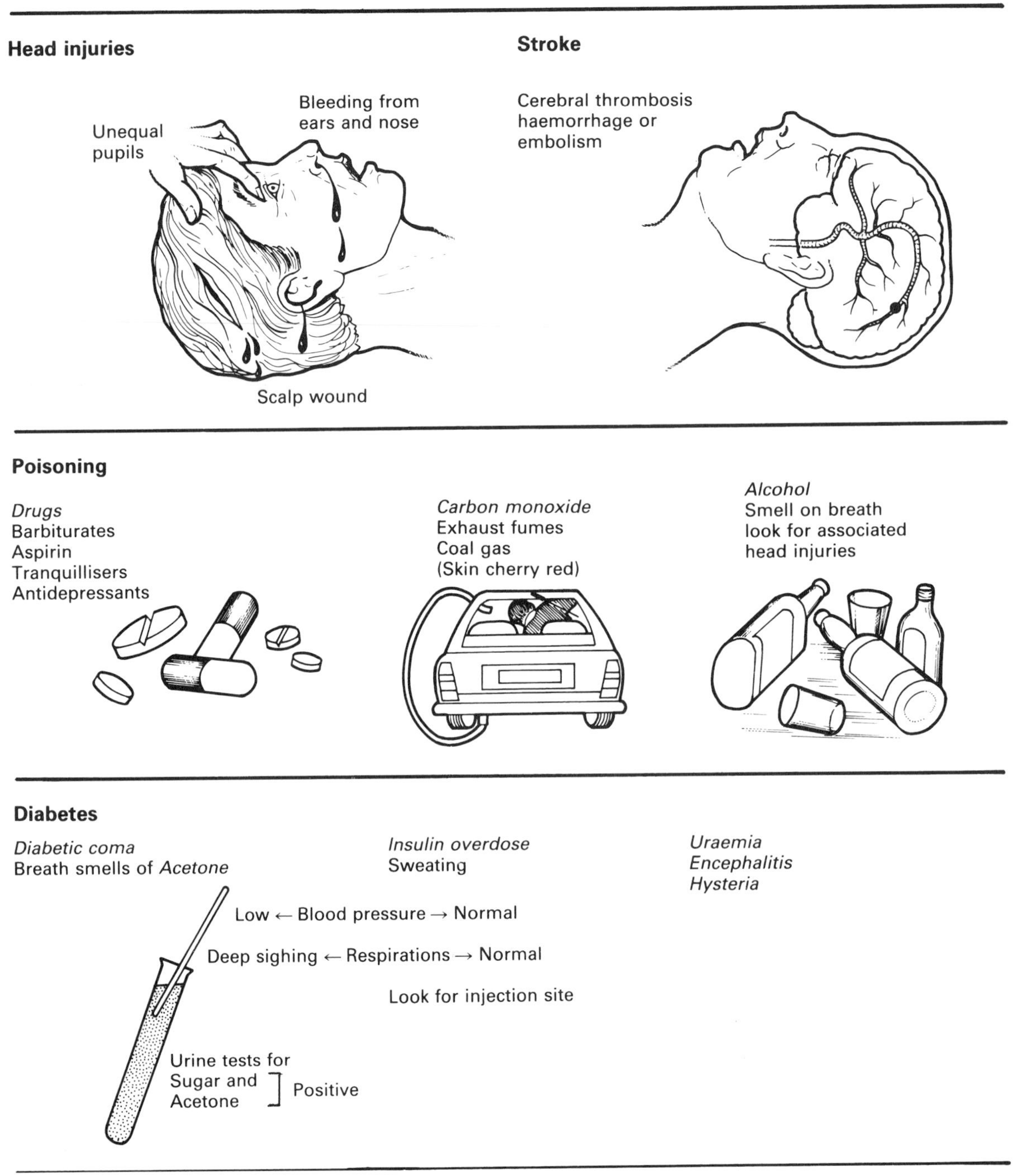

Head injuries

Unequal pupils

Bleeding from ears and nose

Scalp wound

Stroke

Cerebral thrombosis haemorrhage or embolism

Poisoning

Drugs
Barbiturates
Aspirin
Tranquillisers
Antidepressants

Carbon monoxide
Exhaust fumes
Coal gas
(Skin cherry red)

Alcohol
Smell on breath
look for associated
head injuries

Diabetes

Diabetic coma
Breath smells of *Acetone*

Insulin overdose
Sweating

Uraemia
Encephalitis
Hysteria

Low ← Blood pressure → Normal

Deep sighing ← Respirations → Normal

Look for injection site

Urine tests for
Sugar and
Acetone] Positive

Fig. 9.25 Some common causes of coma.

8. Uraemia. The end stage of kidney failure.

9. Myxoedema (see p. 323). If undiagnosed and untreated, coma may ensue.

10. Hypothermia (see p. 20). In the elderly if neglected and undernourished without adequate heating in winter time.

Diagnosis and management of a case of coma

When a patient is admitted to hospital in coma certain routine examinations and investigations are carried out in all cases. The nurse should be fully aware of the importance of all the following points, as when she is undressing the patient she will be able to verify the presence or absence of important details which can help to indicate the treatment of the patient:

1. The history of the case leading up to the coma is most important. The presence or otherwise of an injury, any past history of disease, such as hypertension, diabetes or kidney disease and whether or not the patient has been taking drugs, especially sleeping drugs, are all significant factors. The relatives will be interviewed by the doctor to find out if there has been any emotional crisis likely to lead to a suicidal attempt.

2. Careful examination of the head to find any scalp wounds or bleeding from the ears or nose is necessary. A fractured base of the skull often causes bleeding from the ear, which can be missed unless the ears are carefully looked at.

3. The size and shape of the pupils are important, especially any inequality of the pupils. The latter immediately points to local damage in the brain. The very small pinpoint pupils of morphine poisoning should be looked for. The pupils in hysteria are often widely dilated.

4. The breath should be smelt, the typical sour smell of the alcoholic being easily recognized. The diagnosis of alcoholic coma, however, solely on the evidence of the smell of alcohol from the breath, is most dangerous. A drunken person is very liable to sustain an injury which may be the real cause of the coma. Indeed, the combination of alcohol and head injury is most common. Therefore, in all cases of seemingly alcoholic coma the scalp and ears must be carefully examined for signs of injury and bleeding.

A sweet sickly smell, often likened to sweet pears or apples, is due to acetone in the breath and is characteristic, in particular, of diabetic coma.

5. The character of the respirations is important in diagnosis. Deep noisy respirations are common in diabetic coma. In insulin coma (hypoglycaemia) and in cases of severe injury and haemorrhage, the respirations are shallow. In morphine poisoning, the respiration rate is markedly depressed.

6. The skin is cold and clammy in shock, which would be present in coma due to severe injuries. A moist skin, often with marked sweating, is met in insulin coma while, on the other hand, in diabetic coma the skin is extremely dry. The skin in diabetic coma remains in a fold when it is pinched owing to the dehydration which is always present.

7. The limbs and trunk will be examined by the doctor for any injury, and the utmost care and gentleness used to ensure that any injury present is not made worse by handling the patient. Apart from locating an injury, it is also possible sometimes, even with the patient in a coma, to discern a paralysis of one side of the body. This could lead to a diagnosis of hemiplegia, probably due to cerebral haemorrhage.

8. Examination of urine is done as a routine in all cases of coma. If the cause of the coma is obvious, e.g. a head injury, then the examination of the urine can be delayed till the first convenient moment. In cases of suspected diabetes or poisoning, such as barbiturate or aspirin, or in uraemia, and in all cases where the diagnosis of the coma is not immediately obvious, examination of the urine is carried out immediately, and for this catheterisation will be necessary.

The urine is tested at once for sugar, (acetone) ketones and albumin, although a multistix will also test for blood and protein at the same time, and the remainder is saved and sent to the laboratory with blood samples for further detailed examination. The presence of a heavy glycosuria and acetone immediately gives a diagnosis of diabetic coma in nearly all cases. A urine loaded with albumin would point to a possible uraemia.

By this stage the cause of the coma will be apparent in most cases. In a small number of cases, however, further immediate examinations, such as lumbar puncture and blood urea, electrolyte and sugar estimations, may be necessary to establish the cause of the coma.

Treatment The treatment of coma varies according to the cause and is therefore dealt with in the sections devoted to the causative conditions. The nursing of a patient in coma, whatever the cause, is of particular importance, and the general nursing care of a comatose patient is described under Strokes (p. 207).

Cerebral tumour

Primary tumour

There are different types of primary tumour of the brain, which include:

1. *Glioma.* This is the commonest primary tumour and may range from the very malignant and rapidly fatal to the very slow-growing (see Fig. 2.6).
2. *Meningioma.* This is a tumour growing from the meninges on the surface of the brain and is not usually malignant.
3. *Pituitary tumour.* This grows from the pituitary gland and in many cases can be successfully removed.
4. *Auditory nerve tumour.* Otherwise known as acoustic neuroma, it occurs more often in older people and is of slow growth.

Secondary tumour

Secondary cerebral tumours are due to spread from a primary growth somewhere else in the body, usually the bronchus, stomach, breast or prostate. Secondary brain tumours are more common than primary tumours.

Symptoms and signs Tumours of the brain cause symptoms and signs in two main ways:

1. symptoms and signs due to the increased intracranial pressure
2. symptoms and signs due to the local damage to the brain from the growth of the tumour (localizing signs).

The symptoms and signs of increased intracranial pressure are the same whatever the cause (e.g. tumour, abscess or meningitis), producing the increased pressure within the skull:

1. *Headaches.* These are usually very persistent and severe and are characteristically worse in the morning i.e. after lying down.
2. *Vomiting.* The combination of headaches and vomiting should always lead to the suspicion of a brain lesion.
3. *Papilloedema.* The pressure on the optic nerve causes a swelling of the nerve with blurring of the margins of the optic disc.
4. Drowsiness, passing eventually into a state of coma. This is a comparatively late sign in tumours.
5. Convulsions or fits are frequent.
6. *Slow pulse.* The pulse is usually slow in cases of increased intracranial pressure.
7. Mental changes, such as slowness of action, deficient memory and personality changes, occur at some stage in most cases.

Localizing signs These depend on the area of the brain which is affected by the tumour. As has been seen earlier, different parts of the brain deal with different functions, and a lesion in a particular area will affect the functions of that area, enabling the lesion to be localized. However, there are many areas in the brain which are known as 'silent' areas. A lesion in these areas may produce no particular signs.

Some common localizing signs of tumours in non-silent areas are:

1. In the motor cortex. Fits are very common and in many cases they tend to cause localized convulsive movements of the face, arm or leg. These fits are called 'focal epilepsy'. In addition, a weakness or paralysis in the form of a monoplegia is common.
2. In the visual cortex. A tumour in this area would cause early loss of vision.
3. Of the auditory nerve. Deafness, giddiness and vertigo are common and predominant.
4. The pituitary gland. Disturbances in the endocrine function of the gland, leading to such conditions as hypopituitarism or acromegaly, are often present. The tumour may produce loss of vision by compressing part of the adjacent optic tract.

Diagnosis The diagnosis will be suspected from the signs and symptoms. Investigations will be necessary to provide more precise information as to the presence and location of any tumour. Several procedures are available:

1. X-ray of the skull occasionally reveals erosion of the bone caused by a tumour. X-ray of the chest may reveal a carcinoma of the bronchus, a common cause of cerebral metastases (p. 143).

2. CT scan (computerized axial tomography) and MR (magnetic resonance) scans (see Fig. 9.24). These scanners both use powerful computers to reconstruct images of the brain, slice by slice, and have helped greatly in diagnosis and assessment. They are capable of revealing with accuracy and speed the presence, position and size of a cerebral tumour.

3. Brain scan. Radioactive material (technetium-99m, ^{99m}Tc) is preferentially taken up by a cerebral tumour and its presence detected and recorded by scanning techniques.

4. Cerebral angiography entails the injection of a radio-opaque dye into the carotid artery and X-rays then reveal displacement of arteries by the tumour or an abnormal circulation in the vicinity of the tumour.

5. Electroencephalogram (EEG). This is a record of the electrical activity in the cerebrum, and shows a regular sequence of waves. The presence of a tumour will be revealed by an area of disturbed cerebral electrical activity.

Treatment Surgical removal of the tumour offers the best hope of a cure, but this is usually possible only in benign tumours such as meningioma. Malignant tumours or secondary deposits are seldom amenable to total removal. Surgery, radiotherapy and chemotherapy may be helpful in shrinking the size of the tumour, with relief of headache and vomiting and some improvement of prognosis.

Diseases of the peripheral nerves

Lesions of the peripheral nerves are collectively called peripheral neuropathies. Wounds or other injuries may produce a paralysis of specific nerves. Birth injuries are dealt with on page 231. Peripheral neuropathies may be grouped according to their causes:

1. Trauma
2. Metabolic disorders, such as diabetes mellitus
3. Deficiencies, such as vitamin B
4. Toxins, such as alcohol, arsenic, gold, mercury, lead, organic substances and certain drugs (e.g. cis-platinum, vincristine)
5. Infective and inflammatory disorders, as in acute infective polyneuritis or Guillain–Barre syndrome
6. Carcinoma-related, especially carcinoma of the bronchus
7. Hereditary neuropathies.

Symptoms and signs

1. When larger nerve trunks of the arms and legs are affected, marked diminution of power or even a complete paralysis may result. A typical example of this loss of motor power is a dropped wrist or foot. The muscles affected show wasting.

2. Sensory disturbances are present, usually in the form of pins and needles in the hands and feet. In some cases, however, severe pains in the arms and legs may occur. There may be some degree, varying from mild to severe, of loss of sensation to pain and touch.

3. The tendon reflexes both in the legs (knee and ankle jerks) and the arms may be diminished or absent. All the signs present are typical of a lower motor neuron lesion, with severe loss of power, marked sensory disturbances, wasting of muscles and loss of the deep tendon reflexes.

Some features of neuropathies

1. *Alcoholic neuropathy.* This mainly affects the legs, causing weakness of the feet and incoordination of gait. Sensory disturbances are common and the legs are very tender to the touch.

2. *Diabetic neuropathy.* This usually leads to, loss of sensation in the feet and legs with absent reflexes. Occasionally, pain in the legs can be very severe, especially at night. Autonomic involvement may cause diarrhoea. Proximal limb weakness may occur.

3. *Acute infective polyneuritis (Guillain–Barre syndrome).* The cause of this form of peripheral neuritis is usually an infection, with all the usual symptoms of fever, headache and malaise, which is followed by paralysis of the arms and legs. In some cases, the paralysis may spread to affect the

respiratory muscles with the danger of asphyxia developing. The respiratory function is, therefore, monitored. The cranial nerves may also be involved, particularly the seventh, causing a facial paralysis.

4. *Diphtheritic neuritis.* Serious infections of diphtheria may lead to paralysis of the limbs and the muscles of respiration.

5. *Carcinoma of the bronchus.* This can give rise to peripheral neuritis with weakness of the limbs and incoordination, even before signs in the chest develop. This is not due to secondary deposits, but is probably a toxic effect of the carcinoma.

Treatment of peripheral neuropathy

1. In an acute case, the patient is put to bed. Care must be taken to avoid injury to the affected limbs, and in this respect bed-cradles are very valuable. Particular attention to the skin and pressure areas is most important to prevent pressure sores.

2. The foot-drop, usually present, must be corrected by the use of a foot-board or pillow against the feet, or, alternatively, well-padded light splints may be used. Passive movements to prevent fixation of the joints must be started from the onset.

3. If the case is acute, with a good deal of tenderness and pains in the muscles, active movements will be postponed until the symptoms subside. Analgesics for the relief of pain are usually needed.

4. All the appropriate specific measures will be taken, such as the giving of vitamin B in the vitamin-deficiency cases, control of the diabetes and the withdrawal of any poisons.

5. The use of a respirator will be necessary in those cases of respiratory paralysis due to acute infective polyneuritis.

Sciatica

The term 'sciatica' is given to the common pain which occurs along the distribution of the sciatic nerve. It is most commonly due to pressure on the nerve roots by a prolapsed intervertebral disc (p. 340), but it can be due to other local causes. Hence, sciatica is a symptom which merits careful investigation.

Symptoms and signs The characteristic symptom in sciatica is pain along the distribution of the sciatic nerve. The pain is felt in the back and down the back of the thigh to the ankle and foot. Stretching of the sciatic nerve produces pain, so that the patient avoids any posture or action that leads to this. The ankle jerk may be absent, and in some cases there is a loss of sensation and weakness in the area supplied by the sciatic nerve.

Treatment Treatment will depend on the cause of the sciatica. In the case of a prolapsed intervertebral disc, if bed rest physiotherapy and manipulation fail, surgery may be necessary.

Myasthenia gravis

Myasthenia gravis is a slow progressive disease rare before the age of puberty. It causes a peculiar form of paralysis, which tends to get worse with fatigue or use of the affected muscles and to improve with rest. Characteristically, therefore, the paralysis is minimal in the morning and worst at night. The disease most often affects the eye, facial and shoulder girdle muscles, and less often on the legs. Paralysis of the eye muscles (ophthalmoplegia) leads to squints and double vision. Drooping of the eyelids (ptosis) and weakness of the face muscles cause the peculiar lack of expression and typical myasthenic (snarling) smile. Gradual loss of voice with prolonged speech or difficulty in chewing during the course of a meal are also frequent complaints. Weakness of the arms, especially in combing hair or lifting objects, may be complained of. Weakness of respiratory muscles and of swallowing are the cause of significant morbidity and even mortality, and should be closely monitored.

Myasthenia gravis responds symptomatically to the drugs neostigmine and pyridostigmine, and a profoundly weak patient may be dramatically improved on taking these drugs. Some young patients have been improved by removal of the thymus gland (thymectomy). The condition is auto-immune in origin, so immunosuppressive drugs and plasma exchange may be given to patients with benefit.

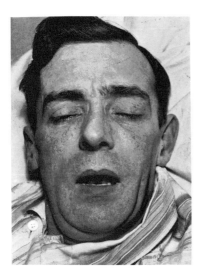

Fig. 9.26 Myasthenia gravis, patient cannot open his eyes or fully close his mouth.

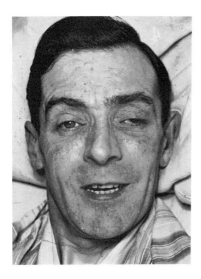

Fig. 9.27 Myasthenia gravis after an injection of prostigmin showing a marked improvement. The typical 'snarling' smile still remains, however.

Myopathies and muscular dystrophies

Diseases which primarily affect the muscles leading to profound weakness and wasting, are called myopathies. Acquired inflammation of the muscles is called polymyositis, and is treated with immunosuppression. Primary degenerative muscle diseases that are inherited and progressive are termed muscular dystrophies. They usually occur, or start, in childhood, and differ in type according to the particular muscles affected. For example, in the facioscapulo-humeral form the face, shoulder girdle and upper arms are mainly involved, with marked wasting (atrophy) and weakness of power in these parts. The normal facial expression being absent, and there is inability to raise the arms above the head.

In *Duchenne's muscular dystrophy* the wasted muscles are replaced by fat, and so may look larger than normal instead of wasted. This form is known as the pseudo-hypertrophic type. It affects boys, and starts at about the age of 4 or 5. The shoulder, pelvic girdle and calf muscles are particularly involved. The child has difficulty in getting about and has a waddling gait. One characteristic feature is the peculiar way in which the child rises from the lying-down position. The child has to roll over on to his face, and then on to his hands and knees, and gradually 'works up' the legs with the hands – the so called 'climbing up his knees' position. These children become wheel-chair bound. Many cases of muscular dystrophy, however, may live in fair health for many years. So far, no treatment has been found to be of any real benefit.

Common diseases of the cranial nerves

The cranial nerves, which arise from the brain and run their course almost entirely within the skull, are frequently affected by diseases of the brain and meninges. Only the more common and important diseases affecting the cranial nerves will be discussed.

The optic nerve

The optic nerve conveys the visual impulses from the retina of the eye to the posterior part of the brain (the visual cortex). The optic nerve is of extreme importance in the diagnosis of certain diseases of the central nervous system. By means of an instrument called an ophthalmoscope, a clear picture of the whole of the retina of the eye, including the actual optic nerve (optic disc), can be obtained.

Normally, the optic disc is seen as a pale circular area with a distinct margin. In cases of increased intracranial pressure, however, oedema or swelling of the optic nerve (papilloedema) develops and the optic disc becomes swollen and its margins blurred. Papilloedema is a most valuable sign of increased intracranial pressure.

Examination of the eye with an ophthalmoscope is of importance, not only in diseases of the central nervous system but in certain other diseases, too, which may show characteristic changes in the retina. Hypertension frequently causes haemorrhages and white spots (exudates) in the retina and, in severe cases, oedema of the optic disc. Diabetes and chronic nephritis also produce changes.

Optic neuritis Multiple sclerosis may cause optic neuritis and is a common presenting feature of the disease. The symptoms are those of loss of visual acuity, visual field, or colour perpection. Optic neuritis may rarely be caused by excessive alcohol and tobacco consumption.

Optic atrophy Atrophy, or wasting, of the optic nerve fibres may follow a severe papilloedema or optic neuritis. The optic disc appears white. Syphilis is especially prone to cause this effect. Total blindness results from complete optic atrophy.

The ocular nerves

The third, fourth and sixth cranial nerves supply the muscles of the eyes responsible for the movement of the eyeball. The iris muscle of the eye, which causes contraction and dilatation of the pupils, is also supplied by fibres that travel with these nerves. In addition, these nerves supply the muscle which raises the upper eyelid.

Diseases which affect the ocular nerves can produce any of the following signs:

1. Drooping of the upper eyelids known as 'ptosis'
2. Squint (strabismus), often associated with seeing double (diplopia)
3. Unequal pupils.

The diseases which most commonly affect these nerves to produce the above signs include diabetes, syphilis, brain tumours, aneurysms, enceph-alitis (inflammation of the brain). Myasthenia gravis, although a disorder of the neuromuscular junction, also causes these symptoms.

The fifth nerve (trigeminal)

A common lesion of the fifth nerve is trigeminal neuralgia, where paroxysms of extremely severe pain occur in its distribution i.e. over the jaw, cheek and forehead. The slightest touch in these areas may bring on an attack.

Treatment of trigeminal neuralgia is often difficult. Bad teeth or sinus infection must be attended to if present. Carbamazepine is often effective in relieving the pain during an attack. In severe cases, separation of the nerve root from a neighbouring blood vessel, or an injection of alcohol into the nerve is necessary to relieve the condition.

The seventh nerve (facial)

A facial weakness is frequently seen as part of hemiplegia, of which the most common cause is a stroke. In hemiplegia, only the lower half of one side of the face is paralysed.

In contrast to this, paralysis of the whole of one side of the face including the forehead is often seen in the condition known as Bell's palsy (Fig. 9.28). The exact cause of Bell's palsy is not known, but it is supposed to be due to inflammation of the facial nerve. The condition usually clears up in a few weeks without any special treatment but occasionally leaves permanent weakness of the affected side of the face. Corticosteroids are sometimes used in the acute phase.

A facial paralysis is sometimes seen after operations on the mastoid, caused by injury to the nerve during the operation. A transitory facial paralysis may arise in infants owing to a birth injury, especially in cases of forceps delivery.

The eighth nerve (auditory)

The eighth nerve has two main functions, one dealing with hearing and the other with the maintenance of equilibrium and proper posture

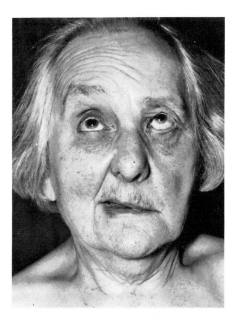

Fig. 9.28 Left-sided facial paralysis (Bell's palsy).

of the body. Diseases of the auditory, or hearing, part of the nerve commonly cause deafness and buzzing in the ears (tinnitus). Diseases of the division of the nerve dealing with equilibrium cause severe attacks of giddiness, during which all objects may appear to spin around. In severe attacks, the patient may fall and vomiting may also occur. These attacks are known as 'vertigo'. Motion sickness (sea-sickness, car sickness), with its nausea, vomiting and vertigo, is caused by the undue motion affecting impulses in the eighth nerve.

Ménière's disease is commonest in elderly people and is associated with tinnitus and progressive deafness. It gives rise to bouts of sudden, terrifying, and incapacitating giddiness and vomiting, which may last for many hours.

Streptomycin, especially if given over long periods, may damage the eighth nerve and give rise to deafness and giddiness.

Tumours of the eighth nerve may cause deafness and can be removed by operation.

The twelfth nerve (hypoglossal)

The twelfth nerve supplies the muscles of the tongue. Paralysis and wasting of the tongue may be seen in motor neurone disease (see below).

When the tongue is protruded from the mouth, the unaffected half of the tongue pushes the tongue over to the paralysed side, e.g. in cases of paralysis of the right side of the tongue, the tongue is pushed over to the right side when it is protruded.

Diseases of the spinal cord

Compression of the spinal cord

Compression of the spinal cord leads to marked motor and sensory disturbances below the level of the lesion. There is loss of sensation below the level of compression, associated with a paralysis of the affected area. Incontinence or retention of urine is present.

The causes of compression of the cord can be conveniently divided into the acute (sudden) and the slow and progressive. In the acute forms, the sensory loss and degree of paralysis are much more complete and severe than in the slow onset types. Fracture-dislocations of the spine, usually in the cervical region, account for most of the acute cases. Haemorrhage and thrombosis in the spinal cord, due to hypertension or syphilis, are more rarely responsible for a similar clinical picture. Transverse myelitis, or inflammation of the cord, has a subacute presentation.

Slow compression of the cord is usually due to one of three main causes: first, to tuberculous disease of the spine seen in young people, secondly, to malignant tumours of the spine in older people, and thirdly, to cervical spondylosis.

In all cases, nursing calls for a great deal of skill to prevent pressure sores and urinary infections. Most patients are treated by immobilizing the spine in a plaster-bed for many months. Suitable cases may be operated on, as in tuberculous caries when a bone graft is done. Cases due to malignant tumours are difficult and only palliative treatment can be given.

Subacute combined degeneration of the cord

This disease is associated with pernicious anaemia and early cases respond to treatment with vitamin B12, given by injection in large doses. It causes a spastic weakness of both lower limbs, with sensory disturbances such as numbness, pins and needles and sensory loss in the legs; the gait is usually ataxic.

Syringomyelia

This malady is due to a defective channel of flow and drainage of the cerebrospinal fluid. This leads to distension of the central region of the spinal cord, which becomes cystic and presses on the various tracts in the spinal cord. It usually starts in early life and slowly progresses, and may sometimes follow trauma.

The main distinguishing features of syringomyelia are a slow paralysis starting usually in the arms and spreading to the lower limbs, with profound wasting of the hands. There is also the characteristic dissociated anaesthesia where pain, heat and cold sensations are lost, but touch sensation is retained. This is due to the crossing of the pain and heat sensory tracts in the spinal cord in the region of the central canal. The touch sensory tracts which do not cross here escape damage. These patients frequently burn themselves from holding cigarettes or matches and also develop ulcers from injuries which they do not feel. Charcot's joints are frequently present.

In some cases, if the diagnosis is made before widespread irreparable damage has occurred, surgical intervention can be undertaken to divert the flow of the cerebrospinal fluid from the cyst to the abdominal cavity via a shunt.

Other common diseases of the nervous system

Multiple sclerosis (disseminated sclerosis)

Multiple sclerosis is now the commonest major disorder of the nervous system in the Western world. Myelin is a fatty material which forms a sheath round nerve fibres and it is this material that is damaged and scarred in disseminated sclerosis. Patches or plaques of sclerosed (hardened) fibrous material are found disseminated through the nervous system replacing healthy white myelin. Hence, disseminated sclerosis is known as a demyelinating disorder of the central nervous system.

It often begins in young adults and runs a prolonged course over many years. The most likely explanation is that it is secondary to a viral infection which settles in the nervous system, and leads to slow and patchy damage of myelin over the years. But so far no particular causative virus has been isolated or identified in humans.

In the early stages the myelin affected is inflamed and damaged but not destroyed. Impairment of function at this stage may be only temporary and apparent recovery occurs. As time goes on fibrosis of the affected areas may take place with permanent destruction of nervous tissues.

Clinical features The early symptoms are:

1. Young adults in their twenties or thirties are most commonly affected.
2. Weakness of one or both legs is a common early symptom sometimes associated with numbness tingling and altered sensation in the limbs. These symptoms vary in severity and often clear up completely for many years.
3. Ocular symptoms. The optic nerves are often involved in the early stages leading to temporary mistiness of vision or even temporary loss of vision in one or other eye. Attacks of double vision are common and sometimes nystagmus (rapid jerky movements of the eyes) can be detected.
4. Unsteadiness of the arms may be noted on making purposeful movements such as reaching out to take a cup of tea.

Further symptoms appear as time goes on, improvement becoming less frequent and incapacity more permanent:

1. The legs become more stiff and the gait more unsteady so that walking becomes difficult or impossible.
2. Unsteadiness becomes more pronounced making arm movement clumsy and uncoordinated.
3. Nystagmus becomes permanent and vision itself may be lost in either eye.
4. The speech becomes slurred.
5. Disturbances of bladder function occur with lack of control and sometimes inability to empty the bladder.

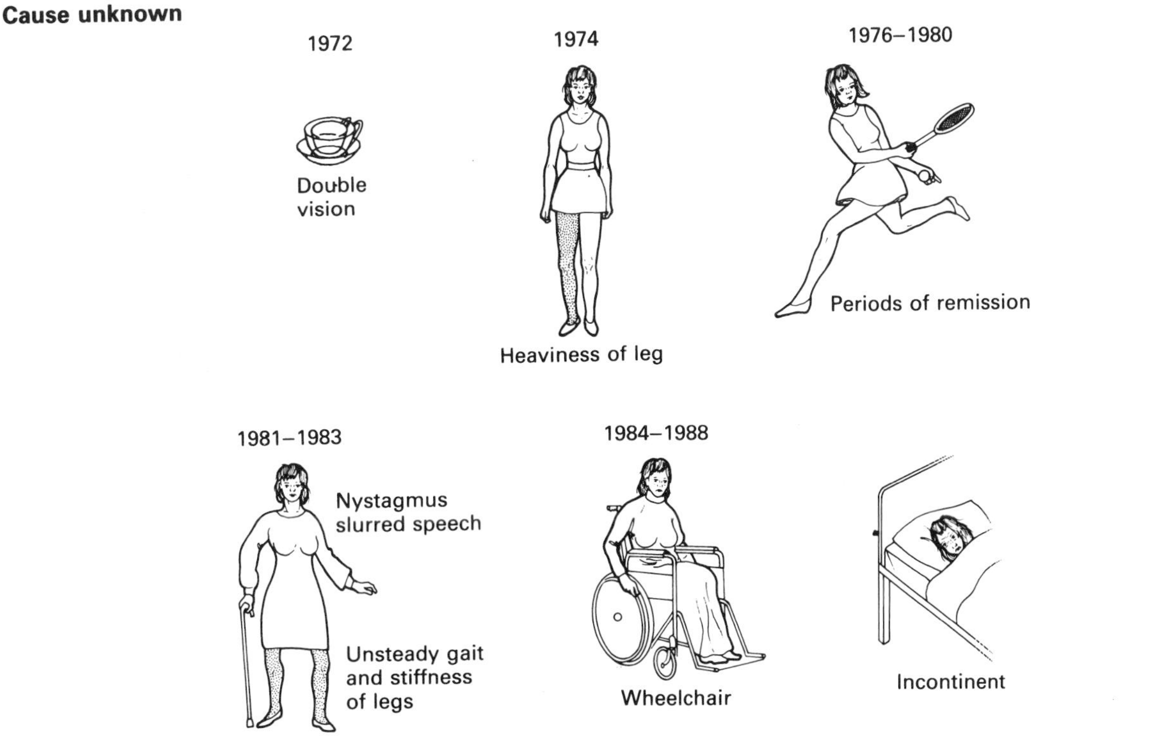

Cause unknown

Fig. 9.29 Multiple sclerosis.

6. Mental changes become evident, occasionally an inappropriate and fatuous cheerfulness (euphoria) but more often emotional instability with bouts of understandable depression.

7. In the later stages of disseminated sclerosis the patient may be confined to bed or a chair with incontinence of bladder and bowels.

Management

1. In the early stages rest is advisable when symptoms appear. Experience has shown that physical activity prolongs symptoms and delays improvement.

2. Corticosteroids (see p. 329) such as a course of intravenous methylprednisolone or ACTH, is helpful in the relief of symptoms during an attack, probably by reducing inflammation of the affected areas in the nervous tissues.

3. Diet has been blamed but there is no evidence that diet plays a part in disseminated sclerosis.

4. When the legs are stiff, drugs such as baclofen or diazepam may be helpful.

5. Physiotherapy can help the patient make best use of what function he possesses. For example, trained use of the upper part of the body can enable a patient with spastic legs to transfer himself from bed to chair.

6. The occupational therapist may recommend the provision of ramps and rails at home to make it possible for the patient to get about. Walking appliances and special utensils for eating may be necessary.

7. Bladder symptoms of urgency and loss of control can be helped by drugs and intermittent self-catheterisation. Occasionally an indwelling catheter may become obligatory.

The diagnosis of disseminated sclerosis is usually made on the clinical signs and symptoms. MRI (magnetic resonance imaging) and examination of the cerebrospinal fluid help make the diagnosis.

It is important to realise that after the initial occurrence of symptoms many patients remain well for years. Hence, although some cases run a down-hill course, it is wrong to take too gloomy a view.

Movement disorders

Parkinson's disease

Paralysis agitans was first described by Parkinson in 1817 and so bears his name. It is a degenerative disorder of the neurones in the substantia nigra, a part of the basal ganglia of the brain, which fail to make dopamine, a neurotransmitter. It usually comes on in later life and can become disabling. A similar condition can be induced by various drugs, particularly the anti-psychotic drugs chlorpromazine or haloperidol. When drug-induced, the disorder is reversible and the symptoms usually clear when the drug responsible is discontinued.

1. There is a characteristic rigidity of appearance and movement (Fig. 9.30). The face tends to be mask-like, showing very little emotion. The patient walks with small shuffling steps; the arms are pressed to the side and do not swing on walking.
2. Tremor. This is very common and is most marked in the hands at rest. There is a constant rolling movement of the fingers and thumb. This tremor may be very severe in some cases, affecting other parts of the body.
3. Speech becomes slurred, soft and monotonous. Swallowing may be affected, causing dribbling.

Diagnosis The diagnosis is usually made clinically from the typical appearance, walk and tremor.

Treatment Various drugs are now available which do much to ameliorate the stiffness and tremor:

1. L-Dopa (levodopa) forms dopamine in the brain and leads to considerable improvement in the majority of patients, allowing them to get about more freely and with less tremor. It is given combined with carbidopa, which can reduce the action and thus the side-effects of L-Dopa in the rest of the body but not its action in the brain.
2. Benzhexol or other anti-cholinergic drugs reduce the tremor and rigidity.

In some younger patients with one-sided disease who have failed to respond to medical treatment and who are seriously disabled, recourse to neurosurgery may be advised. An operation has been devised which may be successful in reducing rigidity and tremor.

Post-encephalitic Parkinsonism The picture of paralysis agitans, with some modifications, is sometimes seen in much younger patients. In these, it is a late complication (often many years later) of a form of encephalitis known as encephalitis lethargica, or, as it was often called, sleepy sickness. This disease, now rare, occurred in an epidemic form in the 1920s.

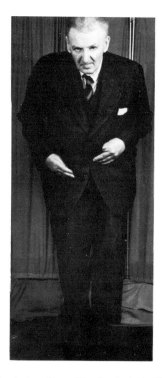

Fig. 9.30 Paralysis agitans. The fixed, rigid attitude of the patient and lack of emotional expression are characteristic of the disease.

Chorea

Chorea is a description of irregular purposeless movements. It may be seen in rheumatic fever, and children who have suffered from chorea may later on develop signs of rheumatic heart disease. This form of chorea occurs rarely in adults, except during pregnancy. There is a rare hereditary form of chorea (Huntington's) which appears usually in adult life and is associated with progressive brain degeneration.

Symptoms and signs

1. Sudden, changing purposeless movements occur in the face, arms and legs, so that the child appears to be continually fidgeting and grimacing. He tends to drop articles held in the hands.

2. There is general clumsiness due to the involuntary movements.

3. The child is often nervous and emotional.

4. There may be evidence of acute rheumatic heart disease, such as a rapid and perhaps irregular pulse.

5. Chorea, when it occurs in women during pregnancy, may take a very severe course with violent movements and mental confusion often bordering on acute mania.

Treatment The child must be nursed with rest as in acute rheumatic fever. As these patients are inclined to be nervous and emotional, the carrying out of all necessary details in these cases will call for the utmost patience and skill.

The clothing should be light and warm, and as the clothing may get thrown off during the choreiform movements. Care must be exercised in the choice of feeding utensils as these may get broken.

There is no specific treatment as yet available. If the choreiform movements are severe, sedatives are useful.

Convalescence, as in cases of acute rheumatic fever, must be prolonged. Constructive toys help the child to regain co-ordinated movements and, in addition, keep him or her amused.

In the adult hereditary form of chorea, the drug tetrabenazine and general nursing form the treatment of this progressive disease.

Motor neurone disease

This is a slow progressive degeneration of the anterior (motor) horn cells and pyramidal tract in the grey matter of the spinal cord, of unknown cause and leading to profound wasting and paralysis of the affected limbs. The disease usually occurs in adults and often starts in the anterior horn cells supplying the muscles of the hands, causing severe weakness and wasting of the hands. The wasting muscles show typical twitchings or tremors known as fasciculation. The pyramidal tracts may be affected in some cases, leading to a spastic paralysis, usually of the legs. It is characteristic of this disease that no significant sensory changes develop.

Respiratory and swallowing difficulties are the usual cause of death in this condition, for which there is only symptomatic treatment.

Diseases of the nervous system in infants and children

Birth injuries

Facial paralysis

A facial paralysis, usually due to forceps delivery, often occurs, but usually clears up completely.

Brachial plexus injuries

The brachial plexus is the main network of nerves which supplies the upper limb. This plexus may be injured at birth in cases of difficult labour.

Two main forms of paralysis occur: Erb's palsy, where the shoulder girdle muscles are particularly involved, and the upper limb takes up a characteristic attitude known as 'porter's tip' position, with the palm of the hand facing backwards and outwards; and Klumpke's palsy, where the hand and forearm are mainly involved, giving rise to marked wasting and the typical 'claw hand'.

Treatment Treatment consists of applying light splints to relax the affected muscles and massage is started early. Active movements are encouraged. Operative measures may be undertaken if there is no improvement within 3 to 6 months.

Intracranial haemorrhage

In cases of difficult labour, such as may result from disproportion or a difficult forceps delivery, trauma to the brain may lead to cerebral haemorrhage which if severe is usually fatal. In some cases, the meninges may be torn and adhesions may then form which block the flow of cerebrospinal fluid. This leads to the development of hydrocephalus, which in infancy is accompanied by gross enlargement of the head.

Severe birth injury may also give rise to paralysis, e.g. a hemiplegia, and, in addition, may be responsible for the development of epileptic fits and mental deficiency.

Spastic paralysis in children (Fig. 9.31)

Owing to failure of the brain to develop properly in the womb, children may be born with various forms of paralysis. Damage to the cortex of the brain involves the upper motor neurons and leads to a form of spastic diplegia known as Little's disease, in which paralysis occurs on both sides of the body. The legs are so stiff and rigid that the child has great difficulty in walking and does so with the legs crossed over each other – 'scissors gait'. Damage of the deeper brain centres may lead to frequent jerky involuntary movements (athetoid type), while involvement of the cerebellum causes an unsteady gait and difficulty in balancing (ataxic type). Seriously handicapped children may have a combination of these disabilities which may be associated with mental subnormality and a tendency to convulsions.

What must be emphasized strongly is that many children with this disorder are both intelligent and capable of training to lead a useful life. Some 1000 cerebral palsied babies are born every year in Great Britain and offer a challenge in education and training to enable them to fulfil their potential abilities.

Hydrocephalus (Fig. 9.32)

Interference with the circulation of the cerebrospinal fluid leads to distension of the brain, and in children this is also accompanied by enlargement of the circumference of the skull

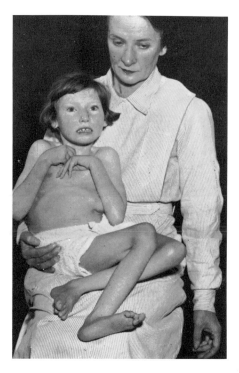

Fig. 9.31 Spastic paralysis showing the characteristic position of the limbs. The child was mentally defective and suffered from fits.

itself. The enlarged head of a hydrocephalic infant or child may be at once apparent. It is a globular or rounded outline and the forehead bulges forward over the eyes. It is important to keep a record of skull circumference.

Causes

1. Congenital. Failure of the brain to develop properly is a frequent cause of hydrocephalus. Congenital hydrocephalus is often associated with other abnormal developmental changes such as hare-lip, cleft palate and spina bifida.

2. Birth injuries. Intracranial haemorrhage is another common cause of hydrocephalus. Difficult labour, especially with forceps delivery, may give rise to intracranial haemorrhage.

3. Meningitis. Adhesions resulting from meningitis may block the circulation of the cerebrospinal fluid and so lead to hydrocephalus.

4. Cerebral tumours. A short-lived hydrocephalus is often seen as a result of a cerebral tumour.

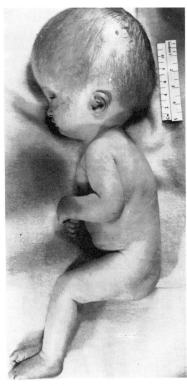

Fig. 9.32 Hydrocephalus.

As with many serious intracranial diseases in early childhood, convulsions and mental deficiency are often present with hydrocephalus.

In some cases where the circulation of the cerebrospinal fluid is blocked, surgical intervention may be needed. Insertion of a plastic tube with a one-way valve in it allows the cerebrospinal fluid to drain away from the distended cerebral ventricles into the peritoneal cavity of the abdomen, thus relieving the pressure causing hydrocephalus. This shunt procedure has much improved the prognosis of this condition. Sometimes, there is malfunction or block of the shunt associated with increased head circumference and signs and symptoms of increased intracranial pressure.

Mental subnormality

Mental disorder can be associated with a wide variety of diseases. It is proposed to give here a brief list of the more common forms of mental subnormality.

Many mentally subnormal cases can be improved by medical treatment or by special training, but severely subnormal patients are incapable of ever leading an independent life.

1. Failure of the central nervous system to develop properly during fetal life results in mental subnormality, and usually physical defects like an abnormally small skull (microcephaly), hydrocephalus or various types of paralysis, e.g. spastic diplegia or Little's disease, are also present. Birth injuries may cause brain haemorrhage and subsequent mental or physical disorders.

2. Phenylketonuria. This is an inherited disorder occurring in families. The baby may be abnormal from birth with vomiting and convulsions and the diagnosis can be confirmed by testing the urine and the blood. This is a rare cause of mental retardation but its importance lies in the fact that the mental changes are preventable if the condition is diagnosed and treated early enough.

The inherited defect is a missing enzyme which normally converts phenylalanine into a harmless protein. Phenylalanine is present in milk feeds and in this condition it accumulates in the blood and causes damage to the brain. The missing enzyme cannot be supplied so the baby must be reared on a special synthetic milk which does not contain phenylalanine. Providing this is begun early enough before brain damage has occurred, the child can develop normally.

The diagnosis can be made by screening the urine for phenylketonoria with phenistix and examination of the blood for phenylala-nine (Guthrie test). The baby's progress can also be monitored by these tests.

3. Down's syndrome is due to a chromosomal defect (trisomy 21) at the time of the conception (p. 12). This relatively common disorder places a great strain on the family, particularly where there are other normal children. The characteristic features can be detected at birth. The eye-slits are narrowed and slanting with an epicanthic fold across the inner aspect, the tongue is thick and fissured and the bridge of the nose is depressed. The hands are broad with a single crease across the palm. There is often an associated congenital heart lesion. Mental subnormality

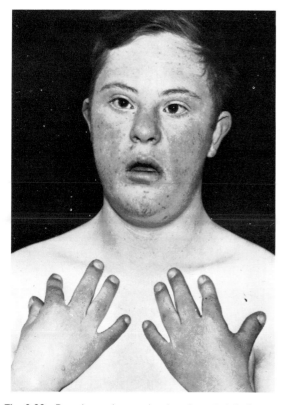

Fig. 9.33 Down's syndrome, showing characteristic features and broad fingers.

may be severe although the temperament may be sunny.

4. Cretinism is due to diminished function of the thyroid gland and unless diagnosed and treated in infancy, leads to stunting of growth and mental development.

Many cases of mental disorder, especially where there is some physical defect as well, are accompanied by convulsions.

Severe cases of subnormality have to be looked after in a suitable institution, but less severe cases are often trained to some useful occupation and even become self-supporting.

10

Diseases of the blood

PHYSIOLOGY

In an adult, about 5 litres of blood are present in the circulation. Blood withdrawn from the body and prevented from clotting separates into two parts, *plasma* and *cells.*

Plasma

Plasma is the clear yellow-coloured fluid in which the cells are suspended. It contains in solution many important substances derived from the food we eat, from the liver and from other organs. These are transported to various parts of the body. Among other substances, plasma contains:

1. The plasma proteins, albumin and globulin. These proteins are a reserve supply of nourishment and become depleted in times of illness or starvation.

2. Prothrombin and fibrinogen. As will be seen, these substances play an essential role in the clotting of blood to prevent undue bleeding after cuts or wounds.

3. Electrolytes. Sodium chloride (salt) and sodium bicarbonate are the principal electrolytes in plasma, which also contains potassium, calcium, iodine, fluorine and iron.

4. Nutrients such as glucose, aminoacids and fatty acids.

5. Vitamins and medications absorbed from the bowel.

6. Hormones derived from the endocrine system.

7. Waste products of metabolism, such as urea and creatinine, for excretion by the kidneys.

Cells

There are three types of cell in the blood: red blood cells (*erythrocytes*), white blood cells (*leucocytes*) and platelets (*thrombocytes*).

1. *Red blood cells* (erythrocytes) are flat cells containing haemoglobin. Haemoglobin is a pigment formed from protein and iron. When haemoglobin combines with oxygen, which it does readily, it becomes bright red giving blood its usual red colour. When oxygen is deficient, haemoglobin is blue and blood is said to be cyanosed.

The main purpose of the red cells is to take up oxygen from the air in the alveoli of the lungs and to carry this oxygen to the tissues in all parts of the body. Waste carbon dioxide from the tissues is taken up by the red cells in exchange for oxygen and this carbon dioxide is breathed out when the red cells in the blood reach the lungs. Thus the red cells bring fresh oxygen to all parts of the body and get rid of waste carbon dioxide. This is part of the metabolic process of burning up fuel.

2. *White blood cells* (leucocytes). There are three main types of leucocyte (which will be discussed later), all concerned with overcoming infection.

3. *Platelets* (thrombocytes) are small round bodies which are able to clump together. If there is any damage to the wall of a blood vessel, the platelets form a plug to seal off any leaks. Platelets also release a substance called thromboplastin important in the clotting of blood.

NORMAL BLOOD FORMATION

Before discussing the diseases that may affect the blood we must first see how blood is normally formed and what constitutes a normal blood count.

Red blood cells

These are formed in the bone marrow which in adults is found in the flat bones, such as the sternum and skull, and in the ends of the long bones. The red cells in the marrow are all in different stages of formation, from the early immature cells to the completely developed mature red cells such as are found in the peripheral blood. Normally only the completely mature red cells pass into the circulation, with all the immature cells remaining in the marrow. In certain diseases, however, these immature red cells may pass out into the circulation, and be seen on the blood film.

Factors necessary for the normal formation of red cells

In order that the red cells may become completely mature and adequate in number various factors are necessary, of which the following are the most important:

1. Vitamin B_{12} (cyanocobalamin). This substance is present in various foods, especially liver, meat, milk, eggs and cheese.

2. The intrinsic factor. Intrinsic factor is normally formed by certain cells in the stomach and is missing in a severe form of gastritis called pernicious anaemia. The intrinsic factor is essential for the proper absorption of vitamin B_{12}.

Vitamin B_{12}, which is absorbed into the body when the intrinsic factor is present, is stored in the liver and released to the bone marrow as required. Vitamin B_{12} is essential for the production of adequate numbers of fully mature red cells. If vitamin B_{12} is missing, the bone marrow will not produce sufficient numbers of red cells and, moreover, many of the red cells produced will be immature. They will tend to be larger than normal (macrocytes) and many of them will contain a nucleus (megaloblasts).

3. Folic acid. Folic acid is part of the vitamin B_{12} complex. It has an action very similar to that of vitamin B_{12}, i.e. it is essential for the development of adequate numbers of fully mature red cells. In the absence of folic acid or if demand is high, as in pregnancy, a macrocytic anaemia will develop.

Haemoglobin

Haemoglobin is the essential component of the

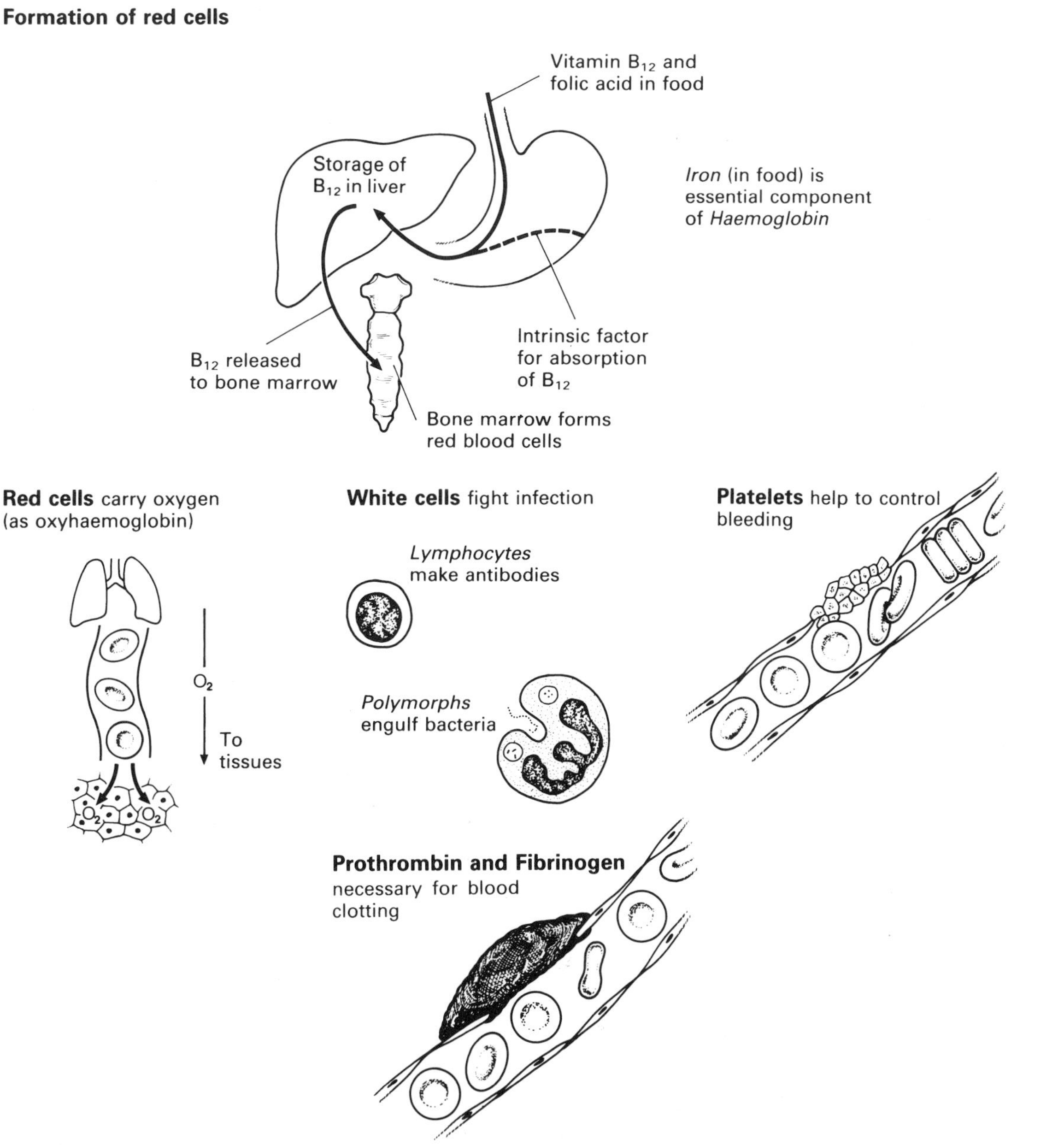

Formation of red cells

Vitamin B$_{12}$ and
folic acid in food

Storage of
B$_{12}$ in liver

Iron (in food) is
essential component
of *Haemoglobin*

B$_{12}$ released
to bone marrow

Intrinsic factor
for absorption
of B$_{12}$

Bone marrow forms
red blood cells

Red cells carry oxygen
(as oxyhaemoglobin)

O$_2$

To
tissues

White cells fight infection

Lymphocytes
make antibodies

Polymorphs
engulf bacteria

Platelets help to control
bleeding

Prothrombin and Fibrinogen
necessary for blood
clotting

Fig. 10.1 The formation and function of various components of the blood.

red cells and it is by means of this that oxygen is carried in the red cells. Haemoglobin contains iron, and if for any reason iron is not available there will be a reduction in the amount of haemoglobin in each red cell, and, as we shall see later, this is one cause of anaemia. This lack of iron can be caused in several different ways:

1. By insufficient iron in the diet. For instance, the diet of normal infants is mainly composed of

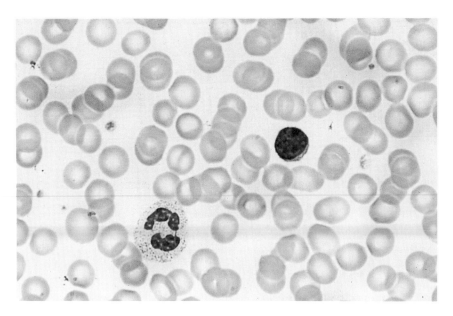

Fig. 10.2 Blood film showing the appearance of the normal red blood cells and the polymorphonuclear and lymphocytic white blood cells.

milk, which contains little iron, with the result that infants commonly suffer from an iron deficiency anaemia in the first year of life.

2. Diseases of the stomach and intestines. These may prevent the proper absorption of iron from the intestinal tract. We shall see later that there are several diseases which are associated with a deficient absorption of iron and so cause anaemia.

3. If there is chronic blood loss (i.e. chronic iron loss).

4. In individuals who naturally absorb iron poorly – the commonest type.

White blood cells and platelets

This topic is dealt with later.

THE NORMAL BLOOD COUNT

The normal blood count in an adult is:

Red blood cells: 5 000 000 per mm^3
Haemoglobin: 10.5 to 14.5 g per 100 ml blood (%)
White blood cells: 5000 to 10 000 per mm^3
Platelets: 150 000 to 400 000 per mm^3

ERYTHROCYTE SEDIMENTATION RATE (ESR)

Blood is drawn from the patient's vein in a special tube. This citrated blood is now drawn up into a long narrow graduated tube up to the 100 mm mark. The tube is held upright in a special container and allowed to stand. The corpuscles gradually settle, leaving clear plasma above. At the end of an hour, the height of the clear plasma is measured off on the tube, and this is known as the ESR. In good health, the corpuscles settle very slowly, so that the ESR is normally less than 10 mm after 1 hour. In various constitutional diseases the corpuscles settle more quickly and the ESR is greater. Thus, in rheumatic fever, for example, the ESR may be 40 mm in 1 hour but as the patient improves the ESR may return to normal. Thus, the ESR is a valuable indication of inflammation and a useful guide to progress.

C-REACTIVE PROTEIN (CRP)

The c-reactive protein is one of the proteins produced in the acute phase of an illness. It is gradually replacing the ESR as an index of underlying disease and as a tool for monitoring disease activity. Its measurement is easy and can be performed on the same blood sample as urea and electrolytes. The protein is made in the liver and will increase within 6 hours of an acute event. It rises with pyrexia, all inflammatory conditions and trauma. It provides a much closer correlation with the clinical state of the patient's illness and, unlike the ESR, it is not affected by the level of haemoglobin. The normal CRP is less than 10 mg/litre; in sick patients it can rise to over 200 mg/litre.

DISEASES AFFECTING THE RED CELLS

Anaemia is defined as a reduction in the haemoglobin level below that accepted as normal for the age and sex of the individual. Anaemia may be due to a number of different causes and often a reasonable diagnosis made by examining a smear of blood suitably stained (*blood film*) under the microscope. If the red cells are small in size (microcytic) and pale in colour (hypochromic), the anaemia is probably caused by lack of iron. When anaemia is due to a deficiency of vitamin B_{12} or folic acid, the red cells are greatly reduced in number but are bigger than normal (macrocytic) and full of haemoglobin (hyperchromic) (see Table 10.1). Measurement of the number of red cells, the size of the red cells and the amount of haemoglobin each cell contains will complete the picture and offers a good idea as to the type of anaemia and its likely cause. Whatever the origin of the anaemia, lack of available haemoglobin causes various signs and symptoms.

GENERAL EFFECTS (SYMPTOMS AND SIGNS OF ANAEMIA)

Many of the symptoms and signs of anaemia are brought about by the deficiency in oxygen supply caused by shortage of the red cells and haemoglobin. The red cells and haemoglobin are the vital agents in the transport of oxygen throughout the body for the supply of all tissues and organs. Signs and symptoms are:

1. Pallor of the skin and mucous membranes.

This is especially seen in the mucous membranes of the lower eyelid and the lips.

2. Weakness, giddiness and fainting. In women, amenorrhoea is commonly present when the anaemia becomes severe.

3. Increased heart rate (tachycardia). To compensate for the deficiency in the amount of oxygen transported, which is caused by the reduction in the red cells and haemoglobin, the heart quickens its rate. This, by making the existing red cells and haemoglobin do more work, may overcome the oxygen deficiency in the tissues and organs in the less severe degrees of anaemia.

4. Dyspnoea and oedema of the ankles. These important signs are seen in severe cases where the heart fails to compensate for the reduction in the carriage of oxygen and, as a result, heart failure develops. As in all cases of heart failure, from whatever cause, dyspnoea is the earliest symptom and is most marked on exertion.

5. If the anaemia is both rapid in onset and severe, all the above symptoms (pallor, weakness, fainting and dyspnoea) will be very pronounced and shock may be present. On the other hand, if the anaemia is more gradual in onset, symptoms may continue to be slight (mainly fatigue and loss of energy) until a profound degree of anaemia is present.

Classification of the anaemias

The treatment of anaemia depends very much on its cause so that accurate diagnosis is essential. There are three main causes of anaemia:

1. anaemia due to loss of blood
2. anaemia due to decreased or abnormal blood formation
3. haemolytic anaemia due to increased blood destruction.

Anaemia due to loss of blood

Haemorrhagic anaemias are probably those most frequently encountered in clinical practice. As can be readily appreciated, any sudden acute loss of blood is likely to result in a reduction in the red

Table 10.1

Type of anaemia	Number of red cells	Size of red cells	Haemoglobin content of red cell	Cause
Hyperchromic macrocytic	Reduced	Larger than normal (macrocytes)	Full (hyperchromic)	Lack of vitamin B_{12} or folic acid
Hypochromic microcytic	May be normal	Small (microcytes)	Very reduced (hypochromic)	Iron deficient
Normocytic	Reduced	Normal (normocytic)	Normal	Acute haemorrhage

cells and haemoglobin. According to the size of the haemorrhage, it may take several weeks or more before the body can replace this loss in both red cells and haemoglobin.

In medical diseases acute haemorrhage is most frequently seen as a haematemesis due to peptic ulcers, and as a haemoptysis from chronic chest conditions, especially tuberculosis and carcinoma. Acute haemorrhage is also commonly seen in maternity and surgical diseases such as post-partum haemorrhage, abortions, injuries, etc. It is only when a sufficient quantity of blood, usually over half a litre, has been lost that any appreciable anaemia occurs. In most cases of acute sudden loss of large quantities of blood, the patient will need treatment for shock. The exact causes producing the clinical symptoms and signs associated with shock are not fully appreciated, but they are certainly caused, in part, by actual loss of fluid from the circulation, which leads to failure of the peripheral circulation. When the blood volume is severely reduced the blood pressure falls, and if the fall is too great the vital centres are affected and shock results. The ideal therapy for shock is immediate fluid replacement to restore the blood volume and raise the blood pressure. It is essential to replace the severe deficiency in the red cells and haemoglobin as otherwise the tissues will lack oxygen. These can be replaced with transfusion of blood. Blood transfusions are essential in all cases of severe acute haemorrhage. A fall in systolic blood pressure to below 100 mm of mercury is an indication that a blood transfusion is likely to be required in a particular patient. In these cases the patient is restless, with marked pallor and a cold clammy skin. The pulse is very rapid, usually in the region of 110, and it may be difficult to feel owing to the low pressure. There is also a marked reduction in output of urine.

The condition of shock with a low blood pressure may occur owing to severe injuries without actual haemorrhage. In these cases, too, it is essential to correct the low blood pressure by transfusions, but here transfusions with plasma instead of with whole blood may be sufficient. Transfusions with saline are useless to restore the blood pressure in severe acute haemorrhage and shock as saline is rapidly poured out of the circulation.

Chronic blood loss also leads to anaemia, and in these cases the haemoglobin is reduced more than the red cells because the red cells can be replaced more quickly than the haemoglobin. The conditions which most commonly give rise to anaemia due to chronic blood loss are chronic haemorrhoids, severe menorrhagia, chronic pep-

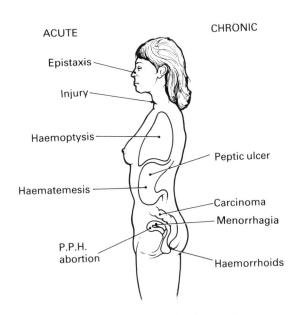

ACUTE   CHRONIC

Epistaxis

Injury

Haemoptysis

Haematemesis

P.P.H. abortion

Peptic ulcer

Carcinoma

Menorrhagia

Haemorrhoids

Fig. 10.3 Some causes of haemorrhagic anaemias.

tic ulcer and carcinoma. The anaemia is managed by treating the cause of the chronic blood loss and by giving iron to manufacture haemoglobin. The bone marrow usually replaces the red cells without special treatment.

Anaemias due to decreased blood formation

This second group of anaemias includes some very common and important types. In our earlier discussion on the red cell and the haemoglobin it was seen that several factors were essential for their proper formation: vitamin B_{12} and folic acid in food, and the intrinsic factor in the stomach and iron being the essential component of haemoglobin. It is clear therefore that either lack of or deficient absorption of any of these factors could lead to deficient blood formation.

Again, from the earlier statements on normal blood formation, it was seen that the blood is formed in the bone marrow. Diseases of the bones, therefore, could interfere with the formation of the blood in the marrow, and in clinical practice we meet with several forms of anaemia due to bone diseases.

Important types of anaemia due to decreased blood formation

1. Pernicious anaemia. Lack of the intrinsic factor.
2. Iron-deficiency anaemia. Deficient intake and absorption of iron, or chronic loss (usually due to chronic haemorrhage).
3. Nutritional anaemia of infants. Lack of iron in the diet.
4. Anaemias of pregnancy. Deficiency due to increased demands for iron and folic acid.
5. Anaemias associated with diseases of the gastrointestinal tract:
   (a) Malabsorption syndrome. Deficient absorption of folic acid, vitamin B_{12} and iron.
   (b) Carcinomas of stomach and bowel causing iron loss due to chronic low-level bleeding.
6. Anaemias due to interference with the bone marrow.
   (a) Drugs and toxic poisons (gold,

chloramphenicol, benzol, chronic infections, X-rays and radioactive substances).
   (b) Mechanical interference (anaemias of leukaemia and carcinomatosis of bone marrow where blood is formed).
   (c) Primary failure of the bone marrow cells (aplastic anaemia).

Pernicious anaemia

Pernicious anaemia is the commonest form of anaemia caused by lack of vitamin B_{12}. As mentioned earlier, vitamin B_{12} is necessary both for the formation of adequate numbers of red blood cells and also for the red cells to become fully mature. Intrinsic factor is normally secreted by the stomach and allows vitamin B_{12} to be absorbed. In pernicious anaemia, antibodies to the parietal cells in the stomach that produce intrinsic factor occur. These antibodies destroy the cells, and without the intrinsic factor vitamin B_{12} is not absorbed from the gastrointestinal tract.

Symptoms and signs

1. This anaemia is commonest after the age of 40 and affects both sexes equally. The onset is gradual and typical remissions occur when the anaemia improves of its own accord.
2. General symptoms and signs of anaemia are present, including pallor and weakness. Their severity naturally varies with the degree of anaemia, but they are usually marked.
3. The patient often complains of soreness of the tongue, which is smooth and inflamed (glossitis).
4. The skin may have a slightly yellowish tint due to a mild degree of jaundice (of the haemolytic type) which, combined with the pallor, gives the pale lemon-yellow colour of pernicious anaemia.
5. The nervous system may be involved with difficulty in walking (ataxia) and pins and needles in the hands and feet. This is as a result of subacute combined degeneration of the spinal cord. This condition is characteristic of pernicious anaemia.

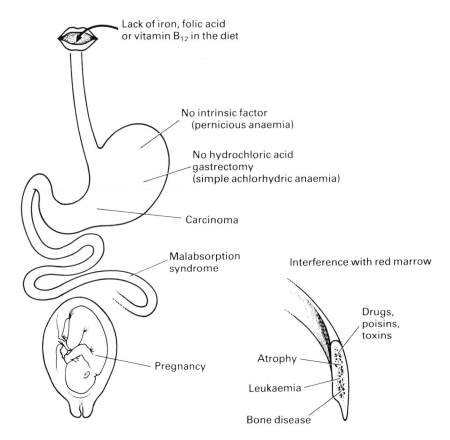

Fig. 10.4 Anaemias due to decreased blood formation – some of the causes.

6. Examination of the patient may reveal an enlarged spleen.

Laboratory tests

1. There is a characteristic blood picture in pernicious anaemia which is always a hyperchromic macrocytic (large cell) anaemia. Immature cells often appear in the peripheral blood and the white cells are reduced in number (leucopenia).

2. A bone marrow puncture is performed from the iliac crest of the pelvis or less commonly the sternum. Examination of the sample under the microscope reveals numerous megaloblasts (abnormal and immature large red cells).

3. Vitamin B_{12} can be measured in the blood. The level in pernicious anaemia is very low.

4. Antibodies to the intrinsic factor can be detected in the blood.

5. Radioactive B_{12} can be administered by mouth and the amount excreted in the urine can be measured (Schilling test). In pernicious anaemia the body is deficient in B_{12} but cannot absorb it unless given a dose of intrinsic factor.

6. Achlorhydria. An injection of pentagastrin normally stimulates a flow of hydrochloric acid from the stomach. In pernicious anaemia analysis of the stomach contents withdrawn by a stomach tube shows no hydrochloric acid (achlorhydria) even after an injection of pentagastrin.

Diagnosis

The diagnosis of anaemia is readily made on the pallor, fatigue and other general signs of anaemia. The diagnosis of pernicious anaemia is made from the typical blood picture, the special

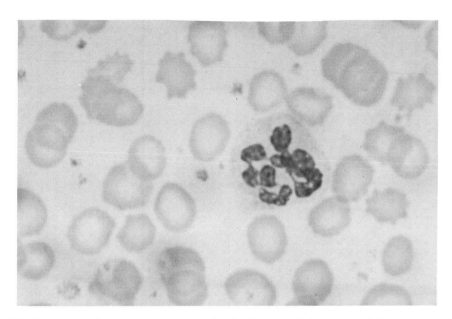

Fig. 10.5 Blood film from a case of pernicious anaemia showing the characteristic larger red cells (macrocytes) and one immature nucleated red cell (megaloblast).

tests mentioned and, if necessary, by a marrow puncture.

Carcinoma of the stomach or intestinal tract often gives rise to effects similar to those of pernicious anaemia, so that careful examination of the gastrointestinal tract by barium X-rays and examination of the faeces for occult blood are necessary in any doubtful case.

Treatment of pernicious anaemia

The essential aim in treatment is to supply the missing vitamin B_{12} (hydroxocobalamin). In the early stages of treatment when there is severe anaemia, 1000 micrograms of vitamin B_{12} are injected intramuscularly once or twice a week until the number of red blood cells and the amount of haemoglobin return to normal. Thereafter a maintenance dose of vitamin B_{12} of 500 micrograms every 3 months is given as the patient will relapse if vitamin B_{12} is stopped. The patient must be warned that vitamin B_{12} will be necessary for the rest of his life. At periodic intervals a blood count is done to ensure that adequate vitamin B_{12} therapy is being given.

If subacute degeneration of the spinal cord is present much larger doses of vitamin B_{12} are necessary; usually 1000 micrograms are given weekly for at least 6 to 12 months and then followed by the usual maintenance doses mentioned above.

Iron-deficiency anaemia

This is the commonest type of anaemia seen in Great Britain and it usually occurs in women in the child-bearing age. It is due to a combination of causes or no cause may be apparent. The diet is often deficient in iron-containing foods, especially meat. Loss of blood at menstruation and the increased nutritional demands during pregnancy further exacerbate the anaemia.

In addition to the general signs and symptoms of anaemia already discussed (pallor, weakness, tachycardia, dyspnoea and oedema), these patients have dry skin and hair, the nails are cracked and spoon-shaped (koilonychia) and the tongue is sore and smooth. Examination of the blood shows a severe reduction in the haemoglobin content (often about 9 g per 100 ml) and the red cells are small and hypochromic.

Treatment

The diet should contain adequate quantities of iron-containing foods. Iron must be taken regularly until the anaemia is fully corrected and is best given as tablets by mouth. There are many satisfactory preparations of iron mixtures and tablets. Ferrous sulphate tablets (200 to 400 mg) can be taken three times a day after meals. They are usually well tolerated but may give rise to nausea or diarrhoea. The stools are always stained black when iron is taken, and this should be explained to patients to avoid unnecessary anxiety.

In exceptional cases where iron cannot be tolerated by mouth, parenteral preparations are available. Intravenous preparations are no longer available in this country because of adverse reactions. An iron sorbitol compound (jectofer) is available for intramuscular injection. An intramuscular injection of 2 ml (100 mg) should raise the haemoglobin level about 4% but is very painful.

Nutritional anaemia of infants

Milk, which is relatively poor in iron content, forms practically the entire diet during the first months of life. An iron-deficiency anaemia, therefore, frequently occurs in infants and is called the nutritional anaemia of infants. Premature infants are particularly likely to suffer from anaemia. In the milder cases the anaemia usually corrects itself at the end of the first year. In more severe cases, however, iron is needed.

Anaemias of pregnancy

During pregnancy an iron-deficiency anaemia is often seen. Various factors combine to bring about this anaemia, including the demands of the foetus for iron and a deficiency of iron in the diet. Less frequently an anaemia similar in type to that of pernicious anaemia (the macrocytic anaemia of pregnancy) is seen. The exact cause of this form of anaemia is unknown, but the anaemia seems to respond best to folic acid therapy.

Anaemias associated with diseases of the gastrointestinal tract

As previously discussed a common cause of anaemia was haemorrhage from a bleeding pep-

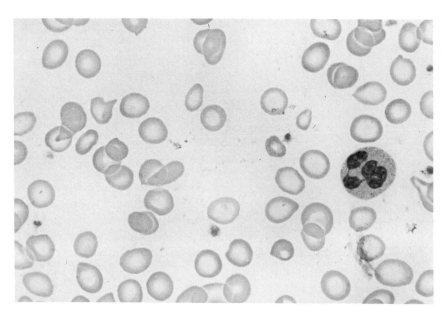

Fig. 10.6 Blood film from a case of iron deficiency anaemia (simple achlorhydric anaemia) showing the characteristic small pale red cells.

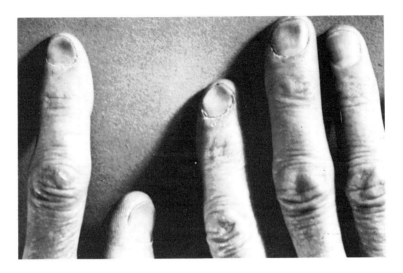

Fig. 10.7 Spoon-shaped nails (koilonychia) from a case of simple achlorhydric anaemia.

tic ulcer or from a carcinoma. There are various other gastrointestinal conditions which may be accompanied by anaemia:

1. In the malabsorption syndrome, in which chronic diarrhoea is a feature, lack of absorption of vitamin B_{12} or folic acid may lead to a macrocytic anaemia similar to that of pernicious anaemia. Alternatively an iron deficiency anaemia may develop from deficient absorption of iron.

2. Carcinoma of the stomach usually causes an iron-deficiency anaemia due to chronic bleeding, but sometimes it also causes a macrocytic anaemia similar to pernicious anaemia owing to interference with the formation of the intrinsic factor in the stomach. A similar anaemia may also arise after the stomach has been removed (gastrectomy) in the treatment of carcinoma or large gastric ulcer.

Removal of large portions of the intestines as carried out for carcinoma or chronic ulcerative colitis, may interfere with the absorption either of iron or of vitamin B_{12} to cause anaemia.

Anaemias due to interference with the bone marrow

Many diseases cause anaemia by suppressing formation of the normal constituents of blood in the bone marrow. This kind of anaemia is seen in:

1. Chronic disease such as rheumatoid arthritis, longstanding renal failure and chronic infection.

2. Drugs such as many of the chemotherapeutic agents, or agents such as phenylbutazone and gold salts used in rheumatoid arthritis.

3. Overexposure to X-rays, radium and some radioactive substances may cause a very severe anaemia. This is so important that people like radiologists and radiographers, who are constantly in contact with X-rays, have a blood examination at periodic intervals. The anaemia due to X-rays and radioactive substances is typically associated with a depression of the white cells. This has been made use of in treating such conditions as leukaemia, where there is a great increase in the white cells. Here radiotherapy can be of value.

4. Extensive bone disease may interfere with the marrow and so depress blood formation. Thus widespread carcinomatous deposits in the bones may cause anaemia. In leukaemia vast numbers of abnormal white cells crowd the marrow to such an extent that red cell formation is greatly reduced. Leukaemia always leads to anaemia for this reason.

5. In some cases the marrow may become

atrophied (aplastic) and a very severe and often fatal anaemia may result. This form of anaemia, known as aplastic anaemia, may be secondary to any of the above poisons (drugs, infections or X-rays), but a primary type of unknown cause also occurs.

Aplastic anaemia (and some forms of acute leukaemia) can be successfully treated by bone marrow transplantation. The marrow is aspirated by needle puncture from the sternum or the iliac crest from a suitable donor and is then transfused intravenously into the patient. A proportion of the healthy transfused marrow cells lodge in the patient's aplastic bone marrow where they proliferate and form new marrow. The patient has to be prepared before this procedure by irradiation or cytotoxic drugs to suppress the immune system and to prevent rejection of the transfused marrow.

Haemolytic anaemias

The third main group of anaemias is due to an increased destruction of the red cells. Normally a red cell has a life of about 120 days, after which it is worn out and destroyed by certain types of cells present in the spleen, liver and the connective tissues, known as the reticuloendothelial system of cells. The haemoglobin is broken down into the pigment bilirubin, which is then excreted by the liver through the biliary passages into the intestines.

In some diseases an over-destruction of the red cells takes place with the result that an anaemia occurs, known as haemolytic anaemia. One of the features of a haemolytic anaemia, is that it is usually associated with a form of jaundice called haemolytic jaundice. It has just been stated that the haemoglobin of the broken-down red cell is turned into bile pigment, bilirubin. Excess of bile pigment accumulating in the blood stream causes jaundice. Therefore in haemolytic anaemias, where there is an excess of bile pigment owing to the excessive breakdown of the red cells, haemolytic jaundice often occurs. In mild haemolytic anaemias, however, the jaundice may be slight or even absent as the body is able to deal with a small excess of bile pigment without jaundice developing.

The most common causes of haemolytic anaemias:

1. Severe infections, especially septicaemias
2. Toxic chemicals and drugs
3. Incompatible blood transfusions
4. Haemolytic disease and the rhesus factor incompatibility
5. Congenital haemolytic anaemias (acholuric jaundice).

Severe infections

Some infectious diseases, especially where the organisms actually grow in the blood stream, cause a haemolytic anaemia. Such diseases are streptococcal septicaemias and malaria.

Toxic chemicals and drugs

Certain chemicals, e.g. lead, cause haemolysis of the red cells. The poisonous venom of some snakes also has this effect. Drugs such as sulphonamides or methyldopa occasionally produce this form of anaemia.

Incompatible blood transfusions

While anaemia is not commonly caused by incompatible blood transfusions, there are other important reactions from giving a patient the wrong blood group.

When a transfusion is given, blood from one person (the donor) is transfused into the blood stream of the patient (the recipient). Unless precautions are taken, the donor's red cells could clump together (agglutinate) and cause serious harm to the recipient. Agglutination of the red cells is due to the presence of certain factors (agglutinogens) present in the donor's red cells which are reacted upon by antibodies in the recipient's serum. Not all donors have these factors in the red cells, and in fact blood can be divided into four main groups (according to which agglutinogens are present):

1. Group O: contains none of the main agglutinogens
2. Group A: contains agglutinogen A
3. Group B: contains agglutinogen B
4. Group AB: contains both agglutinogen A and B.

Naturally, blood containing the agglutinogen A in the red cells does not contain the A antibody in the serum, since this would lead to agglutination of one's own red cells. Hence it is usually safe to give group A blood to a group A recipient or to a group AB recipient. Similarly, group B blood can be given to patients who are group B or group AB. Group AB blood can only be given to group AB patients; on the other hand, group AB patients can usually receive blood from any group without danger of agglutination.

Before a transfusion is given, blood grouping on both donor and recipient is carried out. Unfortunately, this is not enough since other less common factors may be present which also could cause agglutination. A second check, known as cross matching must be made. Some of the recipient's blood is withdrawn and allowed to clot. The serum (clotted plasma) thus obtained is mixed with a small amount of the proposed donor's blood, and if the donor's blood is suitable, i.e. of the right group, no agglutination or clotting should occur.

If, through some mistake or failure to carry out these essential preliminaries, the wrong blood is given, the result is agglutination and destruction

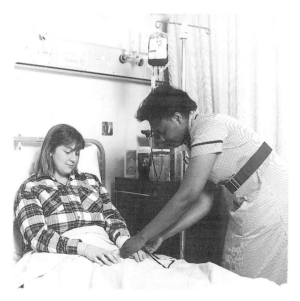

Fig. 10.8 The nurse, having checked the blood with a colleague, connects the unit up to the patient. Regular observation will be necessary over the period of administration.

(haemolysis) of the transfused red cells with jaundice. This is often spoken of as an incompatible or mismatched transfusion. Another effect seen in mismatched transfusions is that the clumped red cells may block the kidneys, when renal failure (uraemia) may result, which can be fatal.

In incompatible blood transfusions the patient becomes restless and has a severe rigor, and there is a rise in pulse rate and temperature. There is usually pain in the chest and back. In severe cases anuria and jaundice develop after a few hours. The nurse must keep a close watch on all patients having a blood transfusion, particularly at the start of each new unit of blood. The pulse, temperature and blood pressure should be checked every half hour so that transfusion can be immediately stopped if any untoward reactions (severe rigors, pain in the back and rise in temperature) occur.

Haemolytic disease and the rhesus (Rh) factor

In addition to the four blood groups mentioned above there is another factor present in the blood of some people which can also cause serious haemolysis and jaundice. This is known as the Rh-factor. Eighty-five per cent of people have this factor and are said to be Rh-positive. The remaining 15% of people lack this factor and are Rh-negative. If Rh-positive blood is given to a Rh-negative person, even though it may be the right blood group (that is, O or A, etc.), Rh antibodies are produced in the Rh-negative recipient which may destroy the Rh-positive blood. It is necessary, therefore, in giving transfusions to ascertain not only the normal blood group of the person but also the Rh factor, and if this is Rh-negative to give only Rh-negative blood.

Rhesus haemolytic disease of the newborn (HDN) At this point it is convenient to discuss the diseases seen in infants due to this Rh factor and associated haemolysis. HDN may result from a number of conditions which have in common the presence in maternal blood of antibodies capable of crossing the placenta and attacking the fetal red cells. It represents a wide spectrum of disease of varying severity. The most serious of the causes of HDN is that due to rhesus factor. There are in fact six components to the rhesus antibody complex, the main one being the D component. Rhesus positive means D-positive, and rhesus-negative means D-negative.

In rhesus HDN, immunization of the mother usually occurs as a result of transplacental haemorrhage, whereby rhesus positive cells from the fetus enter the maternal circulation where they evoke a primary immune response. Such transplacental haemorrhage usually though not exclusively, occur during the third stage of labour, and first pregnancies are not usually affected by rhesus haemolytic disease. In a subsequent pregnancy with a rhesus-positive fetus, further stimulation of the mother's immune system results in antibody production. These antibodies readily cross the placenta and cause HDN. Each pregnancy with a rhesus-positive fetus results in further antigenic stimulation and antibody production, and rhesus HDN tends to increase in severity with each affected pregnancy. When the fetus is rhesus-negative the presence of rhesus antibodies is of no consequence.

Treatment of haemolytic disease of the newborn
In a case of established maternal iso-immunization the aims of treatment are to minimize effects on the fetus by:

1. monitoring the degree of haemolysis by estimating the amount of bilirubin in the amniotic fluid, and delivering the baby early if necessary
2. giving intrauterine blood transfusion if the fetus is clearly distressed and at risk of death prior to delivery
3. using plasmapheresis to reduce the amount of antibody in the maternal circulation; this is rarely used
4. delivering the baby in a unit fully equipped for neonatal intensive care.

Management after delivery Modern management involves delivery of the fetus at the optimal time, and subsequent treatment of the haemolytic anaemia and its complications in a neonatal intensive care unit. Immediate transfusion may be required, so blood tests should be taken at delivery for instant analysis.

Prevention of rhesus HDN The identification of a method of preventing rhesus HDN is one of the most significant obstetrical advances of the last 30 years. It is now possible to prevent maternal iso-immunization by giving anti-D immunoglobulin to susceptible mothers within 72 hours of delivery. This immunization prevents sensitisation of the mothers immune system by fetal cells that have gained access to the maternal circulation during the third stage of labour. A standard dose of anti-D is given intravenously to all

---

Rhesus-negative mother　　　　**Rhesus-positive father**

Rhesus-positive babies

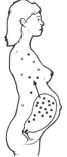

First pregnancy ••••••••
Rhesus Positive Antigens cross the placental barrier and provoke maternal lymphocytes to produce Antibodies ◦◦◦◦◦◦◦◦◦
Baby is usually unaffected but mother goes on and on producing Anti-Rh+ve Antibodies after delivery

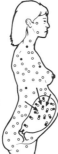

Second and subsequent pregnancies
Anti-Rh+ve Antibodies are now present in mother and production is boosted by Rh+ve Antigens from new baby. Anti-Rh+ve Antibodies cross the placental barrier and react with Rh+ve Antigens in baby Baby is affected (Haemolytic Disease of the Newborn).

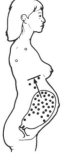

Protection
Mother is given Anti-Rh+ve serum (Anti-D gamma globulin) which depresses her production of antibodies.
Baby is protected

Fig. 10.9

unsensitized rhesus-negative mothers who have delivered a rhesus-positive baby, following abortion, and following ectopic pregnancy.

The administration of anti-D to susceptible women has reduced the incidence of HDN tenfold, but this disorder will probably never be eliminated due to:

1. home delivery not receiving anti-D
2. maternal iso-immunization occurring as a result of transplacental haemorrhage not in the third stage of labour and not covered with anti-D
3. large transplacental haemorrhage that swamps the standard dose of anti-D.

It continues to be essential to screen all antenatal women irrespective of their blood group to detect antibodies capable of causing HDN and to have the expertise to manage such cases.

Congenital haemolytic anaemias (acholuric jaundice)

Congenital haemolytic anaemia is due to a congential defect in the red cells which makes them more fragile than normal and so more easily destroyed. The disease is chronic and usually recognised in childhood, although mild cases may be missed for many years. Recurrent attacks of jaundice of the haemolytic type, with anaemia, and an enlarged spleen are the main features. The diagnosis of the disease can be confirmed by performing a fragility test, when the abnormally increased fragility of the red cells will be evident. The only effective remedy is to remove the spleen. This increases the life of the red cells and so decreases the amount of red cell destruction.

THE HAEMORRHAGIC DISEASES

There are various components of the blood involved in the control of haemorrhage. These include platelets, prothrombin and fibrinogen. The blood vessels themselves also play an important role in controlling haemorrhage, and contraction of the blood vessel (vasoconstriction) usually takes place when a blood vessel is injured. Haemorrhagic diseases are a large group

which have as a predominating feature the presence of haemorrhages. These haemorrhages may occur into the skin to give rise to purple spots which do not fade on pressure and are called purpura (small purpuric haemorrhages are usually known as petechiae). Bleeding may also occur from the mucous membranes, e.g. from the nose (epistaxis), from the bowels (melaena), or from the kidneys (haematuria).

The commoner haemorrhagic diseases can be roughly classified according to the type of underlying interference with the normal mechanism for the control of bleeding:

1. damage to the wall of the blood vessels
2. diminished platelets – thrombocytopenic purpura
3. clotting factor deficiency – acquired, e.g. liver disease
4. clotting factor deficiency – inherited, e.g. haemophilia.

Damage to the walls of the blood vessels

Damage to the walls of blood vessels is the most common cause of purpura and can be divided into the following groups:

Infections

Many infections are associated with purpuric haemorrhages. In some cases small emboli containing bacteria are responsible for the haemorrhages. This is seen in meningococcal meningitis, and in bacterial endocarditis where small emboli cause haemorrhages under the nails (splinter haemorrhages), and in the back of the eye (Roth spots).

Drugs

Many drugs, such as isoniazid, quinine and sulphonamides, may cause purpura – as can the heavy metals used in medicine, such as gold for rheumatoid arthritis.

Vitamin C deficiency

The classical sign of vitamin C deficiency is

haemorrhage due to alteration in the vascular wall, most commonly found in the base of a hair follicle. This is diagnostic of vessel wall damage due to vitamin C deficiency.

Allergic diseases

Purpura is sometimes associated with various allergic manifestations, such as urticaria, oedema of the skin and joint pains. The underlying factor is damage to the lining of the vascular wall which allows leakage of blood and fluid.

Henoch–Schonlein's purpura occurs in young adults and the purpura may be associated with abdominal pain, joint swellings and nephritis.

Senile purpura

This is the commonest type of purpura and is found most often in elderly people, recurrent purpuric spots appearing in the skin. There is little or no upset in the general health and the purpura is of no significance.

Diminished platelets (thrombocytopenic purpura)

One of the functions of the small round bodies known as the platelets (or thrombocytes) is to seal off any lesions or openings in the small blood vessels (capillaries) and so prevent undue loss of blood from a slight injury. The platelets are formed in the bone marrow and, like the red cells, are destroyed by the spleen. Most of the causes, therefore, of this group of haemorrhagic diseases (purpura) are diseases affecting the blood, the bone marrow and the spleen:

1. Leukaemia, by crowding the marrow with abnormal white cells, may depress the formation of platelets in exactly the same way as it may cause anaemia. Purpura, including bleeding from the mucous membranes, may be a feature of some severe cases of leukaemia.

2. Secondary carcinomatosis of the bones acts like leukaemia in causing purpura in that the widespread invasion of the bone marrow by the malignant cells decreases the formation of the platelets. We have already seen that carcinoma-

tosis of the bones causes an anaemia in the same fashion.

3. Aplastic anaemia is due to atrophy of the marrow by poisons, toxins, drugs or unknown causes. Severe purpura with bleeding from the mucous membranes caused by depression of the platelets is often a feature of aplastic anaemia.

4. Drugs, such as quinine, phenylbutazone, sulphonamides and carbimazole, may cause purpura associated with a deficiency of platelets.

5. Thrombocytopenic purpura. Often the cause of the diminished platelets is not known. This is seen most commonly in women and gives rise to severe bleeding from the mucous membranes (nose, bowel, kidneys) and into the skin. Anaemia is present, and the spleen is nearly always enlarged. Careful search for any of the causes mentioned above must be made and also for systemic lupus erythematosis (Ch. 15) in which thrombocytopenia occurs. The treatment depends on the severity of the conditions, and in mild cases treating the anaemia only may suffice. In cases of severity, however, the spleen is usually removed since the spleen may be responsible for excessive platelet destruction. Blood transfusions to control any severe haemorrhage may be necessary. Steroids have been effective in inducing remission or a temporary improvement and so making the patient fit for splenectomy.

Clotting factor deficiency

Coagulation of blood

At the beginning of this chapter the roles of various components of the blood were discussed. It was stated that the substances prothrombin and fibrinogen were concerned with the coagulation of blood. Blood coagulation or clotting plays a major part in the control of haemorrhage. There are many factors involved in the process of coagulation (at least 14), and an in-depth analysis is impossible.

There are two main pathways by which the process of coagulation is mediated:

1. The extrinsic pathway. This is triggered when blood comes into contact with tissue and surfaces outside the blood stream. The anticoagu-

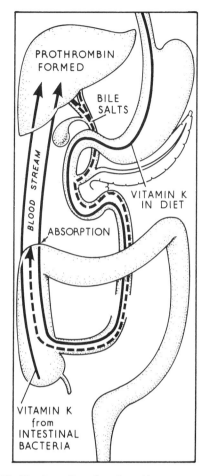

Fig. 10.10 The formation of prothrombin.

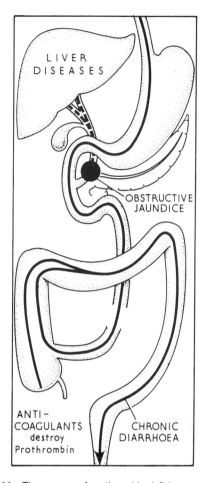

Fig. 10.11 The causes of prothrombin deficiency.

lant warfarin acts on this pathway by blocking it.

2. The intrinsic pathway. This is triggered by damage within the blood stream when cells are damaged and release substances that activate the pathway without an actual breach of the vascular wall. The anticoagulant heparin acts on this pathway by blocking it.

Whichever pathway is activated (and usually both are in action at the same time), once the 'cascade' starts, it continues irrevocably towards clot formation. The end point of the cascade is fibrin formation, which is the basis of the blood clot.

Acquired clotting factor deficiency

Many of the factors in both pathways are pro-

duced in the liver by utilization of vitamin K. This vitamin is present in certain foods, such as spinach, cabbage and egg yolk. Bacteria which are normally present in the bowel can also manufacture vitamin K. For the proper absorption of vitamin K bile salts are necessary.

Causes of deficiency in clotting factors

1. Obstructive jaundice. Here, the absence of bile salts leads to deficient absorption of vitamin K and so, after 6 to 8 weeks, to a fall in the level of clotting factors in the blood. When this is severe, haemorrhages occur. Jaundiced patients are often known to bleed very readily at an operation.

2. Haemorrhagic disease of the newborn. Oc-

casionally during the first week of life haemorrhages, such as epistaxis or melaena, may occur giving rise to the condition known as haemorrhagic disease of the newborn. The cause is prothrombin deficiency brought about by a shortage of vitamin K received from the mother, combined with the inability of the infant during the first week to manufacture vitamin K itself, due to the absence of bacteria in the infants bowel. Premature infants are especially lacking in prothrombin and should be given vitamin K after birth as a routine. Most babies especially those who are breast fed, are now given oral vitamin K at birth as prophalaxis.

3. Disease of the liver. Diseases of the liver may be associated with prothrombin deficiency as prothrombin is manufactured and stored in the liver. Prothrombin deficiency with its resulting haemorrhages is mainly seen in cases of acute liver damage such as may occur in acute hepatitis, and less often in chronic conditions such as cirrhosis of the liver. Paracetamol overdose causes liver necrosis and often grossly deranged clotting.

4. Chronic diseases of the gastrointestinal tract. Chronic intestinal diseases such as ulcerative colitis, and Crohns disease, which cause severe and persistent diarrhoea may lead to a deficiency in vitamin K absorption, sometimes resulting in so severe a prothrombin deficiency that actual haemorrhages may occur.

5. Anticoagulant drugs. Anticoagulant drugs are used in the prevention and treatment of thrombosis and embolism, especially thrombosis of the veins. Anticoagulant drugs interfere with either the intrinsic or extrinsic coagulation pathways, and thus cause a prolonged blood-clotting time. The aim in treatment is to prolong the clotting time of the blood so that thrombosis does not occur or, if already present, does not spread; the risk of a complicating embolism is thus greatly reduced.

In all patients on anticoagulant drugs (such as warfarin or heparin) frequent estimation of the clotting time is essential to control the treatment. Daily routine examination of the urine for red cells is also valuable.

Treatment of clotting factor deficiency

Administration of vitamin K will correct most of the deficiencies. It will not be effective if there is an inherited defect of synthesis, or if the liver is extensively diseased and therefore unable to make use of the vitamin K. It takes some time for vitamin K to correct the deficiency as the liver must manufacture the factors. In emergency cases fresh frozen plasma may be given as this contains all of the factors necessary for clotting. It allows you to control the situation until the liver can make the factors itself.

Inherited clotting factor deficiency

Any of the many clotting factors can be deficient as part of an inherited disorder. In 70% of cases of deficiency factor viii is affected, and deficiency results in haemophilia. Haemophilia occurs in 1 in 7000 of the population. Males only are affected, while females pass the disease on but cannot suffer from it. The severity depends on how little factor viii is in the blood.

Treatment of haemophilia This is managed by giving factor viii concentrate to control bleeding, which can start from early infancy in severe cases. Factor viii is nowadays made artificially by genetic recombinant technology to avoid any risk of infective contamination. Many patients will require frequent blood transfusions, and this puts them at high risk of acquiring transfusion transmitted infections, particularly hepatitis and HIV infection. This risk is minimized but not excluded by:

1. exclusion criteria for blood donors
2. heat-treating plasma
3. testing all donations for hepatitis B and C, and for HIV.

POLYCYTHAEMIA

Polycythaemia is an uncommon disorder of the blood where there is a marked increase in the number of red blood cells and in the volume of the blood. Instead of the normal count of approximately five million red cells per mm^3, the number of red cells may be as high as seven million or more per mm^3. The condition may arise as a compensatory mechanism in diseases where there is incomplete oxygenation of the blood, e.g.

severe chronic diseases of the heart and lungs, especially congenital heart diseases. Certain drugs may also produce this condition. A primary form of the disease, of unknown cause, polycythaemia rubra vera, is more rarely seen. Regular venesection, in which 500 ml of blood is withdrawn, may be undertaken at monthly intervals.

THE WHITE BLOOD CELLS

There are three main types of white cell in the blood:

1. polymorphonuclear white cells or granulocytes (so-called because they have granules present); there are three forms of polymorphonuclear white cell – neutrophils, eosinophils and basophils
2. lymphocytes
3. monocytes.

The polymorphonuclear cells and the monocytes (like the red cells) are formed in the red marrow of the bones, while lymphocytes are produced in the spleen and the lymph glands. The main function of the white cells is to help defend the body against infection. The polymorphs and the monocytes move towards the site of infection and engulf the bacteria.

The lymphocytes act in two ways. B-lymphocytes produce antibodies to counteract bacterial toxins and T-lymphocytes destroy foreign cells by direct contact. The T-lymphocytes are subclassified into T4 (helper) cells and T8 cells according to their main function. The normal total white cell count varies between 5000 and 10 000 per mm^3 in an adult. The polymorphonuclear cells form 65% of this total, the lymphocytes 30% and the monocytes 5%. In most bacterial infections, the white cell count increases, sometimes to more than 20 000. This is known as a *leucocytosis* and shows that the body is responding to overcome the infection. A reduction of white cells below normal is called a leucopenia and occurs in certain infections such as typhoid fever or tuberculosis, probably due to a toxic effect on the marrow itself. When the number of polymorphs is greatly or even completely sup-

pressed, the condition is known as agranulocytosis. This is usually due to the toxic effect of certain drugs and is described later.

Diseases of the white blood cells

Leukaemia

Leukaemia is a disease in which the white cells of the blood are not properly formed and start to increase in numbers in a malignant way. They crowd out the bone marrow and interfere with the formation of the red cells and platelets. This leads to anaemia and haemorrhages. Leukaemia can be classified according to the type of white cell involved.

Myeloid leukaemia is a disease of the polymorphs. Lymphatic leukaemia affects the lymphocytes. Monocytic leukaemia, involves the monocytes, and is the least common. The type of leukaemia is identified by examining the blood and the marrow obtained from a bone marrow aspirate.

It is important to remember that leukaemia is actually a malignant disease of the bone marrow of unknown cause, which leads to a great increase in the number of cells (but these cells are abnormal). Leucocytosis is an increase in the number of white cells as the result usually of infection by organisms such as bacteria. It is the natural response of the body to overcome the infection. Leukaemia can be acute or chronic, the acute form being commonest in children.

Acute leukaemia Acute leukaemia is commonest in children but can occur at any age. The onset is usually sudden with fever, pallor and purpura. There may be bleeding from the nose or from the mouth and general symptoms of severe anaemia with fatigue and loss of strength. When the blood is examined under the microscope, the total white count is usually vastly increased and the cells are immature and abnormal.

The treatment of acute leukaemia has become more successful but more complex, so that children with leukaemia are best treated in special units expert in the latest forms of treatment and the complications arising from them.

The aim of treatment is to use drugs which

destroy all abnormal cells in the blood and bone marrow, without proving too toxic to healthy tissues and cells. In acute lymphatic leukaemia this can be achieved in the majority of cases by using intravenous injections of various combinations of toxic drugs such as vincristine, methotrexate or cyclophosphamide sometimes with the additional use of radiotherapy. This treatment has greatly improved the outlook in acute lymphatic leukaemia; many patients are still healthy more than 10 years after the start of the illness and it is likely that they have a complete cure. The role of bone marrow transplant once the diseased marrow has been eradicated is improving the outlook further. The outlook is less favourable for acute myeloid or acute monocytic leukaemia.

Chronic leukaemia Chronic myeloid leukaemia usually comes on in middle age with gradually increasing tiredness and anaemia. The spleen becomes so greatly enlarged that it may give rise to dragging abdominal discomfort and indigestion. There may be troublesome irritation of the skin.

The diagnosis is confirmed by examination of the blood. The white count may be more than 200 000, the majority of the cells being abnormal polymorphonuclears. Treatment may make the patient more comfortable and prolongs life. Busulphan is a drug which delays proliferation of the white cells and has to be taken regularly, the dose being adjusted according to the white count. When the spleen is very enlarged, deep X-ray therapy may be applied to reduce its size.

Chronic lymphatic leukaemia occurs mainly in men and may run a mild course over many years with few symptoms. The spleen is not greatly enlarged but the lymph glands increase in size. Treatment is, in the main, symptomatic. Chlorambucil is one agent used in it's management.

MYELOMATOSIS (MULTIPLE MYELOMA)

This disorder is caused by a malignant proliferation of special cells called plasma cells in the bone marrow. Plasma cells normally produce protein antibodies and in multiple myeloma large quantities of abnormal protein can be detected in the blood and urine. The cells invade the bones themselves, leading to erosion and spontaneous fractures.

Multiple myeloma is commonest in the elderly and is characterised by bone pains, malaise, anaemia and pyrexia. The sedimentation rate is very high and excessive numbers of plasma cells can be seen in the marrow. There is no curative treatment, but the drug melphelan helps to suppress plasma cell activity. Radiotherapy may relieve the pain of local bone involvement.

AGRANULOCYTOSIS

The term agranulocytosis is used to denote either the complete absence of the granular cells (or polymorphonuclear cells as they are more often called) or a severe reduction in their number, combined with clinical symptoms and signs due to this deficiency. It must be stressed that a leucopenia means a reduction in the white cells which does not necessarily cause harmful results and is not the same condition as agranulocytosis.

The usual cause of agranulocytosis is some toxic depression of the bone marrow, as a result of which the polymorphs are not formed in adequate numbers. Drugs are the commonest cause of this toxic depression, especially the sulphonamides, antithyroid drugs (thiouracil and carbimazole), phenylbutazone, chloramphenicol and gold salts.

In view of the frequent use of phenylbutazone and antithyroid drugs, with their special liability to give rise to agranulocytosis, it is absolutely essential that the early symptoms and signs of this condition should be watched for. The lack of white cells means that there is a lowered resistance to bacteria, so that infection is liable to occur, especially in the throat.

Symptoms and signs of agranulocytosis

1. The commonest early symptom is one of sore throat, which may be very severe, with marked oedema and exudate in the throat.

2. The temperature rises, and if it is already above normal it usually rises further.

3. The patient becomes toxic and lethargic. The pulse is rapid.

Diagnosis

The complaint of a sore throat with fever in a patient on antithyroid drugs should immediately raise the suspicion of agranulocytosis. The drugs must at once be stopped until a white cell count is done and the presence of agranulocytosis confirmed or not.

Treatment

Penicillin is given by injection, perhaps a million units every 4 hours. This is to combat any infection that is present or likely to arise. Penicillin is non-toxic to the white cells so that it can be given with safety.

There is an agent available which stimulates the bone marrow to produce the deficient granulocyte. It is called granulocyte colony stimulating factor (G-CSF). It can reduce the length of time taken to recover normal white cell function.

THE SPLEEN AND LYMPH GLANDS

The spleen and the lymph glands play an important part in protecting the body against infection and are the main sites of production of lymphocytes, which manufacture antibodies. The spleen also filters out damaged red cells, bacteria and parasites which pass through it, and then destroys them. This explains why it enlarges in such diseases as typhoid fever and malaria.

Sometimes it becomes too active and destroys healthy cells, as in thrombocytopenic purpura, when the platelets are destroyed. Removal of the spleen (splenectomy) then becomes necessary. The lymph glands, with their lymphatic ducts, also form a drainage system and act as a local filter to prevent bacteria and malignant cells from entering the general circulation.

Splenomegaly (enlargement of the spleen)

An enlarged spleen is an indication of underlying disease. Some of the causes are:

1. Acute infections. Glandular fever, subacute bacterial endocarditis, tuberculosis, and malaria are among the most common.

2. Chronic infections. Malaria is by far the commonest cause of splenomegaly due to chronic infection. Other causes include syphilis and tuberculosis.

3. Blood diseases. It is in this group of diseases that greatly enlarged spleens are encountered. Leukaemia, especially the myeloid type, is one of the commonest causes. Congenital haemolytic anaemia (acholuric jaundice) and thrombocytopenic purpura are often associated with enlargement of the spleen.

4. Cirrhosis of the liver. Chronic obstruction of the liver occurring in cirrhosis sometimes leads to engorgement and enlargement of the spleen. Distended veins in the oesophagus often bleed, with resultant haematemesis and anaemia.

Lymphadenopathy (enlargement of the lymph glands)

Generally, when disease affects the lymph glands the glands become enlarged. For the sake of convenience we can divide such enlargement into local and general.

Local

Localized enlargement of one group of lymph glands is commonly due to septic inflammation of the tissues drained by those lymph glands. For instance, a septic finger often causes an enlarged axillary gland, while inflammation of the throat may give rise to enlarged cervical glands.

Apart from inflammatory lesions, tumour cells often spread along the lymphatics to cause enlargement of the lymph glands draining the area, e.g. carcinoma of the breast giving rise to enlarged axillary glands. Another frequent cause of localized lymph gland enlargement is tuberculosis, which very commonly affects the cervical glands.

General

The most common causes of a generalized enlargement of the lymph glands include:

1. glandular fever
2. lymphatic leukaemia
3. Hodgkin's disease
4. HIV infection.

We have discussed glandular fever and HIV infection in an earlier chapter, and leukaemia earlier here. The remaining common cause of generalized lymphadenopathy is Hodgkin's disease.

Hodgkin's disease

The cause of Hodgkin's disease is unknown.

Symptoms and signs

1. The disease is commonest in the 20–40 age group, but it may arise at any age. The first sign of the disease is often an enlargement of one group of lymph glands.

2. Any group (or groups) of lymph glands may be affected. Usually the cervical glands in the neck or the axillary or inguinal glands are involved. In some cases, however, the deep internal lymph glands in the thorax or abdomen may be the first to be affected, and here the diagnosis of the condition is often difficult until the superficial palpable lymph glands also become enlarged.

3. The general health may be little affected at first, but as the disease advances weakness, anaemia and loss of weight develop. A characteristic feature of many cases is the recurrent pyrexia, which typically comes in waves lasting 10–14 days and then subsides only to rise again. This undulating type of fever is called the *Pel-Ebstein* fever.

4. Enlargement of the thoracic lymph glands can give rise to the pressure symptoms of cough and dyspnoea, while the enlarged abdominal glands may cause abdominal distension or ascites.

Diagnosis

The disease has to be distinguished from the other causes of enlargement of the lymph glands. Lymphatic leukaemia, which also causes a generalized enlargement of the lymph glands, is differentiated by the diagnostic gross increase in the white cells accompanied by the presence of abnormal types of white cells. Tuberculosis of the lymph glands remains confined to one group only, and the affected glands become matted together and may break down to form a chronic sinus. Hodgkin's glands remain mobile and do not adhere to the skin or break down. Malignant disease of the lymph glands, which is usually due

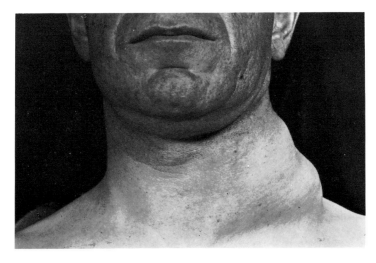

Fig. 10.12 Hodgkin's disease showing enlarged glands in the neck.

to secondary invasion, gives rise to very hard fixed glands, and the primary growth is usually easily found.

The diagnosis of Hodgkin's disease rests on removal (biopsy) of an enlarged lymph gland, usually from the neck, and histological examination under the microscope. The presence in the gland of abnormal cells typical of Hodgkin's disease confirms the diagnosis. The extent to which the glands and the spleen are involved is of importance from the view point of treatment.

CT scanning (computerized tomography), has enabled us to find out the extent of glandular involvement without performing major surgery. In years gone by laparotomy with removal of many glands and the spleen was routine in these patients. Ultrasound is less helpful than CT scan for looking at glands, but MRI (magnetic resonance imaging), may well replace CT as the best investigation in the next few years, when it becomes more widely available. MRI has the major advantage that it does not involve radiation.

Treatment

This will depend on the degree of glandular and splenic enlargement. In the early stages, particularly when the glands involved are not widespread, radiotherapy is the treatment of choice and offers good opportunities for complete cure. Chemotherapy with cytotoxic drugs and steroids may be given in addition to radiotherapy in early cases.

In patients where the involvement of the lymph glands is too widespread to warrant radiotherapy, chemotherapy is used as the sole treatment. The treatment of Hodgkin's disease demands considerable expertise and is best carried out in special oncology units.

11

Diseases of the urinary system

ANATOMY AND PHYSIOLOGY

The urinary system consists of two kidneys, each joined to the bladder by a tube, called a *ureter*, which conveys urine from the kidneys to the bladder for storage. Following contraction of the bladder, urine is expelled through the urethra. The kidneys lie behind the peritoneum on either side of the vertebral column. In an adult they measure approximately 12–14 cm. They are supplied by blood through renal arteries (branches of the aorta), and blood leaves the kidneys through renal veins. Each kidney contains approximately one million nephrons, which act as tiny filters to remove waste materials from the blood. Each nephron has a filter head, or glomerulus. The glomerulus contains a network of thin-walled capillaries which allow fluid and waste products to filter into the glomerular capsule. From there the filtrate passes into the tubule of the nephron. This glomerular filtrate may reach 180 litres a day, and as the volume of urine excreted is about 2 litres a day it can be seen that the tubules re-absorb a very large proportion of the glomerular filtrate. This is important not only to prevent excessive loss of fluid but also to re-absorb important salts and other substances from the urine, but not waste products. The fluid which emerges from the end of the nephron tubule is urine. It drains into the pelvis of the kidney for passage down the ureter. The kidneys have several functions:

1. They remove waste products of metabolism from the body. For example, urea which is a waste product of protein metabolism is excreted in large quantities.

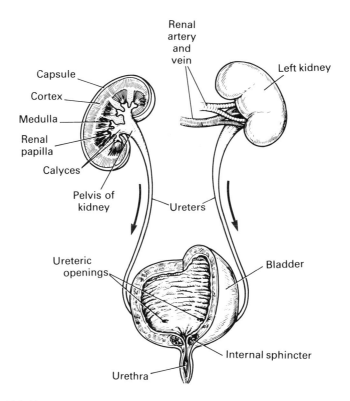

Fig. 11.1 The kidneys and bladder.

2. The kidneys help to maintain a neutral internal environment by preventing the body fluids becoming too acid or alkali. They do this by excreting or retaining hydrogen ions and so maintain the acid alkali reaction of the blood at a constant level.

3. The kidneys regulate the fluid balance by excreting more urine when a large amount of fluid is taken in, and by retaining fluid when more is being lost in perspiration.

4. The kidneys secrete important hormones into the blood stream which include erythropoietin (which stimulates red blood cell production in the bone marrow) and angiotensin (which helps to regulate blood pressure).

5. Vitamin D, which prevents bone disease, becomes fully active after undergoing changes in the kidney. Normal urine contains very little protein as the protein molecules (albumin) are too large to pass through the glomerular filter. If the glomerular filter is damaged, protein can escape and appear in the urine. Sugar appears in the urine if the normal blood levels are exceeded, as

in diabetes, when the excess glucose is too great to be fully re-absorbed.

INVESTIGATION OF KIDNEY FUNCTION

The urine

Important information about kidney function is gained by examining the quantity and quality of the urine (see Ch. 1).

Volume

The volume of urine excreted in 24 hours in a healthy person depends on the amount of fluid ingested and the amount of fluid lost in sweat, stools and in respiration (exhaled breath contains moisture). The kidney maintains the balance so that the total body water remains steady. It is important in severely ill patients and those with kidney disease to record the volume of urine passed over 24 hours on a fluid balance chart,

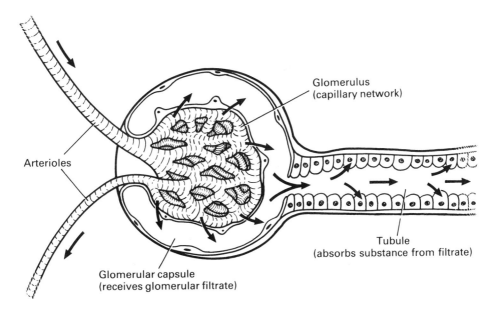

Glomerulus
(capillary network)

Arterioles

Tubule
(absorbs substance from filtrate)

Glomerular capsule
(receives glomerular filtrate)

Fig. 11.2 A close-up diagram of glomerulus and tubule.

together with fluid lost in diarrhoea, vomit or by other means. The fluid losses can be compared with the total fluid input, by mouth or intravenous drip, so that at the end of 24 hours the physician can judge whether the kidneys are maintaining proper fluid balance. Normally, fluid intake will exceed output by approximately 500 ml due to fluid lost in the breath or in sweat, which cannot be easily measured. In renal failure, the output of urine may fall to under 400 ml (*oliguria*) or may cease (*anuria*). Increased volumes of urine (*polyuria*) may occur in some forms of kidney disease where the kidney tubules lose the ability to concentrate the urine, so that large volumes of dilute urine are passed. Polyuria may also occur in diabetes insipidus where the antidiuretic hormone (ADH) is deficient. This hormone normally controls the amount of fluid absorbed by the tubules from the glomerular filtrate. Polyuria is a feature of uncontrolled diabetes mellitus, as the large amount of sugar present in the blood cannot be fully re-absorbed by the kidney and some appears in the urine and draws an obligatory volume of water with it.

Proteinuria

Protein (albumin) in the urine usually indicates

leakage through a damaged glomerular filter and so is present in many types of renal disease, especially those which predominantly affect the glomerulus (glomerulonephritis). Occasionally, healthy young adults show protein in the urine following exercise or prolonged standing (*orthostatic proteinuria*). The simplest method of testing the urine for protein is to dip a stick of Albustix in the urine (Ch.1); a change in colour to green suggests the presence of protein. The amount of protein being lost can be measured accurately by collecting the urine passed over 24 hours and sending it to the laboratory for analysis.

Haematuria

Blood in the urine can arise from the kidney, the ureters, the bladder or the urethra. Heavy bleeding may occur with tumours of the kidney or bladder, renal stones or bleeding disorders, causing the urine to appear red or smoky (macroscopic haematuria). Lesser amounts of blood only detectable with tests may be due to glomerulonephritis or infection of the kidney or bladder (*microscopic haematuria*). In healthy women, blood from menstruation may contaminate the urine. Two tests are available for haematuria. The

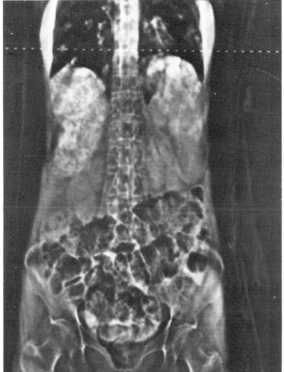

A

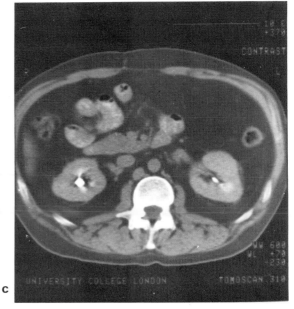

C

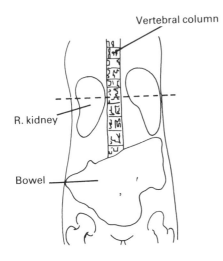

B

Vertebral column

R. kidney

Bowel

Bowel

R. kidney

L. kidney

D

Vertebra

Fig. 11.3 A–D. CAT scan of the whole body from the front, and a cross-section at the level of the kidney.

first may be easily performed in the ward by dipping a test strip (Hemastix) into the urine. If blood is present, the colour changes to blue within 30 seconds. The second is performed in the laboratory by examining the urine under a microscope for the presence of red blood cells.

Pyuria (white blood cells in the urine)

White blood cells can be reliably detected only by examining the urine under a microscope, but if pyuria is severe the urine may be cloudy and may have a fishy smell. Pyuria is due to urinary tract infections: pyelitis or nephritis (infection of the pelvis and substance of the kidney), cystitis (infection of the bladder) or urethritis (infection of the urethra). Tuberculosis, tumours and renal stones may also cause excess white cells in the urine.

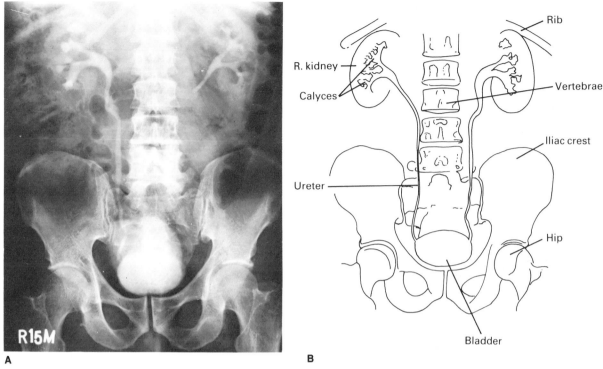

A

B

Fig. 11.4 A, B. Intravenous pyelogram outlining the kidney, ureters and bladder.

Casts

These are small cylindrical protein bodies in the urine which are visible under the microscope. They are formed in the tubules and if they contain cells (cellular or granular casts) they always indicate renal disease, especially glomerulonephritis.

Urine bacteriology

If acute bacterial infection or tuberculosis is suspected, a mid-stream urine specimen must be sent to the laboratory for culture and identification of the bacteria.

Blood urea and creatinine

Urea is an end-product of protein metabolism and so its rate of formation varies with the amount of protein taken in the diet. Creatinine is formed during muscle metabolism, the amount depending on the muscle bulk. Despite fluctuating rates of production, the blood levels of these two substances remain remarkably constant because the kidneys excrete the excess. When the kidneys are not functioning properly, as in acute or chronic renal failure, the blood levels of urea and creatinine increase. In good health, the urea level does not exceed 6.6 mmol per litre (40 mg/100 ml) and creatinine is below 124 μmol per litre (1.4 mg/100 ml). Levels in excess of these figures suggest inadequate excretion due to renal impairment.

Creatinine clearance test

This is a more accurate measurement of renal function as it depends on the rate at which the kidney can excrete creatinine. The urine excreted over 24 hours is collected and a blood sample taken. By measuring the amount of creatinine excreted in the urine and the amount present in the blood, the rate at which creatinine is cleared from the blood can be calculated and compared with normal. The accuracy of the test depends on a full urine collection over the 24 hour period.

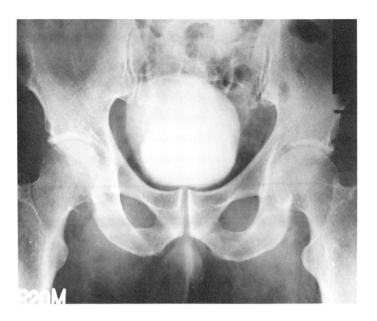

Intravenous urography (IVU), pyelography and renal ultrasound

An IVU is an X-ray of the kidneys taken after an intravenous injection of an iodized oil. The dye is concentrated by the kidney and is opaque to X-rays. Consequently, the X-rays may reveal both normal and abnormal anatomical details of the kidneys, ureters and bladder. A laxative should be given 36 hours before and no fluids should be allowed for 6 hours prior to the IVU, except in patients with renal failure who should not be fluid depleted or given laxatives, as these manoeuvres may worsen renal function.

In patients with suspected obstruction of the lower renal tract an antegrade pyelogram may be performed. This involves introducing a fine-bore needle into the kidney pelvis (under X-ray or ultrasound guidance) and then injecting dye to reveal the site of the obstruction. A fine catheter can also be introduced at this stage to drain urine away from the kidneys so that pressure on the kidney can be relieved, to allow it to function properly.

Similarly, X-rays can be taken by introducing fine catheters into the lower ends of the ureters and injecting dye, a retrograde pyelogram. This has to be done in the operating theatre since it

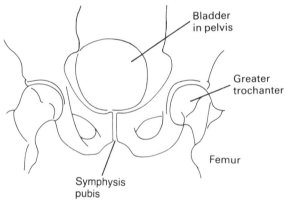

Fig. 11.5 Intravenous pyelogram showing close-up of bladder and pelvis.

involves cystoscopy. Ultrasound is a relatively new technique which involves bouncing sound waves off the kidney. It can be used to measure the size of the kidney and in particular to see if renal cysts or obstructions are present (e.g. when the pelvis of the kidney becomes swollen with urine, hydronephrosis).

Renal biopsy

This procedure involves inserting a special needle (through the skin of the back) directly into the kidney under X-ray screening or ultrasound. It is usually performed under a local anaesthetic with the patient lying prone. Renal biopsy may yield valuable information about the nature of the kidney disorder since the microscopic structure of the glomerulus and surrounding tissue can be examined using a light microscope or electron microscope.

Bleeding may occur after biopsy either around the kidney itself or into the renal tract. The pulse and blood pressure should be closely monitored for 24 hours and urine specimens examined for the presence of blood. The patient should be nursed supine and encouraged to drink at least 1 litre of water over the next few hours.

Other special procedures

Occasionally, other methods may be used to investigate the renal tract. The renal artery may be visualised by injecting dye directly into it through a catheter passed via the femoral artery (renal arteriography). Narrowing of the artery or abnormal vessels associated with kidney tumours can be seen. The renal vein can be investigated in a similar way (renal venography).

Patients with unexplained incontinence or increased frequency may undergo bladder function tests which involve measuring the flow of urine, and recording the pressure in the bladder and urethra.

Hospitals with nuclear medicine departments can use radio-isotopes to examine the site, size and function of the kidney, as well as to look for obstruction and narrowing (stenosis) of the renal artery.

RENAL FAILURE

Renal failure is when the kidneys fail to function normally with a resultant rise in the blood levels of urea and creatinine. The urine output usually, but not always, falls. It can occur suddenly (acute) or gradually over a period of months or years (chronic).

Acute renal failure

There is a large number of causes of renal failure, but they can be grouped into the following categories:

1. Acute tubular necrosis. This is a histological description which is thought to result from two major causes: injury to the kidney because of an impaired blood supply or due to nephrotoxic substances.

There are several causes, including the following:
   a. Severe shock. Here the blood pressure falls so low that the blood flow through the kidneys practically ceases. Shock may result from severe blood loss, heart failure or overwhelming infections (septicaemia).
   b. Mismatched blood transfusion. The haemoglobin which is released from red blood cells is highly toxic to the kidney.
   c. Crush injuries. Severe muscle injury allows myoglobin to escape from the cells and this, like haemoglobin, is toxic.
   d. Drugs. Some drugs, e.g. sulphonamides, gentamicin, are known to damage the kidney.
   e. Poisons. Mercury salts and the weed-killer paraquat, are nephrotoxic.

2. Impaired blood supply to the kidneys. Occulsion of both renal arteries or of both renal veins causes kidney failure. For example, in patients with severe atheroma of the aorta or aortic dissection, the orifices of both renal arteries may be involved.

3. Obstruction. Acute renal failure may result from obstruction anywhere between the renal pelvis and the urethra, but with obstruction above the bladder, both ureters will be involved unless there is only one kidney. A common cause of obstruction is stones in which condition the kidneys are no longer able to excrete urine. Other causes of obstruction include tumours in the bladder or tumours of the prostate or cervix which occlude the flow of urine from bladder to urethra.

4. Intrinsic renal disease including inflammatory diseases of the glomerulus (glomerulonephritis) or the surrounding tissue (acute interstitial nephritis).

Clinical features of acute renal failure

In most patients the cardinal sign of renal failure is the complete, or almost complete, suppression

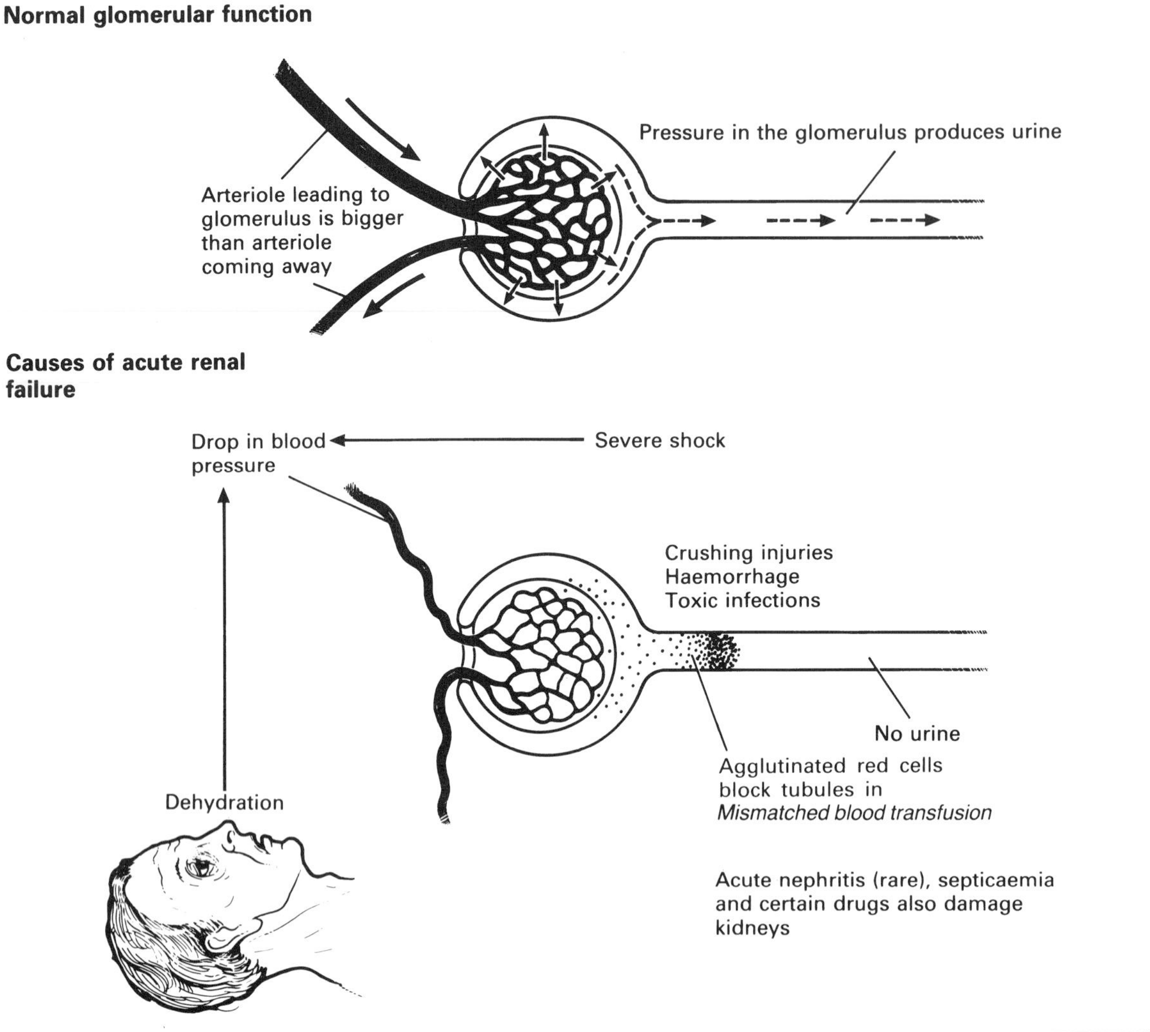

Normal glomerular function

Causes of acute renal failure

Fig. 11.6 The causes of acute renal failure.

of urine flow. Occasionally patients still pass large volumes of urine but it is of poor quality and the blood levels of urea and creatinine rise (polyuric renal failure). If the kidneys do not recover within 7–10 days and the patient is not dialysed, the condition will deteriorate. Vomiting, increasing drowsiness, twitching and, in some cases, convulsions occur.

Treatment of acute renal failure

Prevention (a) Mismatched transfusions. Before giving a blood transfusion, the patient's name, hospital number, the number of units of blood, its group and evidence of compatibility should be checked by two nurses.

(b) Shock. In all cases of shock due to loss of blood, early and adequate transfusions with blood (or plasma) will elevate the blood pressure and prevent renal failure. The aim is to raise the systolic blood pressure above 100 mmHg to ensure an adequate circulation of blood to all organs and tissues.

(c) Dehydration. An adequate fluid input must be provided for all patients, especially the elderly and children, to prevent dehydration. The nurse must not only provide the fluids but must ensure that the patient takes them. Accurate input and output fluid charts will help ensure that sufficient fluids are being taken.

Curative Development of anuria suggests severe damage and the patient needs intensive care during the acute phase until the kidneys begin to function again.

(a) Nephrotoxic substances should be withdrawn and obstruction (which is treatable) ruled out.

(b) Dehydration is corrected with oral or intravenous fluids. When the patient is in fluid balance (neither dehydrated or fluid overloaded), sufficient fluids are given daily to counterbalance the losses from skin and lungs (about 500–800 ml per day), with a further amount of fluid equal in quantity to any gastrointestinal losses or urine passed. Daily weights are essential for accurate fluid balance assessment.

(c) Frequent estimations of blood potassium, other electrolytes, urea and creatinine are necessary during the course of the illness. Potassium may accumulate during the anuric stage causing lethargy, muscle weakness and rhythm disturbances of the heart.

(d) Adequate nutrition with at least 2000 kcal/day is necessary along with supplementary minerals and vitamins. The protein intake is reduced to 60 g per day to prevent overloading the body with urea but once recovery begins, a normal protein intake is allowed.

(e) Dialysis. A patient with kidney failure who does not respond to the above measures will require dialysis to keep as fit as possible, especially if the potassium is very high, if there is fluid overload or if there are uraemic symptoms (hiccups, vomiting, convulsions).

There are two types of dialysis: *haemodialysis* and *peritoneal dialysis*. Haemodialysis involves passing the patient's blood through a kidney machine where waste products are removed. It requires special expertise, is expensive, and the patient must receive anticoagulants during the procedure (which can be dangerous if the patient is bleeding, say from a peptic ulcer). Haemodialysis is preferable for the severely ill patient, especially if he has undergone a recent operation. It corrects electrolyte abnormalities rapidly and

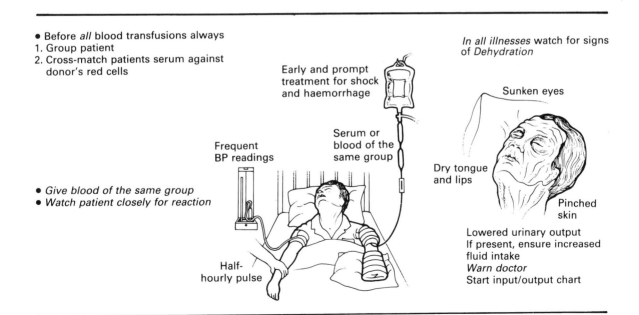

Fig. 11.7 The prevention of acute renal failure.

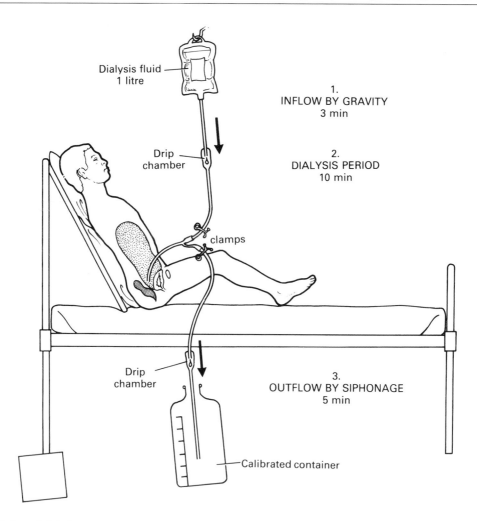

Dialysis fluid
1 litre

1.
INFLOW BY GRAVITY
3 min

Drip
chamber

2.
DIALYSIS PERIOD
10 min

clamps

Drip
chamber

3.
OUTFLOW BY SIPHONAGE
5 min

Calibrated container

Fig. 11.8 Peritoneal dialysis.

carries less risk of infection than peritoneal dialysis.

Peritoneal dialysis involves running dialysis fluid into the peritoneal cavity via a special catheter. The peritoneum acts as a dialysis membrane across which potassium and other waste products can diffuse into the dialysis fluid. The fluid is repeatedly run in and out of the peritoneal cavity in cycles of 30–60 minutes, or longer. It may take several hours to notice an improvement in the patient's well-being. Peritoneal dialysis is simple, cheap and can be carried out in a district hospital. Special attention must be paid to aseptic techniques when changing bags of dialysis fluid and to the peritoneal catheter site, to prevent the development of peritonitis.

When the patient begins to pass urine again, dialysis can be withdrawn. During the recovery phase there is often a marked diuresis, as the kidneys are not able to produce concentrated urine. It may last for 2–3 weeks and it is very important to keep the patient's weight constant by increasing the fluid intake, and by providing adequate nutrition.

Chronic renal failure

About 70–80 people per million (under the age of

70 years) develop chronic renal failure every year. It is more common in men than women.

Causes

Chronic renal failure may follow almost any type of kidney disease and is characterized by a gradually rising plasma urea and serum creatinine. It is most commonly caused by the following:

1. glomerulonephritis
2. hypertensive renal disease
3. reflux nephropathy
4. polycystic kidneys
5. chronic obstruction, including stones
6. analgesic nephropathy
7. kidney disease due to constitutional disorders such as diabetes, myelomatosis, polyarteritis, or systemic lupus erythematosus.

Clinical features

There may be few symptoms and signs, or the patient may be severely ill. Early on there is general fatigue, but as the degree of kidney failure progresses almost every system in the body may become involved, including the following:

1. Gastrointestinal – nausea, vomiting and diarrhoea are frequently present and hiccupping may be a prominent feature.
2. Neurological – drowsiness and twitching occur, progressing to coma and fits in the terminal stages.
3. Cardiovascular – the blood pressure is usually elevated and pericarditis may occur (inflammation of the serous membranes surrounding the heart) causing chest pain.
4. Respiratory – chest infections are common because the immune system is impaired. Pulmonary oedema may develop quickly if fluid overload occurs.
5. Haematological – patients become pale due to anaemia.
6. Skin – itchiness (pruritus) and a yellow tinge to the skin are common.
7. Eyes – patients may complain about dim-

ness of vision due to changes in the retina of the eye (retinitis).
8. Locomotor – bone disease causing bone pains and fractures, muscular weakness and arthritis can all develop.
9. Nephro-urological – the total amount of urine is usually normal or even increased. Albumin may be found in the urine, denoting the presence of a kidney lesion.

Treatment

There is no cure for chronic renal disease, and the aims of treatment are to alleviate symptoms, prevent complications and to maintain kidney function as long as possible:

1. As the plasma urea rises, symptoms such as nausea and vomiting may develop, which may be alleviated by restricting the amount of protein in the diet to 40–60 g a day.
2. The salt and water status of the patient must be carefully monitored by accurate weighing and, if necessary, fluid balance charts. Kidney patients may easily become dehydrated, causing a more rapid decline in kidney function, or overloaded, causing high blood pressure and pulmonary oedema.
3. The blood potassium tends to rise, causing weakness and, if very high, cardiac arrest. This can be prevented by avoiding foods which contain a lot of potassium, such as coffee, fruit and chocolate.
4. If the blood pressure is raised, hypotensive drugs should be given.
5. Anaemia – due to lack of erythropoietin from the kidney, may necessitate a blood transfusion, but these patients generally tolerate anaemia well. Too many transfusions cause the liver to become overloaded with iron.
6. Infections need prompt treatment.
7. Most patients will eventually require long-term dialysis or a kidney transplant.

Long-term dialysis and kidney transplantation

Both peritoneal dialysis and haemodialysis can be performed long-term. Continuous ambulatory peritoneal dialysis (CAPD) as it is called, requires

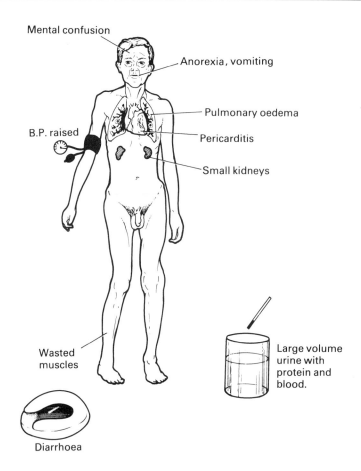

Mental confusion

Anorexia, vomiting

Pulmonary oedema

B.P. raised

Pericarditis

Small kidneys

Wasted muscles

Large volume urine with protein and blood.

Diarrhoea

Fig. 11.9 Chronic renal failure – common clinical features.

the presence of an indwelling peritoneal catheter. The patient is trained to run dialysis fluid into the peritoneum where it is left for several hours before being exchanged for fresh fluid. Three or four such cycles are performed every day, each taking about twenty minutes. The procedure has to be carefully performed to prevent infection.

Haemodialysis involves linking the patient's circulatory system to an artificial kidney machine, by inserting two large needles into a special blood vessel. The blood vessel (or Cimino fistula) is formed by an operation which anastomoses an artery (usually the radial artery in the forearm) to a superficial vein. A single haemodialysis takes 4–6 hours and has to be repeated three times a week. Patients can be trained to dialyse themselves on their own kidney machine at home.

Renal transplantation allows a patient to return to a reasonably normal life-style without having to worry about dialysis. A kidney transplant can be donated by a close relative of the same blood group and tissue type as the patient, or it can be taken from someone who has recently died. Powerful drugs which suppress the immune system have to be given to prevent the kidney being rejected by the patient and are usually successful. Such drugs may also predispose the patient to infection and a careful balance needs to be sought.

GLOMERULONEPHRITIS

Glomerulonephritis is the term used to describe the appearance of the kidney under the micro-scope when the glomeruli are found to be inflamed. There are many different types of glomerulonephritis but the symptoms and signs that they produce tend to overlap, so the only way to be sure of which one an individual patient is suffering from is to perform a renal biopsy.

Glomerulonephritis manifests itself clinically in six ways:

1. blood in the urine (haematuria)
2. protein in the urine
3. acute nephritic syndrome or acute glomerulonephritis
4. acute nephrotic syndrome
5. acute renal failure
6. chronic renal failure.

The first two are asymptomatic. A patient may have more than one feature, for example, blood and protein in the urine along with chronic renal failure. Acute and chronic renal failure have been discussed; glomerulonephritis is one of the causes of acute and chronic renal failure. The acute nephritic and acute nephrotic syndromes are discussed below. In the majority of cases no causes can be found, but occasionally glomerulonephritis may follow an infection (streptococcal sore throat, bacterial endocarditis, malaria), drugs (gold), tumours or constitutional ailments (diabetes, systemic lupus erythematosus).

Acute nephritic syndrome (acute nephritis)

This syndrome is characterized by fever, blood and protein in the urine, oedema of the face (especially around the eyes) and ankles and a high blood pressure. *Typically*, it follows a streptococcal sore throat or skin infection in a child or young adult. The onset is usually fairly sudden. The urine output falls and the urine that is passed is smoky in colour from the presence of blood. Proteinuria is usually very heavy. Casts and red cells can be seen if the urine is examined under the microscope. The high blood pressure may cause severe headaches, vomiting and sometimes convulsions. Rarely, acute renal failure develops.

The disease is usually self-limiting and most patients recover completely. The only treatment that is required in the majority of cases is complete rest, salt restriction, penicillin and sometimes a diuretic or hypotensive drug.

Nephrotic syndrome

This is characterized by three findings:

1. very heavy proteinuria (precisely, more than 3 g in 24 hours)
2. a low plasma albumin due to the loss of albumin in the urine
3. oedema due to the low plasma albumin.

The nephrotic syndrome frequently occurs in children, but adults may also be affected. The oedema is usually most marked in the legs in the early stages, but this may be followed by ascites, pleural effusion and oedema of the face and arms.

The nephrotic syndrome may be caused by several types of glomerulonephritis. The outlook in children is almost always good, but the outcome is less predictable in adults, some of whom may later develop chronic renal failure. Treatment is often supportive as no specific therapy is available for many of the types of glomerulonephritis which cause the nephrotic syndrome. The patient is given a high protein, low-salt diet to counteract the heavy protein losses in the urine and the fluid retention. Diuretics are usually also prescribed. Some patients with nephrotic syndrome are very prone to deep venous thrombosis, so exercise should be encouraged. As in all kidney patients, the weight and blood pressure (lying and standing) must be carefully recorded.

Some patients with nephrotic syndrome, particularly children, have a glomerulonephritis which responds well to steroids. The steroids are given for 6–8 weeks. Some patients relapse within 1–2 years but respond to a further course of steroids. Infections must be treated promptly as both the nephrotic syndrome and steroids lower the patient's resistance.

HYPERTENSIVE RENAL DISEASE

Severe kidney damage, resulting in renal failure, is particularly common in the severe and rapidly progressive form of high blood pressure know as 'malignant' hypertension. Malignant hyperten-

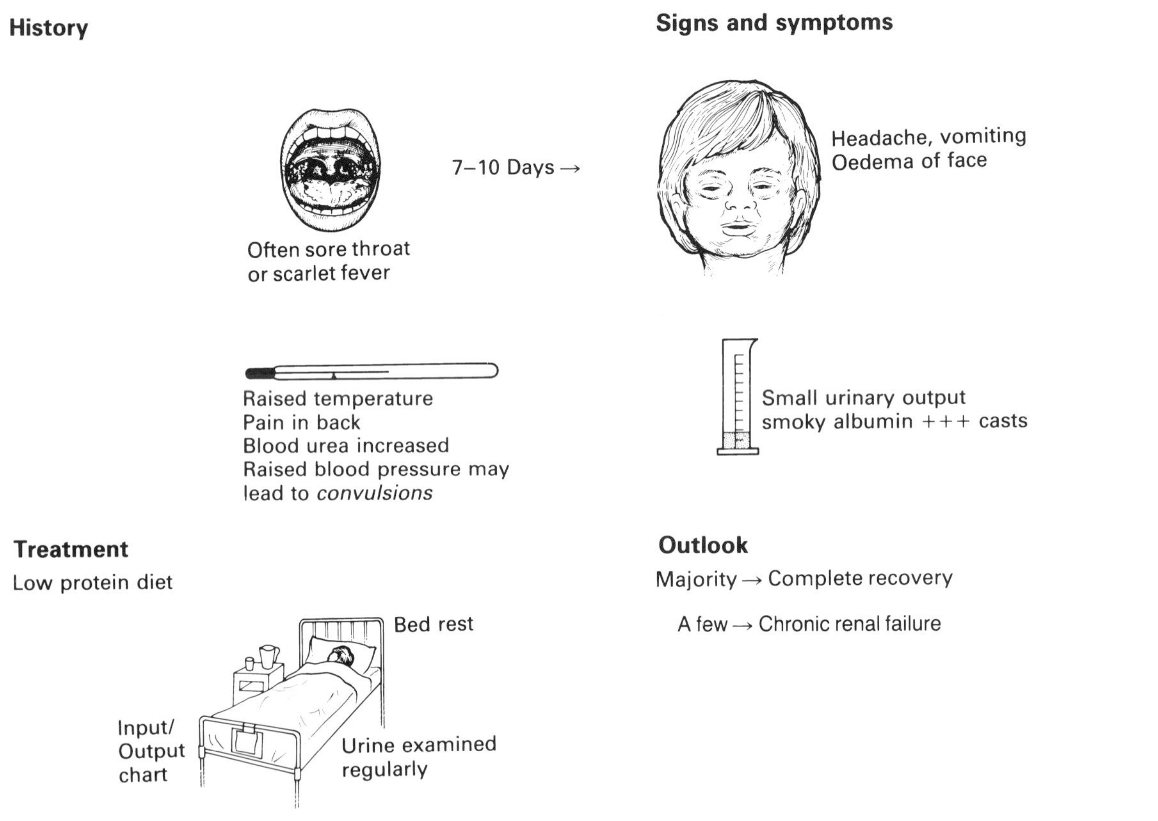

History

Signs and symptoms

7–10 Days →

Often sore throat
or scarlet fever

Headache, vomiting
Oedema of face

Raised temperature
Pain in back
Blood urea increased
Raised blood pressure may
lead to *convulsions*

Small urinary output
smoky albumin + + + casts

Treatment

Low protein diet

Outlook

Majority → Complete recovery

A few → Chronic renal failure

Bed rest

Input/
Output
chart

Urine examined
regularly

Fig. 11.10 Glomerulonephritis.

sion can be quickly recognized by the presence of severe vascular changes in the blood vessels of the retina (hypertensive retinopathy). It has a poor prognosis not only from progressive renal failure but also from cerebrovascular accidents and other vascular problems. Treatment involves controlling the blood pressure with hypotensive drugs and treating the renal failure as outlined above.

URINARY TRACT INFECTION AND REFLUX NEPHROPATHY

Infection in the urinary tract can occur in the urethra (urethritis), in the bladder (cystitis), in the prostate (prostatitis), in the pelvis of the kidney (pyelitis), or in the kidney substance (pyelonephritis). The organism which most commonly causes a urinary tract infection (UTI) is *Escherichia coli*. Most pathogenic organisms are found in normal bowel flora and reach the urinary tract via the urethra.

Acute bacterial cystitis

Acute cystitis is common, particularly in women, as the short urethra predisposes to infection of the bladder. Cystitis is also likely to arise where there is obstruction to urine flow or disease within the bladder, such as stones, tumour or an enlarged prostate. Patients who are paraplegic are prone to bladder infections, particularly if long-term catheters are used; infection can cause kidney scarring in this group of patients, resulting in renal failure. Finally, specific diseases such as gonorrhoea and tuberculosis may cause cystitis.

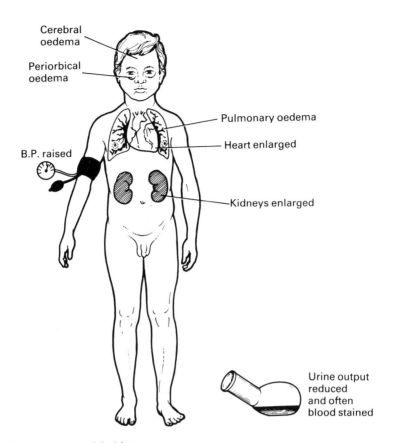

Fig. 11.11 Acute nephritis – common clinical features.

The symptoms of acute cystitis are pain on passing urine (dysuria), frequency and sometimes haematuria. The urine (obtained as an MSU) contains protein, pus and the infecting organisms. Treatment is with appropriate antibiotics and attention to any predisposing factor, such as stones, is necessary.

Acute pyelonephritis

This usually results from untreated bacterial cystitis. Symptoms of frequency and dysuria are associated with loin pain and tenderness, fever and possibly rigors. The white blood cell count is high, indicating a systemic infection. Urine contains protein, pus and a heavy growth of bacteria. The illness may be very severe, especially if the patient becomes shocked as a result of septicaemia.

The patient should be nursed in bed and encouraged to drink 3 litres of fluid a day. Appropriate antibiotics are given, using the intravenous route, in all but the mildest cases.

Reflux nephropathy

The term reflux nephropathy is used nowadays instead of the older term 'chronic pyelonephritis'. Reflux nephropathy describes a particular type of kidney scarring, seen radiologically, where the calyces of the kidney are distorted and the kidney tends to be slightly smaller than normal. Reflux nephropathy begins in infancy and is due to the reflux of urine up the ureter reaching the kidney, so that damage to the kidney substance occurs. It is associated with recurrent urinary infections and, occasionally, leads to renal failure in adult life. There is controversy as to whether very

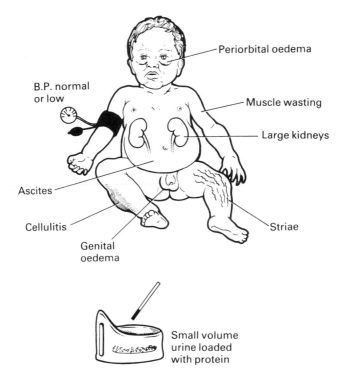

Periorbital oedema

B.P. normal or low

Muscle wasting

Large kidneys

Ascites

Cellulitis

Striae

Genital oedema

Small volume urine loaded with protein

Fig. 11.12 Nephrotic syndrome – common clinical features.

young children with reflux nephropathy should have an operation to prevent it occurring. It is not yet clear whether such operations are beneficial. Infections should however, be treated with antibiotics.

Prostatitis

The prostate gland in men may be a focus of infection and can give rise to fever, dysuria, increased frequency and perineal pain. Bacteria are usually present in the urine. Treatment is with antibiotics.

OBSTRUCTIVE UROPATHY

Obstruction to the flow of urine may occur anywhere in the urinary tract. It may be acute or chronic. Renal failure may develop if both kidneys are affected although one functioning kidney will prevent the development of renal failure.

There are many causes of obstruction at all levels of the urinary tract which include stones, tumours, strictures and an enlarged prostate gland. Sophisticated radiology may be required to diagnose the site and the reason for the obstruction (see above). Treatment, frequently surgical, is aimed at relieving the obstruction. Obstruction allows urine to stagnate in the renal tract, predisposing to infection. Complete obstruction for several weeks or months may cause total destruction of the affected kidney.

RENAL STONE DISEASE

Renal stones may develop as a result of various metabolic disorders which affect the handling of calcium and other minerals by the body. Frequently the reason is unclear. Renal stones usually contain calcium and so are visible on X-rays. In 5% of patients the stones are made up

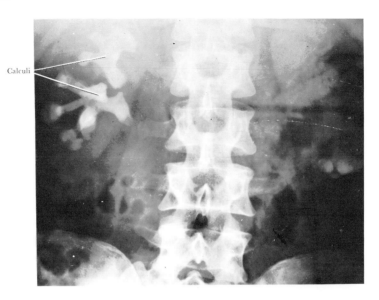

Calculi

Fig. 11.13 Renal calculi. Typical staghorn stones in the right kidney.

of uric acid (e.g. in patients with gout) and these are not visible on X-ray.

Renal calculi may remain silent in the kidney, but if they move into a ureter they can cause renal colic manifested by severe sharp pain along with restlessness, sweating and vomiting. The pain characteristically starts in the loin and radiates downwards and forwards to the groin.

If a stone gets blocked in a ureter it can obstruct the kidney, leading to dilatation of the kidney pelvis and ureter above the stone. Distention of the pelvis and calyces of the kidney is called hydronephrosis and is usually associated with impaired function of the kidney.

Small stones may be passed in the urine; filtering the urine will allow the stone to be isolated and sent to the laboratory for analysis. Surgery is required for stones which are causing obstruction. Patients who have recurrent renal stones can be treated using a variety of drugs and by encouraging a high fluid diet.

INHERITED RENAL DISEASE

There are several inherited renal diseases, the most common of which is adult polycystic disease. In this condition many large cysts develop

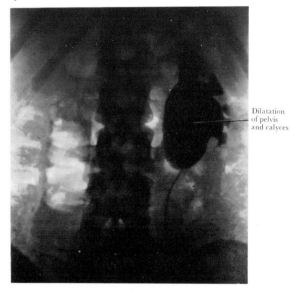

Dilatation of pelvis and calyces

Fig. 11.14 Hydronephrosis of the left kidney outlined by retrograde pyelography.

within the kidney so that the anatomy is distorted and the function of the kidney is upset. Symptoms include haematuria, loin pain, urinary tract infection, high blood pressure and, ultimately, the symptoms associated with renal failure. The cysts can easily be seen on ultrasound. There is no specific treatment for this condition.

TUMOURS

Renal cell carcinoma (hypernephroma, Grawitz tumour)

This is the commonest malignant tumour affecting the kidney and is responsible for 2% of all deaths from malignant disease. It affects mainly adults and is rare in children.

Clinical presentation

This tumour classically presents with painless haematuria, loin pain and abdominal swelling. In addition it may present obscurely as a fever of unknown origin, unexplained anaemia or erythrocytosis (increase in the red cell mass due to erythropoietin production by the tumour), hypercalcaemia, amyloidosis, abnormal liver function tests, a Budd Chiari syndrome (due to growth of tumour into the inferior vena cava) or with symptoms due to metastases. The diagnosis is confirmed radiologically using IVU, renal ultrasound and renal arteriography (see investigations section). All patients must have a cystoscopy to exclude other lesions causing haematuria. Urine cytology may reveal malignant cells.

Treatment

The tumour is removed surgically (nephrectomy). If the patient has only one or two metastases these should be removed as well because the survival rate is good.

Carcinoma of the bladder

Carcinoma of the bladder is common and occurs more frequently in males than in females. There is a high incidence of the tumour in workers in the rubber and dye industries; it has been associated with various chemicals, including naphthylamine. Smoking cigarettes also predisposes to the development of this tumour.

Clinical presentation, diagnosis and treatment

Typically, a patient presents with painless haematuria. Occasionally the advanced disease causes loin pain due to obstruction of a ureter and hydronephrosis, or acute anuric renal failure if both ureters are obstructed.

Diagnosis is made on IVU (which shows a filling defect in the bladder) and cystoscopy. On cystoscopy most tumours appear like warts on the bladder mucosa and can be treated by diathermy (cauterization) through the cystoscope. More advanced tumours are usually treated with radiotherapy. Patients are monitored by check cystoscopy at intervals.

Benign prostatic hypertrophy and carcinoma of the prostate

The prostate is an organ which lies at the base of the bladder around the urethra in males. With advancing age, it tends to enlarge (benign prostatic hypertrophy) and may result in obstruction of the urethra. Occasionally, malignant change occurs. These changes are probably hormonally induced; testosterone encourages the growth of the prostate.

Clinical presentation

Prostatic enlargement causes increased frequency of micturition, difficulty in initiating micturition and nocturia (having to pass urine at night). Sometimes the symptoms progress until no urine can be passed at all (acute retention of urine) and the patient presents as an emergency with a large painful bladder.

Occasionally, patients present with anuric renal failure due to obstruction. Carcinoma of the prostate may present as a result of metastases – usually a pathological bone fracture or general ill health.

Treatment

Patients with prostatic hypertrophy may undergo prostatectomy, usually performed via a special cystoscope. The prostate is removed through the urethra and the operation is called 'transurethral resection of the prostate'. Very large prostates are removed through an abdominal incision in an 'open prostatectomy'.

Carcinoma of the prostate can be treated with stilboestrol, an oestrogen which causes the tumour to regress in many patients. Prostatectomy may also be required for severe obstruction.

12

Metabolism and vitamins

Before considering the specific diseases which affect the metabolism of the body it is first necessary to understand a little about normal metabolism and how it can be upset.

The term *metabolism* is used to define the various chemical processes which occur continuously in the body to allow growth and renewal to take place, and the way the body uses nutrients to provide the energy that it needs. An example of these changes is the breakdown of foods into suitable substances which can be used by the body for the provision of energy and the repair of tissues. The metabolism of the body requires very many different factors if normal health is to be maintained. The essential nutrients and components supplied by foods comprise:

1. carbohydrate (glucose and starch)
2. fat
3. protein
4. non-nutrient bulk (fibre)
5. mineral salts
6. vitamins
7. water.

In addition to an adequate intake of these compounds, metabolism depends on normal functioning of the gastrointestinal tract for absorption of nutrients. The liver is important for many aspects of metabolism, particularly processing of carbohydrates (glucose) and fats. The kidneys are vital for the normal disposal of metabolic waste products, for balancing the salt and water content of the body, and in the production of the hormones, vitamin D and erythropoetin. The muscles are major users of glucose and also store a little glucose (as glycogen) for emergency use. A number of important hormones such as insulin, glucagon, thyroxine, cortisol, growth hormone and adrenalin have profound effects on metabolism and imbalance of these hormones can have deleterious effects. From the above it can be seen that normal metabolism depends on many different factors in the body.

CARBOHYDRATES

Carbohydrates are the least expensive and most freely available type of food. Bread, cereals, rice, potatoes and flour-based foods such as spaghetti are all carbohydrates and form the bulk of the diet in most parts of the world.

Sugar is also a carbohydrate and is obtained from cane and from beet. It is a highly concentrated form of carbohydrate, and is very quickly absorbed from the bowel into the blood stream as glucose. Sugar is used not only as a sweetener in tea, coffee and fruit drinks but it is also present in jams, sweets, chocolates, biscuits and cakes, and it is added to savoury items such as soups and baked beans. Sugar disposes to tooth decay (*caries*), since it encourages the growth of bacteria at the gum margins. In the United Kingdom, the average consumption of sugar is about 55 kg per person annually. It is a very concentrated form of food and a large consumption of sugar promotes obesity. Fruit and milk contain the natural sugars, fructose and lactose.

Carbohydrate is a sugar polymer (many units linked in a chain) and is digested to glucose by the various juices in the saliva, stomach and intestines. The glucose is then absorbed into the blood. Glucose is stored in the liver and muscles in the form of glycogen, and is reconverted into glucose when needed to supply energy for the body.

The body can manufacture glucose in the liver from amino acids to supplement the dietary intake and stores of glucose.

Dietary fibre

Fibre is the term used for the supporting structure of plants and it is present in all parts of the plant. The term *roughage* has also been used. Consequently, fibre is present in vegetables, fruit and the outside of the grain of cereals, including wheat and rye. For the most part, fibre is not digested in the gastrointestinal tract and, since it is not absorbed, it has no energy value. Nevertheless, it plays an important part in the proper functioning of the bowel and produces most of the bulk of the stool. When a food contains a lot of fibre, there is a delay in digestion of its nutrient content, with a resulting slower absorption of products such as glucose and cholesterol.

Modern dietary habits have greatly reduced the intake of fibre in our food. The outer layers of the wheat grain (bran) are discarded in order to produce white flour and white bread. White bread, biscuits, pastry, cakes and puddings made from white flour contain very little fibre. White sugar, refined from beet and cane, is also low in fibre and is swiftly absorbed into the blood stream.

Fibre plays a role in diminishing the risk of developing haemorrhoids, diverticular disease and colon cancer.

A healthy diet should contain adequate fibre or roughage. Wholemeal bread contains the husk of the wheat germ as well as the germ itself and is preferable to white bread. Plenty of fruit and lightly cooked vegetables should be eaten. Wholemeal cereals should be taken at breakfast. Where constipation is troublesome, bran itself can be added to the food, which, combined with an increased fluid intake, increases stool bulk making it easier for the bowel to expel it.

Control of carbohydrate metabolism

In health, the blood concentration of glucose (loosely termed *sugar*) is kept fairly constant. The control of carbohydrate metabolism depends on various factors, including:

1. *Insulin*, a hormone secreted only by small groups of cells called the islets of Langerhans, which lie within the pancreas, plays a most important part in ensuring the proper uptake of glucose by the tissues of the body. Insulin enables the glucose both to be stored in the liver and

muscles in the form of glycogen and to be used as necessary. With a deficiency of insulin, such as occurs in the disease *diabetes mellitus,* glucose is neither burned nor stored effectively, so that it accumulates in the blood (*hyperglycaemia*) and is excreted in the urine (*glycosuria*). On the other hand, too much insulin causes a decline in blood glucose (low blood sugar), which, if severe, produces coma (*hypoglycaemia*).

2. Factors which oppose the action of insulin are collectively termed *insulin resistance,* and when these factors act powerfully a person is said to be insulin resistant. In this situation the body must make more insulin than normal to overcome the resistance. If it fails to make enough extra insulin diabetes may also develop. Factors leading to insulin resistance comprise:

a. *Glucagon,* a hormone also from the pancreatic islets, powerfully raises blood glucose by increasing the production of glucose by the liver.
b. Obesity results in the body being resistant to the actions of insulin particularly in individuals in whom the excess fats are deposited in the adipose tissues in the abdomen, i.e. *upper-body distribution obesity.*
c. Individuals who adopt a sedentary life-style are more insulin resistant.
d. Overactivity of a number of endocrine glands, especially excess adrenalin from the adrenal in phaeochromocytoma, excess cortisol from the adrenal glands in Cushing's syndrome, and excess growth hormone from the pituitary in acromegaly can each increase insulin resistance, raise blood glucose levels and even induce diabetes which may be permanent.

3. Normal liver function is essential for the proper storage of glucose (as glycogen). In some diseases of the liver the metabolism of glucose is upset.

FATS

The fats, next to carbohydrates, are a major energy source in foods. The principal fats eaten in the average diet are:

1. margarine or butter
2. oils and lard, as used in cooking
3. fat in meat
4. milk, cheese and cream
5. processed fat as in chocolate, biscuits and cake.

The diet in Western countries tends to be rich in fat and this is a contributory factor in the causation of *atherosclerosis,* angina, myocardial infarction and premature death. Fat in the diet is composed of glycerol bound to three fatty acids as triglyceride. Some fatty acids have maximum hydrogen bound (*saturated*) and others have few hydrogens (*monounsaturated* and *polyunsaturated*). Saturated fats are chiefly of animal origin such as lard, butter and milk. Polyunsaturated fats are those in many vegetable oils, such as corn oil and sunflower oil. A second type of fat is cholesterol. In the blood, which is a water-based solution, fats will not normally dissolve. They have to be carried by *lipoproteins* to make them soluble in water. It must be remembered that the body can synthesize both fatty acids and cholesterol as well as obtaining them from food.

Cholesterol, and saturated fats from which the body can make cholesterol, can deposit in the arteries and narrow them (*atherogenesis*). Hence, it is recommended that the diet be adjusted so that it contains less total fats, and, in particular, less saturated fats, with mono- and polyunsaturated fats used instead. Sunflower oil can replace lard for frying food, and polyunsaturated vegetable margarine can replace butter, for example.

The fats, after digestion by the intestinal and pancreatic juices, are absorbed to supply energy. Fat is stored throughout the body, thus providing a large reserve for future energy requirements. Fat has a very high energy content, twice that of either carbohydrate or protein, so in fat the body can store the same amount of energy for half the weight as would be the case with carbohydrate.

Factors controlling fat metabolism

1. Bile is necessary for the digestion and absorption of fat, and in obstructive jaundice (in which bile is absent from the intestinal tract) there is defective absorption of fat. The faeces

(stool) then become bulky and pale from excess of fat (*steatorrhoea*).

2. If the intestinal juices, especially the enzyme lipase in pancreatic juices, are absent the fat will not be broken down into a form suitable for absorption and an excess of fat will therefore be excreted in the faeces, again, causing steatorrhoea. Absence of the pancreatic juice is sometimes seen after *pancreatitis*, an inflammation of the pancreas which may develop when gall stones block the outflow of the pancreas gland, and also occurs in alcoholic patients.

3. If the small intestine is damaged deficient absorption of fat is a third cause of excess of fat in the stools and steatorrhoea.

In all these malabsorption syndromes poor absorption of fat and other nutrients leads to wasting and deficient growth.

As well as controlling glucose and carbohydrate metabolism, insulin is important in the control of fats. When insulin is deficient, as in untreated diabetes mellitus, there is excessive release of fats from body stores and these are used for fuel. Some of the final end-products of fat metabolism are, however, the poisonous acids acetoacetate and β-hydroxybutyrate (*ketone bodies*), which are normally burnt down very rapidly. When, however, an excess of fats is being metabolized (as in uncontrolled diabetes) ketone bodies accumulate in the body and the condition known as *ketosis* develops. Large accumulations of acidic ketone bodies are seen in uncontrolled diabetes and are the cause of diabetic coma. Ketoacidosis is discussed further under diabetes (p. 311).

Hyperlipidaemia

The diet in Western countries tends to be rich in fat, and this leads to high blood levels of cholesterol (*hypercholesterolaemia*) and of triglyceride (*hypertriglycerideaemia*). When both occur together this is a *combined hyperlipidaemia*.

Factors causing hyperlipidaemia

1. As an inherited genetic condition (*familial hyperlipidaemia*).
2. In diabetes, hypertriglyceridaemia or

combined hyperlipidaemia are common, particularly if the blood glucose control is poor.

3. In association with excess consumption of alcohol, hypertriglyceridaemia is common.
4. In hypothyroidism, hypercholesterolaemia may occur and it may correct with treatment of the thyroxine deficiency.

People with hyperlipidaemia are at risk of cholesterol deposition in the arteries (*atheroma*), particularly of the heart (*coronary arteries*) where it causes angina, myocardial infarction, and premature death.

Treatment of hyperlipidaemia is by a diet low in fat (30% of energy as fat), with most of the fat as mono or polyunsaturated fat. The diet should be high in fibre. Sugar and alcohol are limited. Energy restriction is required to treat obesity where the patient is overweight. Drug treatment may be required in patients with severe hyperlipidaemia unresponsive to intensive dietary control. Drugs are usually reserved for younger patients, people with very high plasma cholesterol, and individuals with other risk factors for the development of heart trouble, such as a family history or diabetes. Bile acid sequestrants (colestipol, cholestyramine), which bind bile acids in the gut, can lower cholesterol but these drugs may cause gastrointestinal side-effects. The fibrate drugs (bezafibrate, gemfibrosil) and the drug nicotinic acid lower both cholesterol and triglyceride and are useful when both are raised. The statin group of drugs (lovastatin, zimvastatin) can powerfully lower blood cholesterol levels, especially when combined with a low fat diet.

When treating hyperlipidaemia with the aim of decreasing atherogenesis it is most important to tackle all the risk factors present in the patient. Cessation of smoking, reducing obesity, controlling diabetes and hypertension, and encouraging regular exercise are all most important. Attempts to reduce heart disease in the population would be most effective if everyone adopted healthy dietary habits with a low fat intake, rather than just patients who suffer from heart disease or hyperlipidaemia.

The cholesterol in the blood is mostly carried as

low-density lipoproteins (LDL) and this form is particularly harmful. LDL particles have a high content of apolipoprotein B. Another cholesterol fraction is the high-density lipoproteins (HDL), which carry cholesterol away from tissues back to the liver. Thus, HDL is beneficial and protects against atherogenesis. The content of apolipoprotein A is high in HDL. The blood level of HDL is increased by exercise, small amounts of alcohol, and by oestrogen as used in hormone replacement treatment after the menopause. When managing patients with hypercholesterolaemia it is common practice to measure either the LDL and HDL concentrations (or LDL/HDL ratio) or alternatively the apolipoprotein A and B concentrations to assess whether cholesterol lowering treatment is warranted.

PROTEINS

Protein foods supply amino acids which are used by the body to build its own proteins for normal body function. The body's own proteins are continuously renewed by the processes of protein breakdown and protein synthesis. These events occur in the normal course of wear and tear of tissues and growth of new tissues. Apart from this primary function, amino acids from ingested and body proteins can also be used, like carbohydrates and fats, as a source of energy.

The main sources of proteins in a normal diet are:

1. meat and fish
2. cheese and milk   } animal proteins
3. eggs
4. peas, beans and flour.   vegetable proteins

Proteins are made up of twenty different amino acids joined together in a long chain. Some of these amino acids can be made in the body, whereas others which cannot be synthesized in the body are *indispensable*. They must be included in the diet to enable proper renewal of body proteins. Animal proteins, such as meat, provide a balanced complement of indispensable and dispensable amino acids, while vegetable proteins are an adequate but less well balanced source of amino acids.

Ingested proteins are broken down into the constituent amino acids in the process of digestion by the pepsin and hydrochloric acid of the stomach and by the intestinal juices. The various amino acids are then absorbed into the blood stream and distributed to the tissues.

In tissues throughout the body the absorbed amino acids are used to build proteins. Whereas carbohydrates form glycogen and fats (*triglycerides*), the proteins have a variety of different structures, and each protein serves a distinct function rather than acting as an inert energy store. For example, muscle protein is important for movement, liver enzyme proteins for the metabolism of glucose and fats in liver cells, the protein albumin is produced by the liver to provide the oncotic pressure of the blood, and the enzyme proteins of the digestive juices from the pancreas are released into the intestine and break down foods.

Protein structure and synthesis

The structure of proteins depends on the exact order of the different amino acids which make them up. The amino acid sequence is determined from a series of codes kept in the genes in the nucleus of every body cell, a blue-print. The genes are chains of deoxyribonucleotides (deoxyribonucleic acid, DNA) which specify the sequence for every protein, and also provide information to control the rate of production of messenger ribonucleic acid (mRNA). Messenger RNA is produced from DNA by the process of *transcription* where a faithful nucleic acid copy of the DNA is made and then moves out of the nucleus into the body of the cell (Fig. 12.1). In the cell body proteins are built from amino acids, joined precisely in the order specified by the mRNA, a process known as *translation*.

If any error creeps into the DNA code the relevant protein will either be produced with an incorrect sequence of amino acids, or may even fail to be produced at all. It will therefore be unable to do its task in the body. Examples which illustrate this situation are:

1. *Sickle–cell anaemia*, in which haemoglobin has an abnormal sequence and therefore haemo-

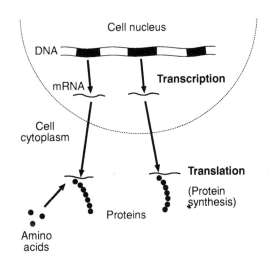

Fig. 12.1 The genetic code is stored as DNA in the cell nucleus. It is copied to messenger RNA by the process of transcription. In the cell cytoplasm the mRNA acts as a template for the production of proteins from amino acids which are joined in a chain in the process of translation.

globin in the red blood cells doesn't work properly if oxygen is very low, making the red cells sickle-shaped.

2. *Cystic fibrosis*, in which chloride-ion transporter proteins do not form properly so that chloride (and water which follows chloride) cannot easily move across cell membranes. In the lung this results in very sticky mucous and patients are at high risk of lung infection.

3. *Duchenne muscular dystrophy*, where the muscle protein dystrophin is not made correctly – with the result that severe muscle weakness develops.

These are genetic diseases, as the abnormal genetic codes are inherited from the patients parents.

The amino acids, unlike carbohydrates and fats, cannot be stored for future use. However, amino acids are released from a number of tissues, particularly muscle protein, in times of need, such as during starvation or in the course of serious illness, infection or after an operation. These amino acids then become available to produce proteins needed during the illness, and muscle is slowly lost (wasting of illness).

The amino acids which are not used for repair and the building up of tissues are broken down

by the liver into urea, which is excreted in the urine.

There is a number of rare genetic diseases each of which is due to the abnormal metabolism of a single amino acid. One example is *phenylketonuria* where phenylalanine metabolism is abnormal, the amino acid builds up to toxic high levels, and mental retardation results. The condition is routinely tested for with a heel blood sample taken from new-born babies.

Factors controlling protein metabolism

Protein and amino acid metabolism is under the control of factors which have widespread effects and others affecting specific proteins only.

Factors with widespread effects

The hormone insulin acts to slow the normal rate of protein breakdown in many tissues. Excess protein is lost in uncontrolled diabetes when insulin is deficient. Growth hormone, from the pituitary gland, generally increases protein synthesis and causes the body to use fats for fuel sparing amino acids.

Factors with specific effects

The body has ways of recognizing the need to produce more of each individual protein and when there is a need it signals synthesis to switch on the required protein. This involves the body first making more messenger RNA for the protein that is needed. An example of the need for synthesis of more particular proteins occurs in the condition anaemia. In this disorder there is an inadequate amount of haemoglobin in the red blood cells which cannot therefore carry enough oxygen to the tissues. This lack of oxygen is sensed by the kidneys which respond by making more of the protein hormone *erythropoetin* which is released into the blood. The erythropoetin then acts on the bone marrow and causes it to switch on synthesis of globin, which, with iron, forms haemoglobin, and also the other proteins needed to make more red blood cells.

Protein-energy malnutrition

Protein-energy malnutrition is a widespread problem in all areas of the developing world. It is particularly prevalent in sub-Saharan Africa. This condition impairs the growth of children and reduces the size of adults. Malnutrition decreases resistance to infectious illness, but protein requirements are increased by infection. The spectrum of protein-calorie malnutrition is as follows:

1. *Nutritional dwarfing* results from prolonged mild to moderate energy and/or protein deficiency and results in a proportional failure of height and weight.

2. *Marasmus* typically occurs in infants and is the result of a severe reduction of both energy and protein. The result is a retardation of growth with the reduction in weight more marked than the reduction of length. The child is emaciated with wasting of muscle and loss of subcutaneous fat. There is typically diarrhoea from gastroenteritis with resultant dehydration, and other infections may also be present such as tuberculosis. Oedema is *not* part of the condition.

3. *Kwashiorkor* occurs when there is insufficient amino acids and protein intake to meet the needs for protein synthesis in the body. Pitting oedema results from the reduction in plasma albumin concentration. In mild cases this affects the feet and ankles but in severe cases it can be generalized and involve the face. The child is emaciated, weak and miserable. Skin lesions include pigmentation, sloughing, excoriation and ulceration, and typically involve the legs and perineal region. The hair becomes fine, straight and sparse. There is angular stomatitis. Anaemia is common. There is often a distended abdomen from ascites, and there may also be hepatomegaly and splenomegaly from associated infectious disease such as malaria. Infection such as gastroenteritis, malaria, measles and tuberculosis can precipitate kwashiorkor and infection is typically present in the condition.

Management of protein-energy malnutrition depends on the immediate correction of dehydration and treatment of infection. Children can take a high-energy, high-protein diet and may require treatment of specific vitamin deficiencies. Prevention in the longer term depends on improving water quality and food sufficiency and safety. It therefore depends on planning of health services and agriculture, and reducing infectious disease. Mothers require education about food hygiene and the value of different foods for children. There needs to be an equitable distribution of an adequate hygienic diet within the population.

ELECTROLYTES (MINERAL SALTS)

To maintain good health many different electrolytes are essential, of which the following are some of the more important:

sodium
potassium
calcium
iron
iodine
fluoride

Sodium

Salt contains sodium and chloride, which are essential constituents of all the fluids of the body. Water is not retained in the body without salt. This is clearly seen in the case of heavy manual workers, for example, miners and stokers, who sweat a good deal and, as a result, lose both salt and water in their sweat. Drinking ordinary water without salt does not replace the lost fluid and they suffer from cramps caused by the lack of fluid. Taking extra salt with water, however, overcomes the cramps.

Oedema is accumulation of water in the tissues. It occurs in congestive heart failure and in the nephrotic stage of chronic nephritis. Diuretics cause excretion of salt in the urine and fluid is therefore excreted as well.

Aldosterone and cortisol (p. 324) are two of the hormones responsible for retaining sodium in the blood. When they are deficient, as in Addison's disease, the loss of sodium leads to loss of fluid. The body becomes dehydrated. The dehydration can be corrected by giving saline and replacement hormones in the form of hydrocortisone and fludrocortisone.

Excessive vomiting, such as may occur in pyloric stenosis or intestinal obstruction, leads to a loss of chloride in the vomit (gastric juice contains a large amount of chloride). In this condition it is necessary to replace the lost chloride as well as the fluid and saline is usually given.

Salt depletion syndrome. Salt restriction and diuretic drugs are used in the treatment of oedema, especially in cardiac, renal and hepatic oedema. The treatment of oedema with potent diuretics can, however, lead to a severe fall in body salt with serious results. It is most important that salt depletion is watched for in all patients on large doses of diuretics. The signs are:

1. The patient becomes lethargic, drowsy and physically weak.
2. Appetite is lost and nausea and vomiting may be present.
3. There is severe reduction in urinary output and in the excretion of urinary chlorides.
4. Abdominal and muscular cramps are sometimes present.
5. Oedema can, paradoxically, be present.
6. The blood pressure falls.
7. The blood sodium is severely reduced. The blood urea is raised.

Potassium

Potassium is an important constituent of all tissue cells. Disturbances in potassium metabolism have been increasingly recognized in recent years. Excess of potassium in the blood (*hyperkalaemia*) occurs to a significant degree in conditions associated with kidney failure, severe oliguria or anuria (p. 261), in the crises of Addison's disease, and during treatment with angiotensin-converting enzyme inhibitors (captopril, enalapril) which are used to treat hypertension and congestive heart failure. Symptoms of potassium excess include marked weakness with numbness and tingling of the extremities. Mental confusion can occur. Heart block develops with a slow and irregular pulse and finally cardiac arrest ensues.

Potassium depletion (*hypokalaemia*) is more commonly met with than potassium excess. The causes of potassium depletion are:

1. The prolonged use of diuretics in large doses.
2. It may develop in any disease or condition with a prolonged low food intake and especially when there is, in addition, excessive intake of sodium. Thus, after major operations, prolonged intravenous saline therapy combined with diminished food intake, is very liable to cause potassium deficiency. Similarly, this deficiency may arise in the recovery stage of diabetic coma, owing to the diminished food intake, intravenous saline therapy and, in addition, the excess loss of potassium in the urine.
3. Excessive vomiting and diarrhoea, especially where there is an inadequate diet.

The symptoms of potassium depletion include severe lethargy and weakness, mental confusion, abdominal distension and finally respiratory and cardiac failure. Heart rhythm irregularity can result, particularly if the patient is receiving the drug digoxin. Potassium depletion is corrected by giving potassium chloride, 8 g per day in divided doses by mouth. In more severe cases intravenous potassium may be necessary.

During prolonged treatment with diuretics such as the loop diuretics (frusemide, bumetanide) and the thiazide group of drugs, especially when large doses are given for prolonged periods, potassium supplements may be prescribed as a routine to prevent potassium depletion. An alternative means of preventing potassium depletion in this situation is to treat concurrently with a potassium-sparing diuretic (e.g. amiloride) or an angiotensin-converting enzyme inhibitor. A close watch must be kept on all patients, particularly elderly patients on prolonged diuretic therapy and not eating, as in these circumstances potassium (and sodium) depletion may easily develop.

Potassium deficiency greatly enhances the toxic actions of digoxin. Particular care must therefore be taken to note any signs of digoxin overdosage, and monitor plasma levels if practical, in patients with hypokalaemia.

Calcium

Calcium, which is present mainly in the diet in

milk and cheese, is essential for health, especially for:

1. formation of the bones
2. formation of the teeth
3. proper functioning of nerves and muscles.

The main store of calcium in the body is in the bones. It can be seen, therefore, that the requirements for calcium are likely to be greatest in childhood when the bones grow, and also in adults during pregnancy and lactation. For this reason, disturbances in calcium metabolism are most often seen during these times of extra need.

Control of calcium metabolism

Parathyroid hormone Disturbances of the hormone secreted by the parathyroid glands (*parathyroid hormone*) have a marked effect on calcium metabolism. Excess of parathyroid hormone (*hyperparathyroidism*), which occurs in tumours of the glands, accelerates release of calcium from the bones. The calcium in the blood rises and an excess of calcium is excreted in the urine.

On the other hand, lack of parathyroid hormone (*hypoparathyroidism*) causes a fall in the level of calcium in the blood. In severe cases this lack of calcium may be so great as to lead to the condition known as *tetany* with its irritability of the nerves and muscles. Lack of parathyroid hormone is occasionally seen after thyroidectomy if the parathyroid glands have been accidentally damaged or removed during the operation. Another cause of hypoparathyroidism is autoimmune destruction of the parathyroid glands.

Vitamin D is necessary for the proper absorption of calcium from the bowel, so that lack of this vitamin causes a deficiency of calcium in the body with consequent effects on the bones. In infancy and early childhood, when the bones are growing, a lack of this vitamin causes the disease known as *rickets*, of which predominant signs are changes and deformities of the bones. A lack of vitamin D is also seen in elderly subjects, in Asian immigrants, and occasionally in pregnant women in tropical countries. Poor diet and the social custom of covering women from public view, and hence sunlight, may cause a marked deficiency of vitamin D leading to the disease *osteomalacia*, the adult equivalent of rickets. Osteomalacia causes microscopic bone changes similar to those seen in rickets but without the deformity. In severe cases there may be a lowering of the blood calcium level with resultant tetany.

Calcitonin is a hormone produced by special cells scattered within the thyroid gland. It has an effect opposite to that of parathyroid hormone since it slows down release of calcium from the bones entering the blood. It is used in the treatment of Paget's disease.

Blood calcium may rise to dangerous levels in patients suffering from *cancer*. This can occur if the cancer spreads to the bones, or in the condition multiple myeloma which originates in the bone marrow. One common means whereby cancer can raise blood calcium levels is by synthesis of the hormone *parathyroid hormone related peptide* which is released by the cancer tissue and which acts in a very similar way to parathyroid hormone itself.

Osteoporosis

Osteoporosis is a thinning of the bones which results in decreased strength and a higher risk of bone fractures, especially of the vertebra in the back, of the hips (neck of femora), and of the wrist. There is thinning of the protein bone structure resulting in less calcium in the bones. The disease is common in older age, particularly in women after the menopause, in whom there is a decline in the level of blood oestrogen. It can arise due to inadequate calcium in the diet throughout life, prolonged lack of exercise which reduces the stresses on the bones, or after treatment with prednisolone or other anti-inflammatory steroid drugs which may be needed to treat asthma among other conditions. Treatment includes a high-calcium diet, regular exercise and hormone replacement treatment with oestrogen may be given in females after the menopause has occurred.

Iron

Haemoglobin, which is present in the red blood cells, is essential for the carriage of oxygen throughout the body and is partly made up of iron. Therefore, in the absence of sufficient iron there is a deficiency of haemoglobin, resulting in an iron-deficiency anaemia.

Deficiency of iron is usually due to insufficient dietary intake, inadequate absorption, or excessive loss due to bleeding. Iron is found mainly in meat, liver, eggs, peas and beans, and a diet which does not contain enough of these foods will lead to an iron-deficiency anaemia. Vitamin C (ascorbic acid) promotes absorption of iron.

In infants whose sole diet is milk, which has a poor iron content, anaemia is common. In women, continued heavy loss of blood in the menstrual flow frequently results in an iron-deficiency anaemia. In many parts of the world, particularly Africa and Southern Asia, iron-deficiency anaemia is very common. This is often due to a combination of a poor diet combined with gastrointestinal bleeding as a result of intestinal parasitosis, such as hookworm infection. Where there is no apparent reason for the occurrence of an iron-deficiency anaemia, a search may be needed for silent causes such as bleeding from a colon cancer.

Iodine

Iodine is essential for the formation of thyroxine, the hormone released from the thyroid gland. Iodine is normally found in many foodstuffs, but the amount depends on the soil and water. Soil and water in areas far from the sea, especially the mountain regions, may lack iodine, and thus the inhabitants of such areas often suffer from iodine deficiency. This is a particular problem in the Andes, Alps and the Himalayas. Iodine deficiency causes one form of enlarged thyroid (go–itre).

Fluoride

Fluoride maintains tooth enamel by remineralizing the early carious lesion and by inhibiting bacteria in dental plaque. There is usually sufficient fluoride in drinking water for this purpose, but in areas where the water contains too little fluoride the teeth of growing children are more likely to develop caries. The addition of fluoride to the water supply, or to salt, milk, or toothpaste, in these areas has yielded encouraging results in reducing the incidence of dental decay in children. A lowered intake of free sugar is beneficial in this respect also.

VITAMINS

Vitamins are factors present in various foods which are essential for the proper maintenance of health. There are many different vitamins, all of which tend to have some specific action on some part of the body's metabolism. Lack of a vitamin usually leads to certain well recognized changes in the body.

Deficiency of a vitamin may arise in several ways. *Inadequate diet* is a frequent cause of vitamin deficiency. Again, even if the diet is entirely adequate, *deficient absorption* from the gastrointestinal tract, because of some disease, may lead to vitamin deficiency. Finally, at certain times there may be an *increased demand* for vitamins, which, if not met, may give rise to vitamin deficiency. It is for this reason that vitamin deficiencies are most frequent during the periods of active growth, during pregnancy, in the course of severe prolonged illnesses and after major operations.

Vitamin A

Action. Vitamin A is necessary for the proper growth of certain epithelial cells of the body, especially those of the eyes, respiratory tract and skin.

Sources. Animal fats, butter, cheese, eggs, milk and liver.

Deficiency of vitamin A results in two related eye diseases and decreases resistance to infection. The eye diseases are:

1. *conjunctivitis* and *corneal ulceration*, also termed *xerophthalmia*, due to improper development of the epithelium of the eye
2. *night blindness*, i.e. great difficulty in seeing in the dark; here, the pigment in the eyes (visual purple) which is necessary for proper vision is not adequately formed.

Vitamin B complex

Vitamin B is not a single vitamin but is made up of several factors, many, though not all, of which are known to have a specific action.

The more important factors in the vitamin B complex are:

1. *vitamin B₁* (also called *thiamine*) – rich sources are yeast, cereals, peas, beans and eggs
2. *niacin*, mainly found in yeast, meat, liver and fish
3. *riboflavin*, chiefly found in milk, eggs, liver and kidney
4. *vitamin B₁₂* (p. 236).
5. *folic acid* (p. 236).

Deficiency of vitamin B complex is usually seen where several of the vitamins in this group are lacking together, but single deficiencies can occur.

Diseases due to deficiency of vitamin B complex

Beriberi The disease *beriberi* is caused by a deficiency of vitamin B₁ (thiamine). It is generally the case, however, that other factors are involved as well, because pure vitamin B₁ will not always cure the disease whereas an adequate diet, especially in protein, usually does.

Beriberi used to be a common condition in eastern and southern Asia but it has now almost entirely disappeared in affluent countries such as Japan and Taiwan. It continues to occur where the staple food is polished rice, as the polishing of the rice removes most of the vitamin B and especially the vitamin B₁. The condition is seen in the sub-Saharan region of Africa in association with generalized nutritional deficiency.

The disease is seen in two forms: wet beriberi, which causes congestive heart failure with oedema, and dry beriberi, which causes a peripheral neuropathy.

In western countries occasional cases of wet beriberi are seen in alcoholics, and these patients may also suffer a confusion state with faulty memory and the neuropathy.

Pellagra Pellagra is nutritional deficiency seen in poor peasants who subsist largely on maize. This diet is deficient in niacin and the indispensable amino acid tryptophan. In the past the

condition occurred in the southern States of America, but it is now found in areas suffering from famine in the sub-Saharan region of Africa. In developed countries sporadic cases are seen in individuals who suffer from chronic alcohol abuse. In these people the general food intake is reduced with energy replaced by alcohol.

The main symptoms of pellagra (remembered as the three Ds) can be divided into the following groups:

1. Gastrointestinal. Severe glossitis, stomatitis and *diarrhoea*.
2. Skin changes. Symmetrical *dermatitis* of the face and hands, with characteristic dark pigmentation in the later stages.
3. Mental. Weakness, anxiety and poor concentration, with *dementia* in severe chronic cases.

Treatment of beriberi and pellagra

Treatment consists mainly of the provision of an adequate diet, supplemented by large doses of combinations of B vitamins.

Vitamin C (ascorbic acid)

Action. Vitamin C is necessary for the proper growth of the capillary endothelium and for the repair of tissues. The main result of deficiency of this vitamin is haemorrhage from the capillaries.

Sources. Oranges, tomatoes, blackcurrant juice, lemons, potatoes and green vegetables.

Deficiency of vitamin C results in the disease *scurvy*. This was once a very common disease, especially among sailors and infants. Sailors on long voyages used to have to live on a diet lacking in fresh foods, especially fruits and vegetables. Infants who are bottle-fed with heated milk also commonly developed scurvy as heating milk destroys all its vitamin C content. As a result of the recognition of the cause of scurvy the disease is now very rare, especially in the infantile form, but it continues to occur in drought-affected populations such as Africa. Unfortunately, it is still seen in old people living on their own and unable to afford or obtain fresh fruit or vegetables. There are two main types of scurvy:

infantile scurvy and *adult* scurvy.

Infantile scurvy

This, as just mentioned, is now rare owing to the widespread preventive use of orange juice or other sources of Vitamin C. Breast-fed babies do not develop scurvy because there is sufficient vitamin C present in human milk to prevent the disease. The necessary boiling or pasteurization of cow's milk, however, destroys practically all the small amount of vitamin C present; as milk is the main if not the sole diet of infants, scurvy will develop in bottle-fed babies given cows' milk unless balanced formulations containing vitamin C are used.

Symptoms and signs The underlying specific lesion which accounts for most of the symptoms is *haemorrhage.*

1. Symptoms usually appear about the age of 8 to 10 months and not before 6 months. As already explained, scurvy never develops in breast-fed babies.

2. The commonest complaint is of severe fretfulness in the infant, especially if the limbs, which may be swollen, are touched. The child stops walking after they have learned to walk, or the age when they start walking may be delayed. The pain and swelling of the limbs is caused by haemorrhages under the periosteum of the bones.

3. The gums are swollen, red and spongy. The teeth if present decay and fall out.

4. Haemorrhages may also occur from the kidneys, bowel or nose. Anaemia is common.

Adult scurvy In adult scurvy the main symptoms are haemorrhages from the nose or into the skin (*purpura*), typically around the hair follicles on the legs. Swelling and bleeding of the gums with general debility and anaemia are also commonly present. There is also pronounced delay in the healing of any wound or ulcers that may be present.

Treatment of scurvy

For adults, as for infants, preventive treatment is important in certain conditions. In chronic gastrointestinal diseases necessitating a strict and prolonged dietary regime, care should be taken to ensure that a sufficiency of vitamin C is given. Extra supplies of the vitamin in the form of ascorbic acid, 100 to 200 mg daily, are often advisable. The treatment of an established case of scurvy is to give large doses of ascorbic acid, 1 to 2 g daily.

Vitamin D

Action. Vitamin D is responsible for the proper absorption of the calcium present in the diet. In its absence calcium is not absorbed from the bowel and the resultant lack of calcium impedes both the normal growth of bone and the normal activity of nerves and muscles.

Sources. The same foods that supply vitamin A, i.e. animal fats, butter, cheese, eggs, milk, liver and fish. However, in addition, to these food sources of the vitamin, sunlight (or ultraviolet light) has the peculiar property of being able to generate vitamin D by its action on the skin.

Lack of vitamin D results in the diseases *rickets* in growing children and *osteomalacia* in adults.

Rickets

Rickets used to be seen in infants brought up in poverty, but a general improvement of nutritional standards, including fortification of margarine, has made the disease much less common in this country. It is still widespread in parts of northern Africa and the eastern Mediterranean, and it occurs not infrequently in Mexico. The lack of sunlight combined with poor diet caused rickets. It is interesting to note, however, that infants in the tropics, because of the continuous sunlight, even if brought up on a poor diet, rarely develop rickets.

Rickets is also seen in infants as a complication of chronic gastrointestinal disease. In this type of disease vitamin D is not properly absorbed from the bowel and this accounts, for example, for the rickets of coeliac disease.

The main changes in rickets are those of disordered bone development caused by the lack of the vitamin, which is essential for normal growth of bone.

Symptoms and signs are as follows:

1. These are first noticed, as a rule, at about the age of 6 months; the infant becomes restless and fretful, sweats a good deal, especially around the head, while respiratory infections are also common.

2. The wrists and ankles become enlarged at an early stage. The child does not stand, crawl and walk at a normal age. The legs become bowed or, alternatively, knock-kneed when the child begins to walk owing to the weight of the body on the softened calcium-deficient bones (Fig. 12.2). The arms, as they are not weight-bearing, are less likely to show such signs.

3. The skull is softened and enlarged, and the typical appearance is one of a square head with a widely patent fontanelle. The spine may be bowed (kyphosis) or twisted (scoliosis).

4. The ribs show a characteristic beading

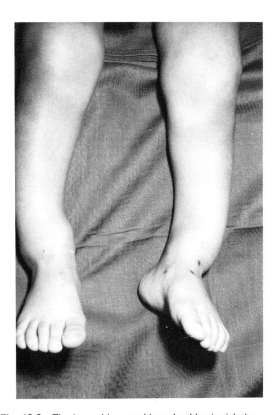

Fig. 12.2 The bowed legs and broad ankles in rickets.

('rickety rosary') owing to the enlarged epiphyseal margins.

5. The muscles and ligaments are flabby and lax.

6. There may be signs of tetany owing to the low blood calcium. Carpopedal spasm and spasm of the larynx with dyspnoea and cyanosis are seen in the tetany of infantile rickets.

Treatment Vitamin D in the form of calciferol completely restores the bones to normal in early cases, and calcium should also be given. In more advanced cases corrective active exercises may be necessary. If the body deformities do not disappear under treatment, splints and operations may be employed to try to correct them.

Osteomalacia

Osteomalacia is a softening and thinning of the bones where the protein structure forms but calcium is not laid down adequately. It is the adult equivalent of rickets. Like rickets it may be due to a diet inadequate in vitamin D and calcium, and where individuals are not exposed to sunlight. It is particularly liable to occur in the elderly and in Asian immigrants. Osteomalacia commonly follows malabsorption of vitamin D and calcium from the small intestine. The long bones and the pelvis become deformed and may fracture. There is a painful muscle weakness, particularly of the muscles of the upper leg.

Vitamin K

Action. Vitamin K is necessary for the formation of prothrombin, which is normally present in the blood and is one of the essential factors in blood clotting.

Sources. Spinach, cabbage, cauliflower and oats. In addition, the bacteria normally present in the bowel can manufacture vitamin K.

Deficiency of vitamin K results in the development of a condition termed a *coagulopathy*. There is a insufficient amount of vitamin K for the synthesis of prothrombin and therefore there is a low prothrombin level in the blood. This can lead to haemorrhage if the deficiency is sufficiently severe. There are limited stores of vitamin K in the newborn who are at risk of severe haemorrhage termed *haemorrhagic disease of the newborn*. Vitamin K is routinely given at birth to prevent the development of this disease.

Bile salts are essential for the proper absorption of vitamin K, and so in *obstructive jaundice* there is deficient absorption of the vitamin. In consequence, in prolonged cases of obstructive jaundice a low prothrombin level with resulting haemorrhages may arise and treatment is needed with vitamin K injections.

In *chronic diseases of the gastrointestinal tract* such as tropical sprue, coeliac disease and chronic ulcerative colitis, or after extensive removal of the bowel, the resultant deficient absorption of vitamin K may lead to prothrombin deficiency and haemorrhage.

Severe *liver disease*, such as may arise in cirrhosis of the liver or severe cases of hepatitis, can prevent the formation of prothrombin in the liver.

Anticoagulant drugs can prevent the normal production of prothrombin and so lead to a prolonged clotting time. *Warfarin* is very potent in this respect and in medicine it is used to produce a prolonged clotting time in the treatment of venous thrombosis.

WATER

Water makes up nearly 70% of the body. It is taken into the body either as fluid or in the solid foods, which themselves contain a considerable amount of water. The amount of water needed in 24 hours is normally about 2500 ml.

Water leaves the body in the following ways:

1. through the lungs in the expired air
2. through the faeces, which contain a small amount of water
3. through the skin, in the sweat
4. through the kidneys, in the urine.

The amount of water which leaves the body via the skin and kidneys varies; the greater the loss through the skin (as seen in very hot conditions) the smaller the excretion by the kidneys. Release of water from the kidneys is controlled by antidiuretic hormone from the posterior pituitary. When the plasma concentrations of salt rises antidiuretic hormone is released to signal the kidneys to retain water and therefore to produce less urine which is more concentrated. This is part of the body's mechanism to balance its water content. The high loss by the skin in high temperatures is a mechanism to cool the body and so prevent a rise in body temperature. In patients with infection and very high fever, large amounts of water can be lost in the sweat each day.

The body uses the excretion of water by the kidneys to get rid of waste products. If urine production by the kidneys is very severely diminished these waste products can accumulate in the blood stream with serious effects.

Thirst. This is one of the ways in which the body shows a need for more fluid. The essential mechanism depends on the total concentrations of all the electrolytes in blood, a measure termed the *osmolarity* of blood. When these increase (high osmolarity) this is sensed by an area of the brain, the hypothalamus, which triggers thirst so that the body knows to drink.

Deficiency of body fluid gives rise to *dehydration* while excess fluid causes *oedema*. In most situations salt is lost or gained along with water.

Water deficiency (dehydration)

Dehydration can be caused by an insufficient intake of water or, more often, by excessive loss of water. Excess loss of water is seen when excessive heat results in marked sweating. Dehydration caused through excessive loss of water by sweating occurs in marathon runners who run in extremely hot conditions. The loss of water and also of salt in the sweat causes cramps.

Other more serious effects of dehydration are also seen in diseases which cause excessive loss of fluid from the body such as:

1. diseases causing severe vomiting and diarrhoea
2. very high fevers, especially in hot climates
3. diabetes mellitus (owing to the excessive quantity of urine produced)
4. use of diuretic drugs

5. severe haemorrhage and burns
6. in prolonged coma, owing to the lack of fluid intake

Effects of dehydration

In the early stages fluid is withdrawn from the skin and tissues in order to maintain the blood volume, whilst to conserve water the kidneys excrete less urine. If the dehydration is not corrected more serious effects follow. The blood volume is reduced and this leads to deficient circulation, especially through the kidneys, which therefore fail to excrete waste products from the body. Acute renal failure (*uraemia*) may then develop, which needs to be rapidly treated.

Clinical recognition of dehydration

1. The patient is lethargic and dull. Thirst is usually present.
2. The skin loses its normal elasticity and if pinched remains in a fold.
3. The output of urine is markedly decreased and the urine passed has a high concentration of salts.
4. The blood urea concentration is raised.
5. The tongue is dry, but this also occurs in mouth-breathing.

The best clinical indication of an adequate fluid balance is the 24 hour output of urine, which should not fall below 1000 ml.

In most cases of dehydration there is a loss of salt as well as of water. During treatment salt plus water is used. This can be given orally or by intravenous infusion as saline, depending on the circumstances. In a case of severe dehydration 3000 to 4000 ml a day are often necessary; in less severe cases approximately 2500 ml. In treating fluid loss due to severe diarrhoea water with salt and sugar is given by mouth.

Excess of water in the body (oedema)

Fluid in the body flows from the blood into the tissues or vice versa. There are four main factors which control this flow:

1. The pressure in the small capillaries and veins tends to force fluid out from the circulation into the tissues. Therefore, anything, that increases the venous pressure tends to force fluid into the tissues. Owing to the force of gravity, increases in the venous pressure are most marked in the lowest parts of the body; as a result the flow of fluid into the tissues is greatest in the most dependent parts (ankle oedema). In addition, fluid also quickly collects in the pleural and peritoneal cavities.

2. Counteracting this venous pressure, which forces fluid out into the tissues, is the opposite action of the proteins in the blood (albumin and globulin). These proteins have the power, called the *osmotic pressure*, of attracting fluid, with the result that they keep fluid in the blood and out of the tissues. Normally, these two opposing factors, the venous pressure and the osmotic pressure, keep a steady balance of fluid within the body. Any upset in either leads, however, to changes in the water balance.

3. A third factor which can affect the amount of fluid in the tissues is damage to the walls of the capillaries, in consequence of which protein may leak through the walls and carry fluid.

4. Salt is another most important factor in oedema. Retention of salt in the body causes retention of water.

Types of oedema caused by the above factors

Cardiac oedema In congestive heart failure there are two reasons why oedema develops. First, there is an increase in the venous pressure which tends, when the pressure is great enough to overcome the opposing power of the blood proteins, to force fluid into the tissues. The oedema forms in the lowest parts of the body, as the venous pressure is greatest in these areas. If there is gross oedema, fluid also collects in the pleural and peritoneal cavities.

Secondly, the kidneys in congestive heart failure fail to excrete salt properly so that salt accumulates in the body. This causes retention of water which in turn causes oedema.

Renal oedema In the *nephrotic syndrome*, owing to a heavy loss of protein in the urine (*proteinuria*) there is a decreased concentration of protein in the blood with a resulting decrease in the osmotic pressure. The decreased osmotic pressure fails to keep fluid out of the tissues and renal oedema develops. The face is characteristically affected, especially around the eyelids.

Hepatic oedema In cirrhosis of the liver the organ fails to make enough albumin to maintain the plasma osmotic pressure. At the same time there is an increased pressure on the portal vein, which drains the gut and carries blood to the liver. The result is a build up of fluid in the abdomen (*ascites*).

Local venous obstruction Obstruction to a large vein will cause increased venous pressure upstream of the blockage, resulting in a localized oedema of the area being drained by the affected vein.

Recognition of oedema

The affected parts are swollen, and pressure on the swollen area causes pitting of the area owing to displacement of fluid. This pitting on pressure distinguishes oedema from the solid swelling of a tumour, or simple fat in the tissues.

Oedema fluid versus inflammatory fluid

One of the most important changes which occurs in acute inflammation is an increased flow of protein-rich fluid (*exudation*) into the inflamed area. When inflammation affects the lung, such as in pneumonia or tuberculosis, large amounts of fluid can collect in the pleural cavity (*pleural effusion*).

Inflammation in the abdomen, for example in cancer which has spread to the peritoneum, results in exudation in the peritoneum and is another cause of ascites.

The fluid which collects as a result of inflammation is called an *exudate* and it is characterized by a high protein content, whilst the fluid in oedema is called a *transudate* and is low in protein.

COMPOSITION OF A NORMAL DIET

The essential nutrients and other constituents of a normal diet have been outlined. It remains to consider nutrition in terms of the different foods that make up the diet, and to view these foods quantitatively. Naturally, the requirements vary between different people according to the amount of energy they expend.

Fundamentally, all food and other essential factors are needed to repair the normal wear and tear of the tissues, and to supply the energy for the bodies metabolic processes and physical activities.

In calculating the food requirements of the body, the amount of energy provided by food can be expressed in the energy units *joules*. Weight for weight, fat produces more than twice as many joules as, either carbohydrate or protein:

1 gram (g) of fat produces 38 kilojoules (kJ)
1 g of carbohydrate produces 16 kJ
1 g of protein produces 16 kJ.

The calorie requirements of an individual will vary according to their age, size and occupation. Thus, a sedentary worker may be satisfied with 7000 kJ (7 megajoules) a day while a heavy manual labourer may need over 12 000 kJ (12 MJ).

In converting these calorific requirements into food it is important that certain amounts of each of the individual foods be eaten to secure a balanced diet. A minimum of 55 g of protein foods a day is needed by a 70 kg adult to replace wear and tear in the tissues. The value on a bodyweight basis is higher for children. During times of stress this may have to be increased.

The amount of fat and carbohydrate in a normal diet varies according to individual taste, social customs and economic status. A high-fat diet is more expensive that a high carbohydrate one. In an average diet the fats usually supply from 90–150 g and the carbohydrates 300–500 g.

A balanced diet must include, however, not only the protein necessary for repairing wear and tear of tissues and enough fats and carbohydrates for energy purposes, but also all the mineral salts mentioned earlier. These will be automatically supplied if a range of ordinary foods are eaten, especially milk, eggs, meat, fish, cheese, cereals, fruit and vegetables. These foods will also supply sufficient vitamins.

In certain periods of life the diet may need supplementing, especially during childhood, during pregnancy and when lactating. For children a generous supply of proteins is needed to allow for growth. For this reason the diet should contain plenty of milk, at least 1 pint (500 ml) a day. Milk also supplies calcium for growth of bones.

Ample quantities of green vegetables, fruit and cereals are important, both for their vitamin content and for their nutritional value.

Prior to conception and during early pregnancy treatment with folic acid is recommended to minimize the risk of neural tube defect. During pregnancy a balanced diet is essential as the energy requirements increase with the growth of the foetus. Vitamins A, B, C, and D are especially important and should be added to the diet. Iron may also be required, particularly if anaemia occurs.

CATABOLIC STATES

In everyday life the body's intake of nutrients is well matched to the needs for energy, growth and tissue repair. When illness intervenes the normal balance can be severely upset.

In a number of illnesses patients are unable to eat so nutrient intake ceases. There may be a simultaneous huge increase in the body's energy needs. In association with infection, burns, surgery, and accident trauma the body may need as much energy as would be the case during hard labour, i.e. up to twice the energy requirement of bed rest. Further, there is a particular need for amino acids to produce the proteins needed to fight infection, for the healing of tissues, and to replace protein lost in exudation fluid. In this situation amino acids are used preferentially as a source of energy. To provide these amino acids muscle protein is broken down much faster than normal and muscle tissue is lost rapidly. The term *autocannibalism* has been used to convey the concept of the body consuming itself in this situation. It can lead to severe debilitation and can prolong recovery after illness.

High levels of the hormones glucose and cortisol combined with low levels of insulin partly account for the development of the condition.

Treatment with large amounts of carbohydrate and protein is relatively ineffective at controlling the condition. Further, this treatment may be difficult to administer as the patient may not desire food or may be unable to eat. It may be necessary to feed the patient via the intravenous route.

TUBE FEEDING

When patients are unable to chew and swallow they will be unable to eat normal solid food. This situation arises when a stroke has occurred which affects the brain stem. These patients are at risk of aspirating food and saliva into the lungs and they may need to be tube fed. They are given liquid food via a soft, narrow-bore tube which is placed to run from the nose to the stomach. A pump is used to slowly infuse the liquid food.

On first inserting the tube it is absolutely vital to ensure that the end of the tube has not inadvertently passed into the lungs via the trachea. Pneumonia, perhaps fatal, would develop if food was run into the lungs. Patients often suffer from diarrhoea when tube feeding commences, due to the rich nature of the feeds. This problem can be minimized by using dilute food for the first few days of feeding.

Tube feeding is indicated in cachectic patients who are unable to eat enough to meet their daily metabolic needs. In this situation the tube feeding may be undertaken at night when the patient is asleep.

PARENTERAL NUTRITION

Parenteral nutrition is the term used for feeding by means of an intravenous infusion. It may be necessary to feed intravenously if there is major disease of the gastrointestinal tract, in particular if the patient needs gastrointestinal surgery, and therefore gastric feeding is not possible. Parenteral nutrition may also be needed in patients who are severely ill, such as in patients with extensive burns.

Parenteral feeds contain fundamentally the

same constituents as a normal diet. However in parenteral feeds the food is in component form, i.e. as glucose and amino acids rather than carbohydrates and protein, respectively. The feeds are strongly hypertonic and very irritant to veins. They are therefore usually given via subclavian catheters ending in the superior vena cava where the rapid blood flow dilutes the hypertonic nutrients. The fluids are sterile and are administered with scrupulous aseptic technique. There are a number of potentially serious problems associated with parenteral feeding:

1. Infection of the intravenous catheter is an all too common problem. Antibiotics are not effective and the catheter has to be removed.

2. Mechanical problems may occur which relate to the catheter. *Pneumothorax* may occur if the lung is punctured. Subclavian vein thrombosis may result if the cannula causes a large thrombus to form.

3. High blood glucose levels may result requiring the use of insulin.

4. Patients can readily develop specific nutritional deficiencies and to prevent this happening vitamins and trace elements are routinely given.

5. The monetary cost is high.

OBESITY

Energy balance is the total quantity of energy produced from the food eaten less the amount of energy needed by the body for resting energy, for exercise and for the energy in metabolic processes such as growth and tissue repair. When more food is consumed than needed the energy balance becomes positive and the excess energy is stored in the body as fat. When a significant excess of fat accumulates in adipose tissue this is termed obesity.

The condition obesity is defined as a weight 20% or more above an acceptable range based on sex and height. Another way of quantifying obesity is based on the *body mass index* (BMI). This index is calculated from the body weight in kilograms divided by the square of the height in metres (kg/m^2). A BMI of 30 or more indicates obesity, whereas a BMI between 25 and 30 indicates overweight. Conversely a BMI between 19 and 25 indicates normal weight for height.

Obesity is not only a social stigma in Western countries, it also presents a hazard to health. It predisposes the individual to diabetes, hypertension, gall bladder disease, gout, heart disease, hyperlipidaemia, hirsutism, osteoarthritis, and colon and breast cancer. Fat people do not live as long as those who are of normal weight. Their activity and enjoyment of life may be restricted by their excessive weight. The unfavourable metabolic effects of obesity and premature death are more frequent when the excess fat tissue accumulates in the abdomen as *upper body fat distribution obesity* (apple-shaped individuals), as opposed to an accumulation of fat on the thighs as *lower body fat distribution obesity* (pear-shaped individuals).

The cause of obesity is almost universally due to an excessive food intake in relation to the body's normal energy needs. Only rarely is there a major decrease in energy needs to less than normal. Careful studies of energy balance show that obese people actually consume more food than thin people but *report* eating less food than they actually consume. However, they often eat less than they would like, or expect, to eat and so do not understand why they are overweight.

Obesity tends to run strongly in families due to a hereditary tendency. Additionally, some families make a habit of overeating and may take less exercise. Many people turn to food for solace when they are anxious, unhappy or bored. There are strong sociological pressures with obesity stigmatized in some cultures and situations but normal in others. Sometimes women put on weight excessively during pregnancy, perhaps because they think mistakenly that they must eat enough for two. Obesity occurs in some patients with depression but weight loss is more common in this condition.

There are some uncommon but important glandular causes for obesity:

1. Patients with an underactive thyroid gland may become obese and find it very difficult to lose weight, even if they follow a strict diet. These individuals have a decreased metabolic

rate. They require treatment with thyroxine in addition to their weight-control diet.

2. Excessive cortisol, either in Cushing's syndrome or given as treatment, leads to obesity of an unusual kind; the face and trunk are obese but the legs and arms are spared.

3. In poorly-controlled overweight diabetic patients who are treated with insulin there is often a marked increase in weight. The insulin treatment is blamed for the problem but it arises because the patient feels better; he eats more and at the same time stops losing glucose (and hence energy) in the urine. The problem is therefore really due to them eating excessively.

Treatment

Diet The only successful way to reduce weight is to eat less. Patients are usually reluctant to accept this comfortless doctrine, hoping for magic tablets or injections.

In a weight-reducing diet energy from fats in particular is severely restricted and energy from carbohydrate, protein and alcohol is reduced. Dietary fibre is increased to prevent constipation and to increase satiety. Sugar, chocolates, biscuits, cakes and jams are rigidly minimized. Protein foods such as fish, chicken, and low-fat cheese can be eaten in moderate amounts, with substantial quantities of green vegetables and salads which have a low energy content. Reducing diets appear frequently in magazines and lay journals, varying in energy content from 3.5 to 5.0 kJ (1000 calories) per day.

Great self discipline is required, particularly in continuing the diet long-term. Attempts at weight loss fail frequently, especially where the individual is not highly motivated. After successful weight loss it is all too easy for the weight to be regained. New eating habits must be acquired that can be adopted long term.

Appetite suppressants Various drugs are available which to some extent may control hunger and so help the obese patient to eat less. Appetite suppressants including fenfluramine, mazindol and diethylpropion can help curb appetite if it becomes a problem when the patient is established on the diet. Amphetamine and related drugs are habit-forming and should not be pre-

scribed. Similarly thyroxine should only be given in the occasional case where the patient is clearly deficient in thyroxine.

Exercise Regular exercise is helpful in preventing the development of obesity but it is of limited effect in treating established obesity, and is effective then only when used with an energy-controlled diet.

Success in reducing weight can only be achieved and sustained if the patient is highly motivated. They may benefit from support to maintain their motivation if they join a slimming group or are seen regularly by a dietitian.

ANOREXIA NERVOSA

This is a condition usually occurring in adolescence and in women under 25. It is characterized by *amenorrhoea*, weight loss, and behavioural changes.

Affected individuals are obsessed with taking low-energy foods such as diet drinks and raw vegetables. They have an abnormal perception of their food intake and weight, stating that they have eaten well when they have taken almost nothing and saying that they are fat when they are clearly emaciated. They are usually preoccupied with exercise programmes and they engage in regular intense exercise. There may be an underlying serious psychological disturbance.

Treatment must be started as early as possible, ideally before there is a major loss of body weight as a decrease to 25% less than ideal weight can be dangerous. Treatment can be most effective when carried out by a team specialising in the condition and able to offer psychological support. In more severe cases the patient is best admitted to hospital. Where the condition has continued for more than a year the ultimate outlook is less favourable.

ACIDOSIS AND ALKALOSIS

The hydrogen ion concentration, i.e. $[H^+]$, in the blood normally remains constant such that the blood is always slightly alkaline. It never becomes acid as death would result. Even a slight change leads to profound and serious consequences.

There is a complicated mechanism for maintaining [H$^+$] constant. Acids are formed in the process of metabolism but the body continues to get rid of them in several ways. Carbon dioxide, which is an acid, is expired by the lungs, whilst the kidneys also excrete any excess acid.

Acidosis

Acidosis means the accumulation of excess acids so that the blood [H$^+$] rises. Acidosis arises chiefly in the following conditions:

1. Failure of the heart to pump effectively, either because of reduced blood volume as occurs in haemorrhage or due to severe heart disease, results in shock and poor oxygenation of the tissues. There is increased accumulation of lactic acid which lowers [H$^+$]. Treatment is directed at improving the circulation with intravenous fluids and blood transfusion in the case of haemorrhage.

2. Diabetic ketoacidosis. In this condition excessive breakdown of fats occurs owing to the deficiency of insulin. This results in an accumulation of acid ketone bodies. Treatment is with insulin, fluid and electrolyte replacement.

3. Renal failure. Here the kidneys fail to excrete the acids formed during normal metabolism. This is an indication for dialysis.

4. Respiratory failure. If there is lung disease or drugs have been taken which depress respiration the lungs may fail to excrete carbon dioxide such that it accumulates resulting in acidosis. Mechanical ventilation may be indicated if drug treatment is ineffectual.

Alkalosis

The opposite to acidosis, alkalosis, is most usually seen as a result of:

1. Prolonged vomiting. Here the alkalosis is due to the excessive loss of the hydrochloric acid in the gastric juice. Pyloric stenosis with its persistent vomiting is often accompanied by alkalosis.

2. Hysterical overbreathing, where the alkalosis is caused by the loss of the acid, carbon dioxide.

The main chemical result of alkalosis is tetany, which is discussed on p. 328. The treatment of alkalosis is to remove the cause and to give calcium for the tetany.

13

Diabetes mellitus

Diabetes mellitus is a common disorder characterized by an excess of glucose in the blood (commonly, but imprecisely called blood sugar). When it develops in middle age, the symptoms may be mild and may pass unnoticed in the early stages. When it occurs in children or young adults, however, the symptoms are more severe and can lead to diabetic coma if the disease is not diagnosed and treated. Whether the symptoms are mild or severe, excess glucose in the blood can do great harm over the years and can lead to complications with serious damage to the eyes, kidneys, blood vessels and nervous system. Hence even when the symptoms are mild, it is important to diagnose diabetes as soon as possible and institute treatment that will restore the blood glucose to normal.

Cause

Sugar, and all carbohydrate foods (such as bread, potato and rice) are broken down in the bowel and absorbed into the blood as glucose. Glucose is then carried to the liver where it is stored as glycogen by the action of insulin. Only enough glucose is left in the blood for the provision of normal metabolism. Hence insulin plays a very important part in regulating how much glucose is available in the blood for energy, and how much is stored away in the liver as glycogen.

Insulin is a hormone produced by special collections of cells in the pancreas known as the islets of Langerhans. The islets of Langerhans release a lot of insulin into the blood stream after a large carbohydrate meal has been eaten, since large quantities of insulin are necessary to store excessive glucose in the liver.

In diabetes, the islets of Langerhans are damaged. Not enough insulin is produced, and instead of excess glucose being stored in the liver, it simply accumulates in the blood. When the sugar in the blood rises above a certain level or threshold, the kidneys excrete the excess sugar in the urine. Hence, large quantities of urine are passed to get rid of the excess sugar. This excessive urination soon leads to thirst, while the continuous drain of glucose from the body depletes the tissues of their vital energy supplies. In severe cases, since carbohydrates are no longer available for adequate metabolism, fat is used instead. Improper fat metabolism leads to the formation of toxic ketone bodies and it is the excessive production of these toxic acids (ketosis) which may lead to diabetic coma.

In persons hereditarily disposed to diabetes, persistent overeating and obesity in middle age may lead to the onset of the ailment, perhaps because fat makes the tissues insensitive to the action of insulin. Sometimes the onset of diabetes is precipitated by an infection, by an accident or by pregnancy.

In children, diabetes develops without obvious cause and usually without anybody else in the family suffering from the disorder. More children develop diabetes in the winter months than in the summer and it is thought in these cases that a virus infection might be responsible by damaging the islets of Langerhans. Diabetes sometimes follows mumps, for example. Other viruses, at present unidentified, could have the same effect.

Symptoms and signs

In mild cases developing in middle age (maturity onset diabetes) there may be no obvious symptoms and the ailment is first diagnosed as the result of a routine examination for sugar in the urine.

In more severe diabetes, especially in children or young adults, the symptoms are more pronounced. There are four cardinal symptoms:

1. Polyuria. Excessive output of urine occurs during the night as well as in the day. In small children, bed wetting is common.

2. Thirst. Consequent on the polyuria and dehydration, there is a constant desire to drink.

3. There is a loss of weight, often despite the fact that the patient is eating well.

4. Lassitude and loss of energy occurs; if the diabetes is not diagnosed, this may lead to drowsiness or even coma (see later).

Other lesser symptoms are often present:

1. Particularly in elderly women who are obese, irritation of the genitalia (pruritus vulvae) is caused by local deposition of sugar from the urine. This may be severe and disturbs the sleep.

2. Paraesthesia (tingling) may occur in the fingers and feet.

3. Aching and cramps are common in the legs.

4. Temporary blurring of vision: excess sugar causes changes in refraction in the eyes.

5. Minor infections such as boils or unhealed cuts are liable to occur.

Diagnosis

The diagnosis is suspected by the clinical picture and confirmed by finding excess sugar (glucose) in the urine and blood.

Urine (a) The output is increased. (b) The urine is pale in colour but has a high specific gravity (1030 to 1040) due to the glucose contained. (c) The tests for sugar are positive. (d) Ketone bodies (acetone) may be present in more severe cases.

Blood (a) Normally, the fasting blood sugar is about 4.5 mmol per litre (80 mg/100 ml) and this rises to about 6.5 mmol per litre (120 mg/100 ml) after a meal. In diabetes, the fasting blood sugar may be over 11 mmol per litre (200 mg/100 ml) and even higher after food. (b) In doubtful cases, a glucose tolerance test may be performed. The suspected diabetic is advised to eat a normal diet on the days preceding the test, but must have no food or drink on the morning of the test. They are given a drink containing 75 g of glucose and blood is then taken for the measurement of glucose every half an hour. The test takes two and a half hours. Normally the blood sugar does not rise above 10 mmol per litre (180 mg/100 ml) even when the levels peak after one and a half hours. The blood sugar returns to the fasting level

Table 13.1

	Young patients	Middle-aged or elderly patients
Onset	Rapid: with loss of weight, drowsiness, polyuria and thirst	Gradual: symptoms slight or absent
Weight	Loss of weight;thin	Usually obese
Blood sugar	Very high	High
Urine	Sugar and acetone	Sugar
Coma	Liable to coma if neglected	Coma very unusual
Treatment	Full diet; insulin	Restricted diet; sometimes tablets
Pathology	Destruction of islets of Langerhans (no insulin produced)	Reduction of islet functions (some insulin production continues)

of 4.5 mmol (80 mg) at the end of two and a half hours. The peak and fasting levels of blood glucose are raised when diabetes is present.

TYPES OF DIABETES

There appear to be two main types of diabetes, as follows.

Insulin-dependent diabetes (sometimes known as juvenile-onset or type I)

This form of diabetes occurs mainly in children and young adults, though it can develop at any age. The symptoms (thirst, polyuria, loss of weight and lassitude) usually become severe and the patient or his parents are soon obliged to seek medical advice. The urine contains sugar and acetone. Patients of this type need insulin and a full diet. They do not respond to tablets. They are prone to diabetic coma if they neglect themselves or if they develop an infection such as pyelonephritis or gastroenteritis.

Non-insulin-dependent diabetes (sometimes known as maturity-onset or type II)

These patients are usually middle aged or elderly and symptoms may be absent or mild. In women, pruritus vulvae is common. Thirst and polyuria develop gradually. The urine contains sugar but not acetone. It is very unusual for this sort of patient to go into coma and insulin is not often needed.

The patient must adhere to a low-energy diet in order to lose weight. In most cases, once a normal weight has been achieved, the blood sugar levels return to normal and no sugar can be found in the urine.

In patients of this type, who are not overweight and who do not respond to dietary restriction (or occasionally for overweight patients together with a reducing diet), tablets are available which reduce the blood sugar to a normal range (see later).

TREATMENT OF DIABETES

Treatment will depend on the type of diabetes.

Insulin-dependent diabetes

In severe diabetes of this type, the initial treatment is often carried out in hospital (in diabetic outpatients or as an inpatient) since patients have to be instructed as to their diet, self-injection of insulin and how to test blood (and urine) for sugar. Patients are more likely to co-operate if they understand the nature of their complaint, and although there are many books on diabetes available for the public, nothing can take the place of a friendly and reassuring explanation as soon as possible after diagnosis. This is particularly important in children, when parents must be able to co-operate.

Dietary regime

In normal people the supply of insulin from the

Type	Urine	Treatment
Middle-aged or elderly over-weight 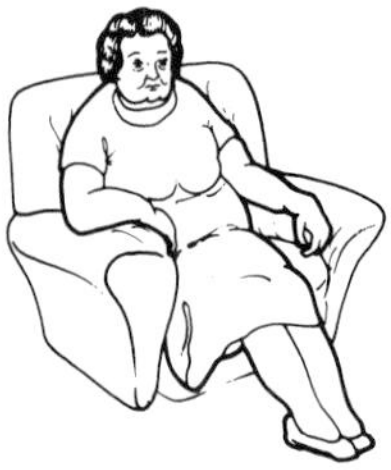	Sugar but no acetone	*Must lose weight* Reducing diet 800–1200 calories daily
Not young, normal weight moderate symptoms 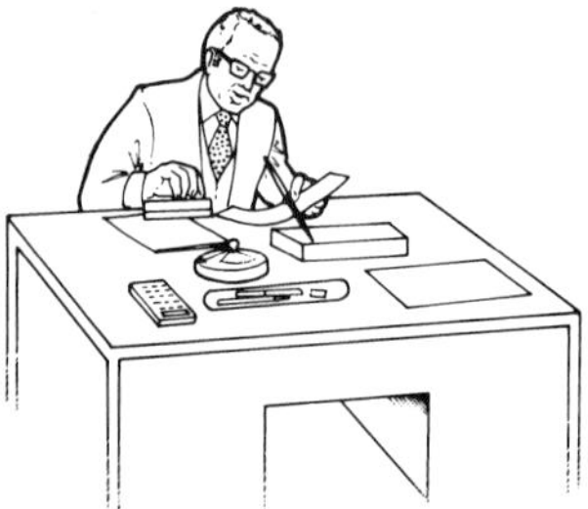	Sugar but no acetone	*Tablets* Adequate diet 1500–1800 calories daily
Young under-weight marked thirst and polyuria 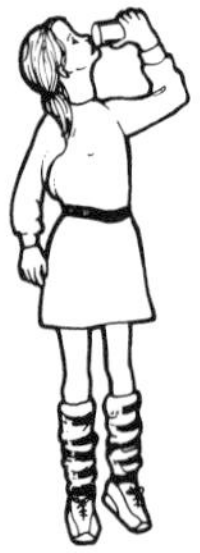	Sugar and acetone	*Insulin* Full diet according to size and activity 1800–2800 calories daily

Fig. 13.1 Types of diabetes.

pancreas is regulated by the food eaten. If no food is taken, very little insulin is secreted. Following a large carbohydrate meal, the pancreas produces considerable amounts of insulin. In diabetics this mechanism is lost. *A fixed amount of insulin is injected each day and hence the diet must not be allowed to vary much in quantity.* The

principles of the diet in patients taking insulin must include:

1. A diet sufficient in quantity to enable the patient to undertake their activities, to satisfy their appetite and to maintain their weight at a proper level. A girl of slight physique leading a sedentary life may require a diet of 8000 kilo-

joules (2000 calories). A man doing a heavy labouring job may need a minimum of 11 500 kJ (2800 calories).

2. Roughly half of the dietary energy should come from carbohydrates (particularly complex carbohydrates), no more than one third of the energy from fats (with a maximum of 10% from saturated fats), and about 10–15% of the dietary energy from protein. Plenty of fresh fruit and vegetables should be eaten.

3. Meals must be spaced during the day. Thus, in addition to the three main meals of breakfast, lunch and dinner, there should also be snacks in the middle of the morning, in the early afternoon and at bedtime.

4. Meals must be taken at regular times. Delayed meals may lead to hypoglycaemic attacks (see later).

It can be seen that the type of diet recommended to the diabetic is almost identical to that recommended to the general public as a healthy diet for life.

Arranging the diet

A diet is chosen suitable for the patient's size and activities, say roughly 8800 kJ (2200 calories). This will contain:

304 g carbohydrate	= 5060 kJ	(1210 calories)	= 55% of total
78 g protein	= 1300 kJ	(310 calories)	= 15% of total
25 g saturated fat	= 920 kJ	(220 calories)	= 10% of total
48 g remaining fat	= 1840 kJ	(440 calories)	= 20% of total
Total	= 9120 kJ	(2180 calories)	

Tables and charts are available which set out the composition and energy values of common articles of food, and so a diet can be composed to suit the taste of the individual. In practice, many diabetic clinics provide their patients with an outline diet, similar to that shown in Table 13.2, and a list of alternatives as in Table 13.3. Note also:

1. Protein foods are exchangeable. Meat can be exchanged for equivalent amounts of cheese, fish or eggs, for example. However, fish and poultry

should be eaten in preference to red meat or dairy products.

2. The fat content of the diet should be made up mostly from mono and polyunsaturated fats, with as small an amount as possible of saturated fats. This means choosing low fat spreads, cheeses and milks wherever possible.

3. It is a good idea for much of the carbohydrate to be rich in fibre, since the quality of the food is just as important as the quantity. Food choices in this respect include wholewheat biscuits and crackers, wholegrain breakfast cereal, products made from wholewheat flour or pasta, brown rice, beans and pulses. Bread can be

Table 13.2 Specimen outline diet: 8400 kJ (2100 calories)*.

Breakfast (51 g carbohydrate)
Fish or alternative
Bread, 75 g
Margarine, 12 g
Skimmed/semi-skimmed milk for tea or coffee, 50 g

Midmorning snack (19 g carbohydrate)
Skimmed/semi-skimmed milk for tea or coffee, 50 g
Bread, 25 g
Margarine, 6 g

Dinner (47.5 g carbohydrate)
Lean meat, 75 g
Green vegetables
Boiled potatoes, 125 g
Milk pudding (skimmed/semi-skimmed milk 175 g, rice 12 g)

Tea (35 g carbohydrate)
Bread, 50 g
Butter, 12 g
Salad, etc.
Skimmed/semi-skimmed milk for tea, 50 g

Supper (51 g carbohydrate)
Low-fat cheese, 50 g or alternative
Salad or green vegetables
Bread, 62 g
Margarine, 12 g
Fruit, one portion
Skimmed/semi-skimmed milk for tea or coffee, 50 g

Bedtime snack (20.5 g carbohydrate)
Skimmed/semi-skimmed milk, 175 g
Two crispbreads

* A list of alternatives is provided for each item on the diet.

exchanged for appropriate quantities of potato, wholewheat crackers, fruit or vegetables. Using a portion of 10 g of carbohydrate as a standard, the equivalent values of various common carbohydrate foods are set out in Fig. 13.2.

Thus it can be seen that once a diabetic patient has grasped the principles of the diet and has learned the food values of the common items of

Table 13.3 Diet guidelines for diabetics

Foods to encourage	In moderation	Foods to avoid
High fibre Wholemeal bread Brown rice Wholegrain breakfast cereals Wholewheat pasta Lentils Dried peas and beans Fruits and vegetables Wholewheat biscuits and crispbreads	Milk, Cheese, Butter, Margarine, Lean meat, Eggs, White bread, Rice and Pasta	*High sugar* Jam, honey, marmalade, sugar, treacle, tinned fruit, fizzy drinks, fruit squashes, cakes, puddings, sweet biscuits, sweet alcoholic drinks, instant desserts and mousses, ice creams, sweets, sugar-coated cereals
Low fat Skimmed milk Cottage cheese Fish Lean chicken Low-fat plain yoghurt Low-calorie squashes Tinned fruit in water Oxo, marmite, Bovril Tea, coffee Sugar-free sweeteners		*High Fat* Lard, suet, dripping, fried foods, crisps, cream, mayonnaise, sauces, salad dressing, pâté, condensed milk, chocolate

food, the diet can become both interesting and varied. In the early stages, food should be weighed until the patient is confident of his or her ability to recognise the weight of the various food components without the need to weigh. Nevertheless, many diabetics prefer to weigh all items of food just to make sure. It must be remembered that the amount of fat in a meal and the type of carbohydrate eaten will significantly effect how quickly the blood sugar rises after a meal. With time, diabetics become more experienced in the effects of different types of food on blood sugar levels.

Insulin

Although in the past insulin was prepared directly from the pancreas glands removed from cattle and pigs after slaughter, most diabetics now use human insulin. This is prepared in two different ways. Either insulin from pigs (porcine insulin) is altered to human insulin (for example human Actrapid insulin), or more commonly it is synthesized by bacteria (for example, humulin Lente). Human insulin is not regarded as foreign by the body, so it will cause less reaction at the injection site and less insulin may be required. Although there has been much publicity claiming that patients who change to human insulin have less warning of hypoglycaemic attacks, and so may get dangerously low blood sugars, the majority consensus is that this is not true. Almost all diabetics who require insulin should now be using human insulin.

Insulin is destroyed by the gastric juices with the result that it cannot be given by mouth, and has to be administered by subcutaneous injection. Clear insulin, known as soluble insulin, when injected subcutaneously relatively quickly leads to a fall in the blood sugar, but its effect only lasts a few hours. Hence, various forms of insulin have been prepared which prolong its action to last all day. There are now many different types of commercial insulin available, differing from each other in various ways.

Source. Most insulin used now is human insulin, although porcine and beef insulin is still available it is used by a very small minority of diabetics.

Strengths. Insulin in the United Kingdom, America, Canada and Australia is available as 100 units per ml and the syringes are calibrated appropriately. In other countries, and particularly in Europe, insulin is available as 40 units per ml, so that a greater volume has to be injected for the

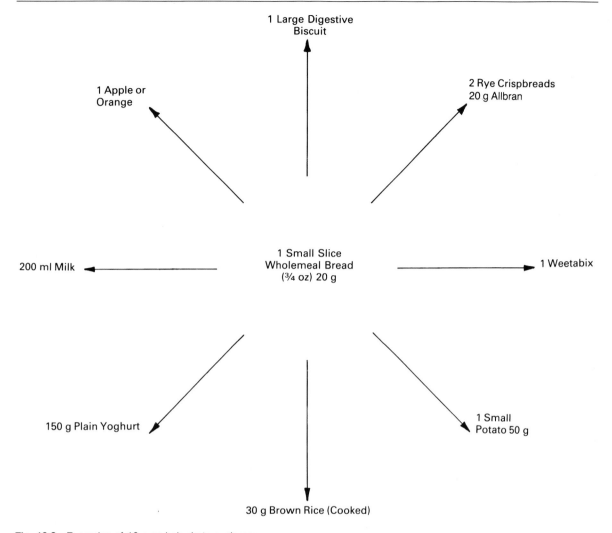

Fig. 13.2 Examples of 10 g carbohydrate exchange.

same amount of insulin. It always pays to carefully check the strength of insulin stated on the bottle and the markings on the syringe.

Duration. The duration varies according to the preparation used (Table 13.4):

1. Soluble insulin. This is clear insulin and its effects last about 6 hours. In order to control diabetes on its own it must be given at least twice a day. It can be given intravenously in the treatment of diabetic coma. Humulin S and Actrapid are preparations of soluble insulin. These short-acting insulins can be mixed with certain of the longer-acting insulins in the same syringe. Thus, soluble insulin can be mixed with

isophane insulin: the soluble acts quickly until the isophane begins to exert its effect.

2. The medium or intermediate insulins, if injected in the morning before breakfast, exert their maximum effect at lunchtime and early afternoon. The effect is less marked overnight and consequently a second injection is often necessary before the evening meal. Two examples of these intermediate-acting insulins are Humulin I and Semitard.

3. The long-acting insulins such as Ultratard or Protamine Zinc are useful as a single injection in the morning. They are suitable for diabetics who have easily controlled blood sugar and do not need a large dose.

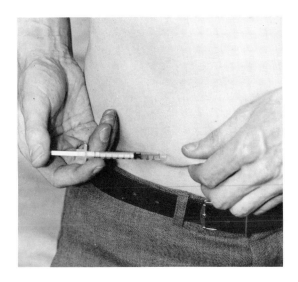

Fig. 13.3 Injecting insulin with disposable syringe.

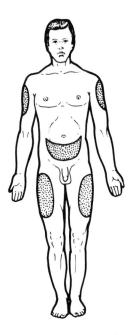

Fig. 13.4 Sites suitable for insulin injections.

4. Ready-mixed combinations of short- and long-acting insulins are also available. These have a wide range of duration of action depending on the proportion of short and intermediate insulin present. Some examples of these include:

Humulin M1 (10% humulin S, 90% humulin I)

Humulin M4 (40% humulin S, 60% humulin I)
Mixtard (30% velosin, 70% insulatard)

Injecting insulin

Unfortunately, there are over 20 different preparations of insulin available, depending on the duration of action (and its source). Hence it is important to check that the patient is using the correct insulin as has been prescribed. Although in 1983 it was decided to standardise the strength of insulin so that all preparations contained 100 units per ml, older strengths (for example 40 units per ml or 80 units per ml) may still occasionally be used and this too should be checked. Syringes are sized either 1 ml (100 units) or 0.5 ml (50 units) and are now usually made of plastic. Glass syringes were used previously, and had to be kept in industrial methylated spirits and carefully dried before drawing up the insulin. Plastic syringes are disposable but can safely be re-used on several occasions. They should be kept empty in the refrigerator between injections. New diabetics needing insulin must be fully instructed on the following points:

1. the preparation and strength of insulin to be used
2. the dose to be injected and how often during the day
3. the technique of giving the subcutaneous injections and the sites suitable for injection (Figs 13.3, 13.4)
4. the care of the syringe and needle.

The insulin pen

Pen syringes are an increasingly popular method of injecting insulin. They offer convenience together with good control. Insulin is supplied in a cartridge which fits into the pen (Fig. 13.5). The amount of insulin given is regulated by a dial or a system of clicks, which is invaluable for diabetics with poor eyesight. The pen containing insulin can be carried around as a whole, so injections can be easily and unobtrusively given, if necessary, in public places such as restaurants, schools or even business meetings! A common regime is to give short-acting insulin three times daily

Table 13.4 Some insulins available

Preparation	Type	Type of action	Maximum effect	Duration of action
Actrapid	Human	Short	About 2–4 h	Up to 8 h
Humulin S	Human			
Velosulin	Human, Porcine			
Humulin I	Human	Medium	4–8 h	Up to 24 h
Semitard	Human			
Monotard	Human			
Lente	Human, Bovine			
Insulatard	Human			
Ultratard	Human	Long	6–12 h	30 h or longer
Humulin Zn	Human			

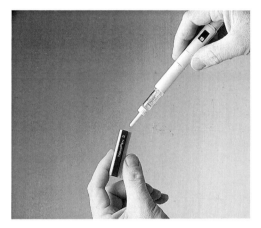

Fig. 13.5 The insulin pen with insulin cartridge loaded.

before meals, with an intermediate acting insulin at bedtime.

Infusion pumps

Most diabetics are well controlled on one or two injections of insulin each day, the morning injection before breakfast and the evening injection before the evening meal. However, particularly where control is difficult, a portable pump is now available at special centres. The pump is carried by the patient on a waist belt and contains a reservoir of insulin. The insulin is delivered continuously by the pump through a cannula attached to a winged needle inserted under the skin. By this means, a steady flow of insulin is maintained throughout the day and night and this flow can be boosted before meals. The insulin in the reservoir and the subcutaneous needle have to be renewed every few days and regular medical supervision is necessary.

Hypoglycaemia

When the blood sugar level falls too low, symptoms of hypoglycaemia occur. Some diabetics, sometimes called 'brittle' or 'unstable', are particularly liable to these attacks despite all precautions. Hypoglycaemia is most likely to occur:

1. when meals are delayed or irregular
2. when unusual exertion or exercise is undertaken
3. when the insulin dose is excessive.

The earliest symptoms of hypoglycaemia are sweating, mental confusion, a feeling of hunger or weakness, palpitations and trembling. An astute nurse should be on the lookout for these symptoms in a diabetic patient taking insulin, especially before meal times or if the patient is behaving in an peculiar fashion. The patient may have a vacant look, they will be pale and sweating, with a rapid pulse. It is most important to institute treatment immediately since otherwise the patient will go into hypoglycaemic or insulin coma. After measuring glucose levels using blood glucose strips, the patient should be persuaded to take a glucose drink without delay, and only if they become too stuporous to swallow is it necessary to administer glucose by intravenous injection. Every diabetic patient taking insulin should be aware of the early symptoms of hypoglycaemia and must always carry lumps of sugar or glucose sweets to prevent this happen-

Table 13.5 Diabetic coma

Symptoms and signs	Diabetic coma	Insulin coma (hypoglycaemia)
1. Onset	Gradual. History of severe thirst and polyuria: abdominal pain and vomiting	Sudden. Patient previously well and active, taking insulin
2. Infection	Usually present (e.g. tonsillitis, enteritis, pyelitis)	Not usually present
3. Respirations	Deep, sighing. Breath smells of acetone	Quiet regular breathing
4. Skin	Dry, inelastic. Tongue dry and shrunken	Sweating, moist shrunken
5. Blood pressure	Very low; rapid thin pulse	Normal. Full pulse
6. Urine	Sugar and acetone	No sugar or only a trace

ing. Diabetics should carry a card or bracelet stating that they are diabetic and if found confused or unconscious must be offered a glucose drink if conscious or sent to hospital as an emergency.

When patients are admitted to hospital in hypoglycaemia or 'insulin coma', it is often not known whether the patient is a diabetic. Search should be made for evidence of insulin injections in the thighs or lower abdomen. The patient is usually sweating, with dilated pupils and normal blood pressure. The breathing is quiet and there is no evidence of dehydration or collapse. The blood glucose will be low and the urine, if it can be obtained, is free from sugar. This condition should not be confused with diabetic coma (Table 13.5). Glucose must be injected intravenously and the patient soon regains consciousness. Nevertheless, in some cases who have been allowed to remain in coma for many hours, permanent brain damage may result and recovery will not take place despite elevation of the blood sugar level to normal. This danger explains the importance of prompt treatment in the early stages.

Glucagon is a hormone secreted by special cells in the islets of Langerhans and has exactly the opposite effect of insulin. It causes the liver to produce more sugar and so the blood sugar rises. Glucagon is available in a powder form and when dissolved in sterile water, it can be injected subcutaneously.

When the blood sugar is low and the patient cannot be given intravenous glucose for any reason, an injection of glucagon (2 mg) subcutaneously will elevate the blood sugar in about 15 minutes. In a comatose patient, there is a return of consciousness and glucose can then be given by mouth.

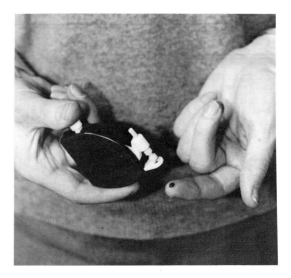

Fig. 13.6 Self testing for blood sugar. Apparatus (Autolet) for drawing blood.

Blood and urine testing Many patients test their own blood for sugar. The pulp of a finger is pricked with a lancet and a blob of blood transferred to a special strip such as Dextrostix. The blood is washed off after a minute and the colour on the strip is compared with a colour chart. More accurately the strip can be placed in a special machine (such as Glucometer) and this gives a reading of the blood sugar level (Fig. 13.7).

It is also possible to test the urine for sugar, since the amount of sugar in the urine gives a rough guide as to the sugar in the blood. Clinistix or Diastix may be used for this. However, it is much more accurate to test the blood directly, and levels of glucose in the urine do not always reliably reflect the levels of glucose in the blood.

Testing the blood (or the urine) gives the

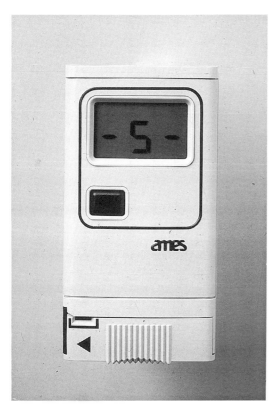

Fig. 13.7 Machine for automatic reading of blood sugar levels from measuring strip.

patient information as to whether or not the diabetes is well controlled. Patients needing insulin may have to adjust the dose or type of insulin if the control is poor with high blood sugars. Badly controlled diabetes over years leads to complications.

Diabetics needing tablets

Many adult patients who develop diabetes can be controlled without recourse to insulin. These diabetics are not overweight, but they are not thin or wasted. The urine contains sugar but no acetone.

Dietary regime

The diet should just be adequate to maintain weight at the normal standard for the patient's age and height. In practice, most patients in this category require a diet varying from 6000 kJ (1500 calories) to 8000 kJ (2000 calories), which is less than is usual for diabetics taking insulin.

Tablets or oral hypoglycaemics

There are two types of tablet used in the UK, sulphonylureas and biguanides:

1. Several types of sulphonylurea tablets are in common use to bring down the blood sugar. These compounds stimulate the pancreas to produce more insulin, and this explains why they are ineffective in the more severe type of diabetes where the pancreas is incapable of producing any insulin at all. Tolbutamide and glipizide have a short duration of action and are normally taken twice a day. Glibenclamide has an intermediate strength of action. Chlorpropamide and tolazamide have a longer action and once a day is effective. All these tablets are well tolerated and seldom give rise to hypoglycaemia or other ill effects. Unfortunately, they become ineffective if the diet is not adhered to, and should not be used as an excuse to overeat. They often give rise to an increase in weight.

2. Metformin is a biguanide and probably helps to lower the blood sugar by reducing the peripheral sensitivity to insulin. It is not as effective as the sulphonylureas and often causes nausea and stomach upsets. However, metformin helps to keep the weight down and is often prescribed in patients who are overweight.

Overweight diabetics

These patients usually need neither tablets nor insulin, provided they are willing to reduce their weight by restricting their food intake. Overeating places a strain on the pancreas, and if the supply of insulin is limited diabetes will result. Hence the diet must be so restricted that the patient loses weight. Depending on the degree of obesity, the diet will vary from as little as 3500 kJ (800 calories) a day to 5000 kJ (1200 calories) a day. Once the weight is reduced, the blood sugar falls to normal, the urine becomes free from sugar and the symptoms disappear. The patient must always keep to a diet, though not necessarily as severe as the original one.

Complications of diabetes

The immediate aim of the treatment in diabetes is to keep the diabetic fit, feeling well and free from troublesome symptoms. The ultimate aim is to reduce the risk of various complications which tend to occur after diabetes has been present for many years. It is believed that the incidence of complications can be reduced by keeping the blood sugar level as near normal as possible, and this means careful adherence to the diet and careful adjustment of the dosage of insulin. The diabetic patient should attend his doctor or hospital clinic at regular intervals to ensure that the blood does not contain more glucose than can be avoided. Unhappily, complications, especially in the eyes, kidneys and nerves, can occur even in diabetics who have done their best to keep to their regime. These complications are as follows:

1. Increased chance of coronary heart disease and stroke. Diabetes increases atheroma in the vulnerable coronary and cerebral arteries. Ischaemic heart disease is the main cause of excess deaths in diabetics.

2. Retinopathy. Degeneration of the retina at the back of the eye occurs in a high percentage of patients who have had diabetes for 20 years or more. Haemorrhages may occur and may be of sufficient severity to lead to blindness (Fig. 13.6, 13.7). Eyes should be examined once a year as, if used in good time, photocoagulation by laser beam can prevent retinal haemorrhages.

3. Nephropathy (Kimmelstiel–Wilson syndrome). The kidneys are damaged by long-standing diabetes and this kidney disease may ultimately lead to kidney failure with albuminuria, oedema of the legs, high blood pressure and uraemia. This is frequently a cause of death in diabetes. The earliest sign is microalbuminuria.

4. Neuropathy. Involvement of the peripheral nerves leads to loss of the reflexes, pain in the legs, wasting of the muscles and weakness of gait.

5. Peripheral arteriosclerosis. Particularly in elderly patients, hardening of the arteries of the

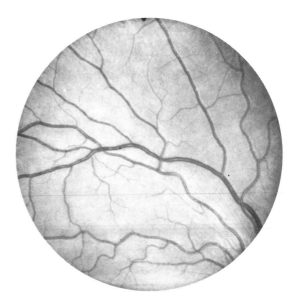

Fig. 13.8 Normal retina seen through ophthalmoscope.

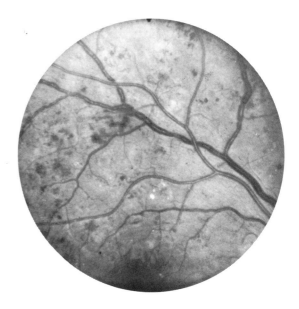

Fig. 13.9 Retina in severe diabetes with numerous small haemorrhages.

legs leads to an impoverishment of the blood supply to the feet. Any minor damage to the toes takes a long time to heal and is prone to infection; this dangerous sequence may lead to gangrene, with consequent amputation of the whole leg (Fig. 13.10). Hence, all diabetic patients, but particularly elderly diabetic patients, must be urged to look after their feet. They must make sure that there are no holes in their stockings and that they have good well fitting shoes. They must keep the feet warm but avoid roasting them before too hot a fire. They must avoid cutting the toe nails too short or digging into the corner of the toes. It is often best for a regular foot toilet to be undertaken by a trained chiropodist.

6. Infections. Diabetic coma is often ushered in by an infection such as tonsillitis, pneumonia, pyelitis, appendicitis or phlebitis. Treatment of the infection must be vigorous and immediate (see below).

7. Pregnancy. Diabetic mothers tend to have large babies, often weighing more than 4.5 kg (10 lb) at birth. These babies are sometimes stillborn, and are very oedematous. Since the damage is done in the last month of pregnancy, many obstetricians perform a Caesarian section at the 38th week to avoid this risk. The diabetes must be carefully controlled throughout the pregnancy and if control is good, there is every reason to expect a healthy baby.

Diabetic coma (diabetic-ketoacidosis)

Before the days of insulin, young people who developed diabetes nearly always died in diabetic coma. Nowadays, with earlier diagnosis and effective treatment, diabetic coma is uncommon. Sometimes elderly or mentally slow people delay reporting to the doctor when symptoms develop; they become more drowsy and are found in coma. In patients already known to have diabetes, coma is nearly always due to an accompanying infection, such as pneumonia, pyelitis or gastroenteritis. The patient may feel too ill to eat, and may mistakenly omit the usual injection of insulin. The blood sugar rapidly rises, ketosis occurs and coma is often preceded by vomiting.

Symptoms and signs of diabetic coma (Fig. 13.9)

1. At first drowsiness with great thirst and polyuria, followed by unrousable coma.

2. Deep sighing respiration with the breath smelling of acetone.

3. Cold extremities, sunken eyeballs, shrivelled tongue, dry skin and a low blood pressure; these signs are due to dehydration (loss of fluid).

4. The blood glucose level is very high.

5. Urine contains heavy amounts of sugar and ketones.

Treatment of diabetic coma

The successful treatment of diabetic coma demands constant supervision and close cooperation between nurses, doctors and laboratory staff. Many patients still die with this condition. The basic requirements are administration of insulin and the adequate replacement of fluid and electrolytes, with frequent monitoring of the clinical state, and the biochemistry of the blood and urine. A special chart must be kept of the fluid and insulin administered, of the urine passed and the results of the blood tests.

1. These patients are seriously dehydrated, having passed large quantities of urine in the hours or days preceding the onset of coma. Vomiting may have caused further loss of fluid. Fluid must be administered intravenously by drip, and in most cases isotonic saline is given initially. The first litre can be given rapidly, perhaps within half an hour; thereafter, the infusion can be run at a slower rate as judged by

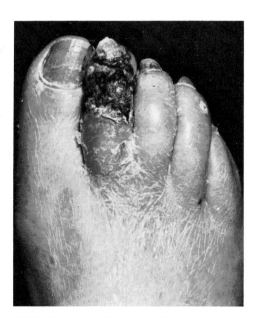

Fig. 13.10 Gangrene of the toe in diabetes.

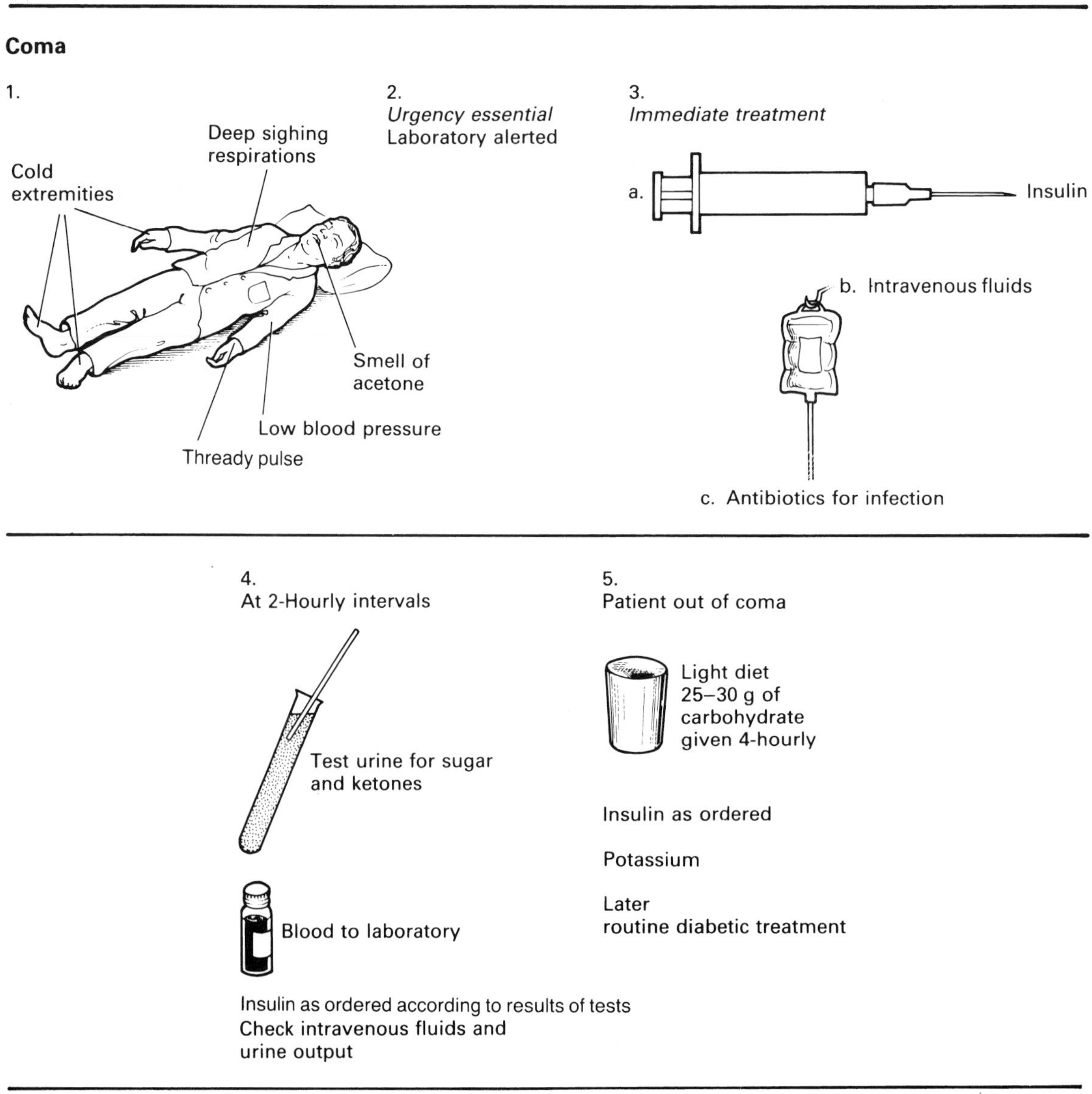

Coma

1.

Cold
extremities

Deep sighing
respirations

2.
Urgency essential
Laboratory alerted

3.
Immediate treatment

a.   Insulin

b. Intravenous fluids

Smell of
acetone

Low blood pressure

Thready pulse

c. Antibiotics for infection

4.
At 2-Hourly intervals

Test urine for sugar
and ketones

Blood to laboratory

Insulin as ordered according to results of tests
Check intravenous fluids and
urine output

5.
Patient out of coma

Light diet
25–30 g of
carbohydrate
given 4-hourly

Insulin as ordered

Potassium

Later
routine diabetic treatment

Fig. 13.11 Treatment of diabetic coma.

the patient's progress. When ketoacidosis is very severe, alkaline solutions (sodium bicarbonate) may be administered.

2. The best way to give insulin is by continuous intravenous infusion and insulin can conveniently be added into the saline bottle. Thus 20–40 units soluble insulin can be added to each bottle, the amount regulated by the results of repeated blood and urine sugar estimations. A more accurate method of delivering insulin is by means of a constant rate infusion pump attached by a fourway tap to the intravenous tube. This can deliver insulin in saline at a steady rate of 6 units every hour and is independent of the rate of the drip. An alternative method is to give insulin every hour by intramuscular injection, usually 20 units as a start and then 10 units every hour.

3. Whatever the method of administering in-

sulin, regular estimations of the blood sugar and electrolytes are essential to guide progress. The aim is to get the blood sugar to a near normal level within 4–6 hours.

4. As the blood sugar falls, there is a tendency for the blood potassium to fall too low so that it may be necessary to add potassium (KCl) to the infusion.

5. The onset of coma may have been precipitated by infection. For example, there may be evidence of pneumonia or of a renal tract infection. Appropriate chemotherapy may be necessary, often given intravenously by adding to the drip.

6. Urine should be tested every 2 hours and for this purpose a retention catheter may be needed. The urine is tested for sugar and acetone.

7. Where there has been frequent vomiting, it is best to empty the stomach by using a stomach tube.

Progress

1. As the patient gains consciousness and the blood sugar and electrolytes return to normal, the drip can be maintained at a slow rate. It should not be discontinued until it is clear that the patient is able to take adequate fluids by mouth without nausea.

2. A regime of subcutaneous soluble insulin can be started, usually three times a day for the first few days.

3. A light diet should be given with frequent small feeds. The energy content is not important at this stage.

14

Disorders of the endocrine system

The endocrine system consists of a series of endocrine glands and special cells which manufacture *hormones* and pass them directly into the blood stream. Hormones are chemical messengers. When released into the blood, hormones exert important regulatory effects on the metabolism and function of the cells of the body. The endocrine system, like the nervous system, helps determine the way in which the body reacts to the environment. The outer world is perceived by our five senses: sight, hearing, taste, smell and touch. These senses relay impulses to the cells of the nervous tissue of the brain.

The hypothalamus

The hypothalamus is composed of groups of special cells lying at the base of the brain. It lies above the pituitary gland and is connected to it by a stalk containing blood vessels and nerve fibres. Under the influence of neurotransmitters from the cerebral neurones, the cells of the hypothalamus produce a number of local hormones which it transmits to the pituitary gland. Some of these hormones stimulate the cells of the pituitary gland (*releasing hormones*), others prevent them from acting (*inhibitory hormones*). Many of these hormones have been isolated and some are in clinical use. TRH (*thyrotrophin releasing hormone*), GnRH (*gonadotrophin releasing hormone*), and ACTH (*adrenocorticotrophin*) are some examples of hypothalamic hormones now in regular use to test pituitary and other endocrine gland function.

The pituitary gland

The pituitary gland produces growth hormone and controls the action of three other very important endocrine glands. The thyroid, adrenal cortex and the gonads are all controlled by the pituitary gland. However, not all endocrine glands are under the influence of the pituitary gland. The parathyroid glands and the adrenal medulla are independent of the action of the pituitary gland. In addition, there are many collections of endocrine cells lying in the pancreas (*the islets of Langerhans*), in the wall of the bowel and in the kidney which produce hormones in response to metabolic changes in the body state, uninfluenced by the pituitary. Any part of the endocrine system, the hypothalamus, the pituitary or any of the endocrine organs or cells can be affected by a tumour or some other disease. This leads to a change in the hormone pattern of the body, with either hormone excess or deficiency and associated profound constitutional disturbances.

PITUITARY GLAND

The pituitary gland lies in a bony hollow at the base of the skull (pituitary fossa). It is controlled by the hypothalamus to which it is connected by the pituitary stalk. It has two quite separate divisions, or lobes, the anterior and the posterior.

Hormones of the anterior lobe

1. *Growth hormone.* An excess of this hormone gives rise to gigantism in young people and acromegaly in older people. Lack of growth hormone in children causes short stature, and in extreme cases dwarfism.

2. *Gonadotrophins.* These are necessary for the normal functioning of the testicles in the male and ovaries in the female.

3. *Prolactin.* This hormone stimulates and maintains milk production after pregnancy. Excess production by tumours causes milk secretion (galactorrhoea). It also causes irregular menstruation in the female and testicular failure in the male when present to excess.

4. *ACTH.* This stimulates the adrenal cortex to produce cortisol, which is essential to maintain our electrolyte balance and metabolic rate.

5. *Thyrotrophin-releasing hormone (TRH).* This regulates the production of thyroid hormone by the thyroid gland. If deficient the thyroid gland fails to produce thyroxine.

PITUITARY DISEASES

These result from either hormone excess or deficiency. In addition there may be symptoms and signs of a pituitary tumour such as headache or visual disturbance.

Growth hormone excess

Depending on whether the growth plate (epiphyses) of the bones have closed, the patient will have gigantism (before closure) or acromegaly (after closure).

Gigantism

In childhood or adolescence, a tumour of the pituitary may develop with excess production of growth hormone. Since the epiphyses (growth plate) of the bones have not yet fused, tremendous increase in size results with some of the patients reaching eight or nine feet tall.

Acromegaly

Once the epiphyses have closed, the excess growth hormone produced by the tumour causes a generalized bony overgrowth, without an increase in height. This results in an increase in foot and hand size. The face becomes broadened with characteristic coarse features and thickened skin. In particular there is prominence of the lower jaw (prognathism). The hands are said to be spade-like and the patient said to have a 'pillow' handshake, due to the soft tissue overgrowth in the hand.

Diagnosis Measurement of the level of growth hormone in the blood is very helpful. However it can be elevated in normal people who are anxious. In the latter group the level of growth

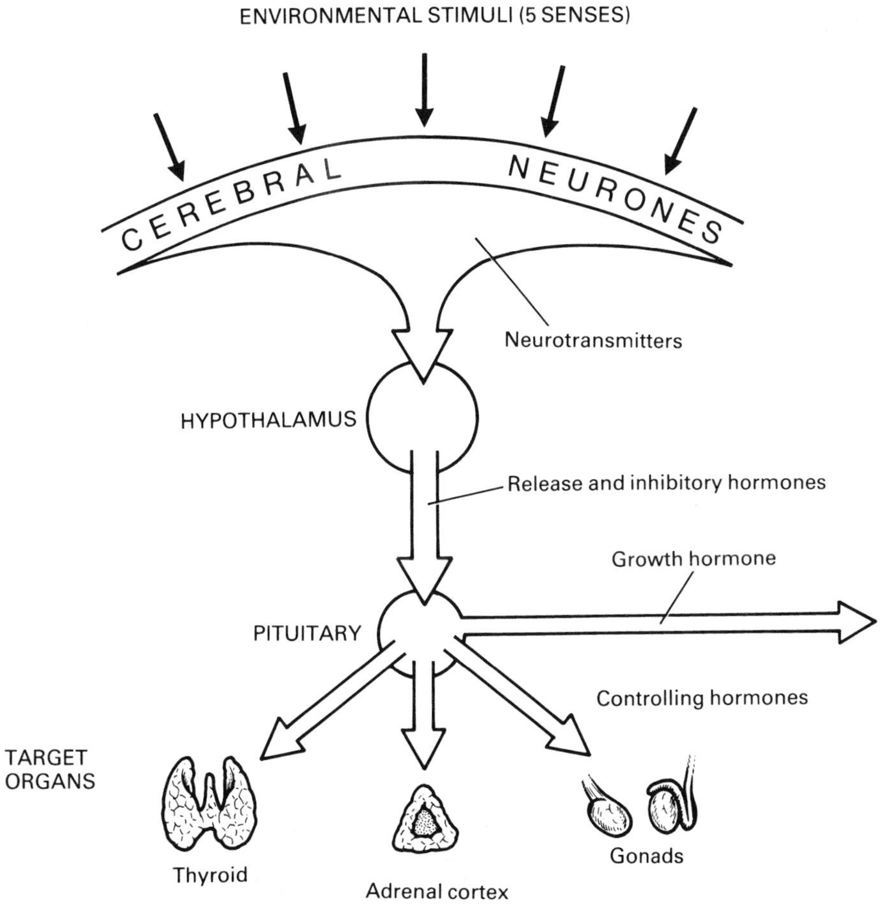

ENVIRONMENTAL STIMULI (5 SENSES)

CEREBRAL NEURONES

Neurotransmitters

HYPOTHALAMUS

Release and inhibitory hormones

Growth hormone

PITUITARY

Controlling hormones

TARGET ORGANS

Thyroid

Adrenal cortex

Gonads

Fig. 14.1 Outside stimuli release neurotransmitters in the brain; these then act on the endocrine system.

hormone will return to normal if they are given a glucose load orally. In those with tumours, it will not.

Radiological investigations are extremely helpful. A plain X-ray of the skull may show an increase in the size of the pituitary fossa. However, in recent years computerized axial tomography (CAT or CT) scanning, and magnetic resonance imaging (MRI) have revolutionized our ability to visualize these tumours which can be as small as 1 mm and cause significant problems.

Treatment This may involve:

1. Surgery. Where there are visual symptoms, surgery must be performed. If the tumour can be localized then surgery is still preferable to remove just the tumour. When it is not possible to find the tumour within the pituitary then either the

whole gland can be removed or the patient can be given radiotherapy to destroy the tumour. With all forms of treatment the possibility that the patient will need replacement of their pituitary hormones subsequently must be remembered. Deficiency should be looked for both clinically and with blood tests at follow up.

2. Octreotide. This drug is now in routine use in acromegaly. It acts by inhibiting secretion of growth hormone from the pituitary and preventing its action in the periphery. It is increasingly being realised that it has similar effects on many other hormones and is being used in other situations where there is hormone excess. It must be given by subcutaneous injection, usually three times a day. It is very expensive, with an average cost for a patient with acromegaly being £6000 per year.

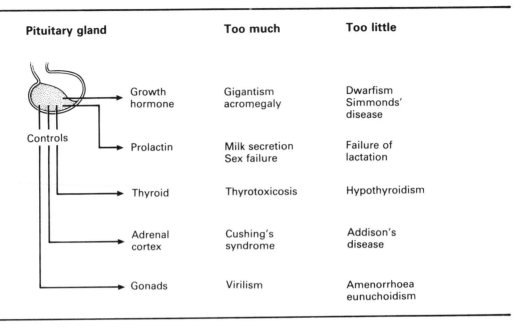

Pituitary gland		Too much	Too little
	Growth hormone	Gigantism acromegaly	Dwarfism Simmonds' disease
Controls	Prolactin	Milk secretion Sex failure	Failure of lactation
	Thyroid	Thyrotoxicosis	Hypothyroidism
	Adrenal cortex	Cushing's syndrome	Addison's disease
	Gonads	Virilism	Amenorrhoea eunuchoidism

Fig. 14.2 Actions of the anterior lobe of the pituitary gland.

Prolactinoma

This is the commonest tumour of the anterior pituitary. They are usually very small (microadenomas), and often asymptomatic. As mentioned earlier, excess prolactin can cause galactorrhoea and amenorrhoea in women, and impotence and infertility in men. The main reason to treat them in the absence of visual symptoms (which requires immediate intervention) is infertility. In this instance prolactin suppressing drugs, such as bromocryptine, are very effective.

Hypopituitarism (Simmonds' disease)

This is due to destruction of the pituitary gland. The commonest causes are compression by a tumour or necrosis following a large haemorrhage. Whatever the cause the thyroid, adrenal cortex, and gonads all fail to function properly. If it occurs in a child then the child fails to grow, due to the growth hormone deficiency.

Symptoms and signs

There is progressive loss of the pituitary function.

Interestingly the loss tends to occur in order of increasing importance (loss of prolactin secretion is early while the much more important thyroid and steroid hormones are the last to be lost).

The main clinical manifestations are of hormone deficiency, with:

1. Marked lethargy and malaise, due to steroid and thyroid deficiency.
2. Loss of sexual functions with amenorrhoea and gonadal atrophy.
3. Low blood pressure, again due to steroid deficiency.
4. In long-standing hypopituitarism the patient has smooth skin and loss of axillary and pubic hair, giving a characteristic appearance of premature ageing.

Diagnosis

Clinical suspicion is essential to make the diagnosis. There may be a history of postpartum haemorrhage, or another form of bleeding. If, following this, the menses have failed to return or breast milk has not been produced then one should consider the diagnosis. In the case of a

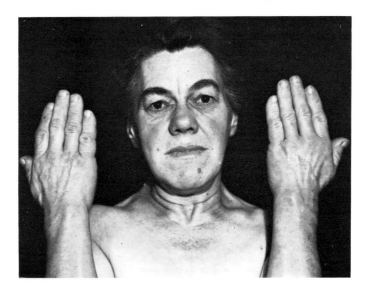

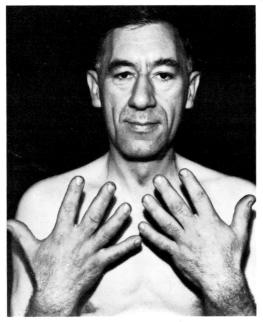

Figs 14.3, 14.4 Two patients with acromegaly. Note the heavy features, the larger lower jaw and the broad fingers and hands.

man if impotence has developed then once again the diagnosis should be entertained. The appearance of the patient is an important clue, with the smooth hairless skin.

Confirmation of the diagnosis is by testing the ability of the pituitary to secrete hormones in response to stress (in the form of hypoglycaemia), or in response to the hypothalamic factors such as TRH or GnRH. A low level of cortisone production by the adrenal gland indicates that the pituitary is not producing ACTH and this helps to confirm the diagnosis.

Treatment

This depends on replacing those hormones that are deficient. This is done with hydrocortisone tablets (20 mg in the morning and 10 mg in the evening as this is the way our adrenal gland produces steroid, a lot in the morning and less in the evening), thyroid hormone, and either oestrogens or androgens depending on the sex of the patient.

Dwarfism

In childhood growth hormone deficiency results in short stature. If this is combined with other hormone deficiencies, in particular sex hormones, then the child fails to develop any secondary sex characteristics. In this situation the patient retains the hairless body and high-pitched voice of childhood. It is important to realise that pituitary problems cause very few cases of short stature.

More common causes include:

1. malnutrition (commonest cause worldwide)
2. chronic infections in childhood, e.g. cystic fibrosis
3. malabsorption, e.g. coeliac disease
4. congenital heart disease
5. inherited, e.g. achondroplastic (circus) dwarf

Diabetes insipidus

This occurs following damage to the posterior lobe of the pituitary. One of the main products of this lobe is antidiuretic hormone (ADH), also called vasopressin. This acts on the kidneys to prevent loss of fluid. Without this ADH, the patient is unable to concentrate their urine and looses lots of dilute urine. These patients are very thirsty, and often get up several times at night to drink jugs of water they put ready by their bed.

The commonest cause is following surgery to the pituitary, or a head injury. Treatment is now available with a form of the hormone as a nasal spray, which needs to be taken once or twice each day. This long-acting form of the hormone is called desmopressin or DDAVP.

THYROID GLAND

Anatomy and physiology

The gland is situated in the lower portion of the neck. It consists of two lobes either side of the trachea, joined by a central segment that bridges across the trachea (called the isthmus). The main role of the thyroid is to produce the hormone called *thyroxine*. The main substance required for manufacture of thyroxine is iodine. This hormone controls the rate of metabolism in the body. Too much thyroxine leads to an increase in basal metabolic rate, with weight loss, irritability, and palpitations. This condition is known as *hyper-thyroidism* or *thyrotoxicosis*. Too little thyroxine leads to the opposite, and a condition known as *hypothyroidism*.

Either underactivity or overactivity of the gland can be associated with enlargement. An enlarged thyroid gland is called a *goitre*.

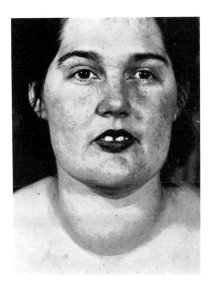

Fig. 14.5 Simple (non-toxic) goitre.

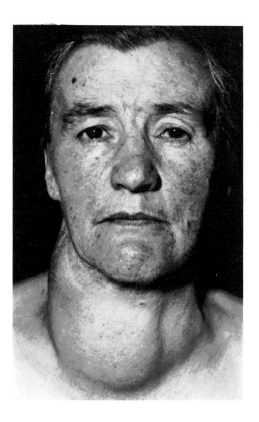

Fig. 14.6 Non-toxic goitre. The goitre was removed because it was causing pressure symptoms.

Diseases of the thyroid gland

Goitre

This is defined as an increase in size of the thyroid gland. There are various forms of goitre:

1. Simple (non-toxic) goitre. Here the gland is behaving normally. There may be a nodular feel to the gland, but there is no sign of hyper- or hypothyroidism.
2. Toxic goitre. Here the enlargement of the gland is associated with signs of overactivity of thyroxine. It can be:
    a. diffuse toxic goitre (Graves' disease)
    b. nodular toxic goitre
3. Malignant goitre.

Simple non-toxic goitre

This is a common condition that is endemic in some areas where iodine is deficient in the water supply. Such areas include Switzerland, some areas of America and some regions of England. Derbyshire was once famous for its high prevalance of goitre. Simple goitre is common at certain times of life, in particular pregnancy and puberty. In most cases there is no need for treatment. The occurrance of simple goitre has been reduced by the addition of iodine to water supplies where this is deficient. Treatment may be required if:

1. it continues to grow and causes pressure symptoms, such as difficulty swallowing or difficulty breathing
2. it causes severe cosmetic problems.

In these instances surgical removal of all or part of the gland is the definitive approach. It must always be remembered that a simple goitre may become overactive or indeed malignant.

Type of goitre	Hormone secretion	Signs and symptoms	Treatment
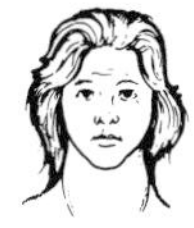 Simple	Normal	Sometimes local pressure symptoms	Iodine Thyroxine Removal if persistent
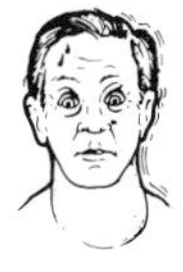 Toxic	Increased	Irritability Loss of weight Sweating Tremor Exophthalmos Tachycardia	*Medical* Carbinazole Thiouracil Radioactive iodine *Surgical* Partial thyroidectomy
Malignant	Normal	Goitre hard Local pressure symptoms Secondaries	Total thyroidectomy
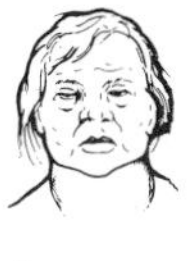 Myxoedema (Hashimoto's disease)	Decreased	Skin thickening Loss of hair Slow pulse Slow mentality Constipation Fatigue	Thyroxine

Fig. 14.7 Types of goitre.

Toxic goitre

This is defined as a swelling of the thyroid gland associated with oversecretion of thyroid hormone. There are two main types of toxic goitre:

1. Diffuse. Here there is generalized enlargement of the gland, it occurs in younger people and is also known as Graves' disease.
2. Nodular. Here the enlargement is focal with one or two nodules being responsible for the excess hormone being produced. It tends to affect older patients.

Thyrotoxicosis is the over-production of thyroid hormone by the gland. This increases the metabolic rate of the body. Associated symptoms and signs include:

1. anxiety, irritability
2. weight loss despite a good appetite
3. sweating and heat intolerance
4. tremor (very fine and seen best with the hands outstretched)
5. tachycardia and subjective palpitations
6. exophthalmos. This is the characteristic prominence of the eyes seen especially in the diffuse type of goitre; it can occur long before or after any problem with the thyroid hormone production is manifest
7. diarrhoea is also a feature.

Diagnosis In the presence of the classic symptoms and signs a clinical diagnosis can be made. This is confirmed by measuring the circulating level of thyroxine which is usually elevated appropriate to the degree of symptoms.

Treatment This is either medical or surgical.

Medical

Antithyroid drugs. These include carbimazole and thiouracil. They are effective in controlling symptoms, but take some days to act. For this reason they are often combined with a beta blocker in the first instance which provides more immediate control of the symptoms. The main serious side-effect of these drugs is depression of the white cell count. This can lead to overwhelming infection and death. The first sign of this low white cell count is often a sore throat and patients must be well warned to stop the drug in the event of this and to make arrangements to get a full

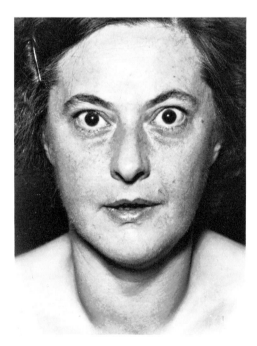

Fig. 14.8 Primary toxic goitre (Graves' disease) showing the characteristic staring, apprehensive expression and the enlarged thyroid.

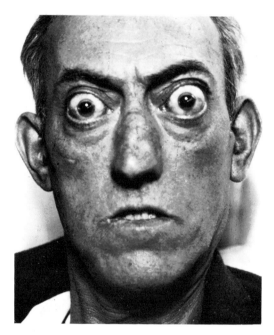

Fig. 14.9 Severe exophthalmos in a case of primary toxic goitre (Graves' disease).

blood count done immediately.

Radioactive iodine. As iodine is taken up by the thyroid gland this, if radiolabelled, will damage the thyroid and make it less active. This will have the effect of returning the thyroid towards normal activity but may obviously cause the thyroid to become underactive. In this case hormone replacement is required after the radioactive iodine.

Surgical A total or partial thyroidectomy is performed when:

1. medical treatment has failed to control the overactivity
2. pressure symptoms have occurred due to the size of the gland.

Most patients will have a pre-operative course of antithyroid drugs to reduce the risk of the operation.

Malignant goitre

This is unusual. Pressure symptoms are common, and the goitre tends to be hard and painful. It spreads to bones often before detection. The treatment is surgical if possible. This may be combined with radioactive iodine.

Thyroid hormone deficiency

As hormone excess causes increase in metabolic rate, so deficiency causes a decrease in the metabolic rate. This causes myxoedema or hypothyroidism in adults and cretinism in young children.

Myxoedema (hypothyroidism)

Causes
1. Post surgical removal of the gland.
2. Following treatment with antithyroid drugs or radioactive iodine.
3. Destruction of the gland by abnormal antibodies in the circulation; this is called Hashimoto's disease.

Symptoms and signs
1. Weight gain, lethargy and malaise.
2. Dry, coarse, thickened skin.

3. Loss of hair.
4. Slow pulse (bradycardia).
5. Memory loss. It is essential that all patients with possible dementia are checked for hypothyroidism.
6. Cold weather intolerance.
7. Constipation is a prominent feature.

Diagnosis A typical history and clinical appearance make the diagnosis easy. It can be confirmed by a low serum thyroid hormone level. In addition the pituitary gland tries to keep the thyroid gland going by producing extra TSH (thyroid stimulating hormone), which is accordingly elevated in the blood.

Treatment This consists of replacing the deficiency with oral thyroxine. The dose is individual and must be titrated against both the thyroxine level and the TSH level in the blood. Care must be taken to avoid over replacement and thus symptoms of thyrotoxicosis. In the elderly the increase in metabolism may unmask angina.

Cretinism

Causes This is usually due to atrophy of the

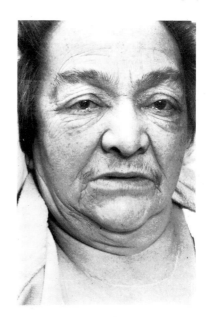

Fig. 14.10 Myxoedema showing the characteristic puffy and bloated appearance. The condition developed after thyroidectomy for a toxic goitre. (The scar in the neck is still visible.)

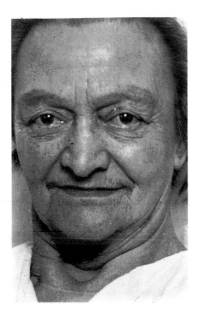

Fig. 14.11 Myxoedema after thyroid therapy showing the marked improvement. (Same patient as in Fig. 14.10.)

child's thyroid, the precise cause of which is unknown.

Symptoms and signs

1. Symptoms begin within 6 months, but are not present at birth.

2. Failure of growth in both physical and mental terms. If undiagnosed the child becomes a mentally deficient dwarf.

3. The abdomen is distended and they have a flat nose, dry skin, scanty hair, and a coarse tongue.

Diagnosis The clinical appearance is confirmed by the low thyroxine and raised TSH levels in the blood. This test is performed in all newborn infants 10 days after birth. This test involves pricking the heel and collecting a blood sample. It is called the *Guthrie test* and also looks for other reversible causes of mental retardation in addition to hypothyroidism.

Treatment It is most important that cretinism should be recognized as early as possible as early treatment can result in a complete cure. If, however, treatment is delayed too long then some permanent mental deficiency may remain. As in myxoedema, thyroxine is prescribed though naturally in much smaller doses applicable to a child.

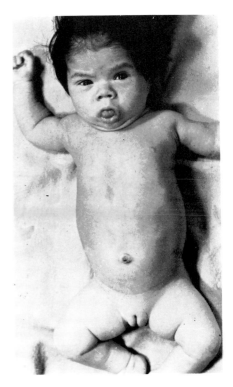

Fig. 14.12 Cretin, aged 8 months. The appearance with the thick, protruding tongue is typical, as is also the umbilical hernia.

ADRENAL GLANDS

The adrenals are divided into two main parts, the cortex and medulla.

The cortex

The adrenal cortex secretes many different hormones, which can be classified as follows:

1. *Cortisone.* This important hormone has many actions. It plays a part in the control of carbohydrate metabolism and can convert protein into glucose. It affects the output of sodium. It controls the processes of inflammation and allergy, and this property explains its use in the treatment of many diseases.

2. *Aldosterone.* This hormone regulates mineral metabolism, particularly sodium and potassium. If present in excess the body retains excessive

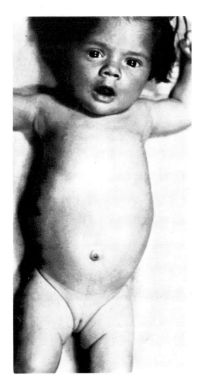

Fig. 14.13 Same patient as in Figure 14.12. Three months after starting thyroid therapy.

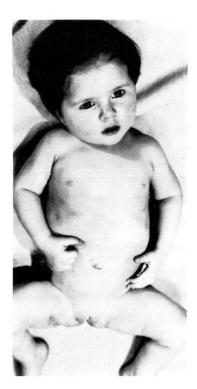

Fig. 14.14 Same patient as in Figure 14.12. Eleven months after starting treatment; the child's health is now normal.

sodium and excretes too much potassium.

3. *Sex hormones.* These include the various androgenic hormones, which have a masculinizing effect and also tend to cause bodily growth. The other main sex hormones are the oestrogens.

Corticotrophin (ACTH) is the pituitary adreno-corticotrophic hormone which stimulates the adrenals to produce cortisone and allied hormones.

The medulla

The medulla secretes two hormones, adrenalin and noradrenalin. These are very powerful hormones and are used in the treatment of some diseases.

Diseases of the adrenal cortex

1. *Addison's Disease.* This leads to lack of the hormones produced by the cortex, particularly those involved with salt control.

2. *Hyperplasia* or tumours with overproduction of the hormones.

Addison's disease

Causes

1. Atrophy of the gland probably due to destruction by abnormal antibodies.

2. Tuberculous disease producing widespread gland destruction.

Symptoms and signs

1. There is profound weakness which, in later stages, may be so severe that the patient is unable to get about. Generalized wasting is also a fairly early feature.

2. There is a characteristic pigmentation of the skin and mucous membranes. Brown patches are often seen on the lips, in the mouth and around the nipples. The pigmentation may also be more generalized and is particularly prominent in areas exposed to sunlight, in areas under pressure from a belt or constricting garment or in scars.

3. Nausea, with attacks of diarrhoea and vomiting, is very frequent.

4. A low blood pressure, often with a systolic blood pressure of less than 100 mmHg.

5. Changes in the blood biochemistry are characteristic. The amount of sodium and chloride is usually diminished and the potassium raised, especially during the acute stages. The fasting blood sugar is often low.

6. The level of cortisol (cortisol is secreted by the adrenal cortex) is very low in the blood in Addison's disease and does not rise when ACTH (which normally stimulates the gland to produce cortisol) is injected. This is used as a test in the diagnosis of Addison's disease.

Course of Addison's disease If undiagnosed and untreated, patients with Addison's disease gradually deteriorate and suddenly collapse, the so-called acute adrenal crisis or Addisonian crisis. This is often precipitated by vomiting and diarrhoea or a chest infection. The blood pressure falls to dangerous levels, the pulse becomes rapid and thready and the extremities are cold. Death will follow unless treatment is instituted.

Treatment

1. Patients with Addison's disease can be maintained on hydrocortisone 30 mg daily. Their symptoms resolve on this. Some will require a small dose of fludrocortisone to maintain salt balance in addition to the hydrocortisone.

2. An Addisonian crisis will require aggressive monitoring, often in an intensive care bed. Intravenous hydrocortisone is given at high doses initially, but then gradually reduced. Prevention is critical. Warning the patient that in the event of an infection they should increase their dose of steroid is the key.

Cushing's syndrome

This is the clinical picture resulting from excess cortisone. It can be caused in different ways:

1. a tumour of the pituitary gland which produces excess ACTH and so stimulates the adrenal cortex to produce too much cortisone
2. a tumour (adenoma) of the adrenal cortex which produces excess cortisone
3. some forms of lung cancer (bronchial carcinoma) produce excess ACTH
4. steroid therapy; cortisone or prednisone if given in large doses over long periods of time.

Clinical features
1. Obesity. This is characteristically central with thin extremities (the so-called Lemon on a stick phenomenon).
2. Acne, hirsutism, and purple striae on the abdomen and buttocks.
3. Hypertension.
4. Diabetes.
5. Osteoporosis.
6. Proximal muscle weakness and mental depression.

Diagnosis Normally cortisone is formed and released into the blood overnight, so that the blood levels of cortisone are higher in the morning than in the evening (diurnal variation). In Cushing's syndrome the blood levels of cortisone are high and are unaltered day or night. When the diagnosis is confirmed in this way, further investigation is necessary to establish the cause. The level of ACTH in the blood can be measured and will be high if the cause of the disorder is in the pituitary but will be low if there is an adrenal growth. X-ray of the skull will show if the pituitary fossa is enlarged, which would suggest a pituitary tumour. X-ray of the chest might reveal a bronchial carcinoma. A plain X-ray of the abdomen can be taken to see if there is an adrenal tumour with calcification. Operation might be indicated either on the skull to remove a pituitary tumour or on the abdomen to remove an adrenal tumour.

Adrenogenital syndrome (virilism)

Here, there is chiefly an excessive secretion of the sex hormones, although the other adrenal cortical hormones may also be affected.

Clinical features
1. The most predominant signs are seen in women, who develop masculine characteristics with excessive growth of hair on the face (hirsutism). The voice deepens and muscular development resembles that of a man. The sex organs undergo striking changes, with enlargement of

the clitoris. Amenorrhoea is present and acne is also a feature.

2. In adult males there may be few striking changes, but generally the picture is similar to that described under Cushing's syndrome where excess sex hormones are responsible for many of the features.

3. In young boys there is very early sex development with growth of hair on the face, enlargement of the penis and pronounced muscular growth – a condition called *precocious puberty*.

4. If excessive adrenal activity occurs in intrauterine life it produces in girls the picture of virilism. The child may be mistaken for a boy. Pre-natal adrenal steroid oversecretion in boys causes marked enlargement of the external genitalia.

Diagnosis Male hormones (androgens) are found in excess in the blood and are excreted in the urine as 17-ketosteroids and these are found in excess.

Treatment Treatment depends on whether an actual tumour or merely hyperplasia is present. Tumours, which are more likely to be present in adults than in children, are removed. If hyperplasia only is present, as is probable in young children, hydrocortisone is given and this will suppress the activity of the adrenals.

Diseases of the adrenal medulla

Phaeochromocytoma

The commonest disease known to affect the adrenal medulla is a tumour called a phaeochromocytoma. This tumour produces an excess of the normal secretion of the medulla – adrenalin. The main effect of this overproduction of adrenalin is severe hypertension, which characteristically occurs in paroxysmal attacks. During these attacks the patient complains of very severe headaches, sweating and vomiting and the blood pressure is markedly raised. When the diagnosis is suspected, special chemical tests can be used to detect excessive amounts of derivatives of adrenalin (catecholamines) excreted in the urine. The treatment of choice is surgery, which can only be

performed when adequate therapy to block the effect of the adrenalin and noradrenalin has been instituted. Without this many peroperative problems may arise – especially severe hypertension.

PARATHYROID GLANDS
Anatomy and physiology

The parathyroid glands are four in number and are situated directly behind the thyroid gland. The main function of the parathyroids is the regulation of the calcium and phosphorus content of the bones and blood. The main functions of calcium are:

1. the formation of bone (any disturbance in the level of calcium can lead to improper development of and deformities in the bones)
2. the control of the irritability of muscles and nerves
3. as a necessary background factor for many enzyme and cellular processes.

The proper absorption and usage of calcium is regulated in three main ways.

1. Vitamin D controls the absorption of calcium from the bowel. The calcium absorbed is important for the bones to help in their proper formation and calcification. Lack of vitamin D, as one would expect, leads to marked changes in the bones (rickets in children and osteomalacia in adults).

2. The parathyroid hormone (parathormone) regulates the flow of calcium between the bones and the blood. Excessive secretion of the hormone causes a withdrawal of calcium from the bones into the blood with the result that the bones become soft, spongy, deformed and liable to fracture. On the other hand, deficiency of parathormone leads to a low level of calcium in the blood, which is one cause of the clinical syndrome known as tetany (this will be discussed later).

3. Calcitonin is secreted by the parafollicular cells of the thyroid gland. It opposes the effect of parathormone and increases deposition of calcium into the bones from the blood.

Diseases of the parathyroid glands

Tumours of the parathyroid glands may lead to overproduction of parathyroid hormone. Underproduction is usually due to damage of the glands (which lie behind the thyroid gland) during operation on the thyroid.

Tumours

These are very rare. The excess of parathyroid hormone causes a condition known as *hyperparathyroidism*

Symptoms and signs of hyperparathyroidism

1. Excessive calcium in the blood. This is the earliest occurrence and may be without symptoms for some years. When more severe it usually causes weakness and loss of appetite and weight. Generalized muscle and joint pains are common. In severe cases there may be nausea and vomiting.

2. Changes in the bones. As parathyroid hormone causes excess removal of calcium from the bones, high levels make them become soft. In addition they are liable to fracture.

3. Excretion of calcium into the urine. Because of the presence of excessive calcium in urine kidney stones develop, and in severe cases these may block off the kidneys. This would result in signs of renal damage and uraemia. In some cases the kidney stones are small enough that they pass down the urinary tract and out in the urine. This is often associated with severe pain and visible blood in the urine (haematuria).

Diagnosis The diagnosis is usually made on the above symptoms and signs, and by estimating the level of calcium and parathyroid hormone in the blood, which are persistently raised above normal.

Course and treatment Unless the condition is treated the patients will eventually become bedridden due to the bony abnormalities, and they may die from renal failure. The treatment is for a surgeon to explore the parathyroid glands in the neck and remove the tumour. If this is done early a complete cure is possible.

Injuries during operation on the thyroid gland

The condition which most commonly affects the

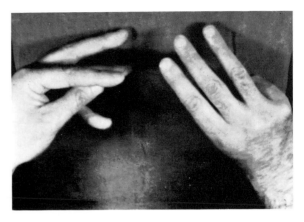

Fig. 14.15 Tetany showing the characteristic position of the hands in carpopedal spasm.

parathyroid glands is accidental injury during operations on the thyroid. The main effect is to produce a deficiency of parathyroid hormone which results in a low serum calcium and its clinical manifestation – tetany. In most cases, however, the tetany is transient because the remaining undamaged parathyroid glands enlarge and respond to doses of vitamin D and calcium which raise the blood calcium level.

Tetany

In the discussion on the action of the parathyroid hormone we saw that undersecretion of this hormone can lead to a low blood calcium level and so to the condition of tetany. This can be caused in several different ways:

1. Undersecretion of parathyroid hormone. This cause is rare and is usually the result of injury to or accidental removal of the parathyroids during operations on the thyroid gland.

2. Lack of vitamin D. Vitamin D is necessary for the control of absorption of calcium from the bowel. If vitamin D is lacking hypocalcaemia may result and thus tetany.

Symptoms and signs

1. Painful cramps occur in the hands and feet. The hands take up a characteristic cramped position, with the thumbs pressed into the palms and the fingers hyperextended. This is known as carpopedal spasm. Pressure on the arms will

bring on the carpopedal spasms and this reaction is referred to as *Trousseau's sign*. It is very important to check this in patients who have had their thyroid removed, as Trousseau's sign may be the first indication that the parathyroid gland was damaged.

2. Convulsions, which are particularly common in children.

3. Laryngeal spasm. Sudden spasm of the larynx occurs causing cyanosis and stridor.

4. Chvostek's sign. Tapping on the branches of the facial nerve in the face produces twitching of the muscles of the face especially the corner of the mouth. This is due to the irritability of the nerves which is present in tetany. It indicates the same problems as Trousseau's sign.

Treatment This will depend on the cause, but relief of low-calcium spasm can be obtained by slow intravenous injection of calcium gluconate. When the parathyroid glands are not functioning prolonged treatment with vitamin D (calciferol) will be necessary and regular estimations of blood calcium levels are required to regulate the dose.

Hyperventilation and tetany

The commonest cause of tetany is overbreathing. This causes a complex change in acid–base balance because the patient is blowing off too much carbon dioxide which is an acid. The result is an alkalosis which causes calcium to leave the cells of the body temporarily. This results in tetany. It is treated by re-breathing into a bag which prevents the carbon dioxide from escaping.

THE USE OF HORMONES IN CLINICAL MEDICINE

Hormones are used not only to replace the natural hormones where these are deficient, but also in the treatment of other disorders.

Cortisone and allied steroids

Cortisone is one of the most important steroid hormones produced by the adrenal cortex. These steroids control the processes of inflammation

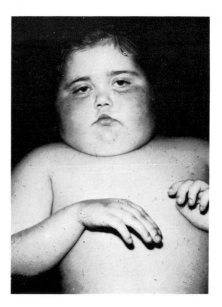

Fig. 14.16 Nephrotic syndrome treated with large doses of prednisolone to protect the kidneys. The bloated moon face is due to prolonged steroid treatment.

and allergy, and so hydrocortisone is often prescribed to suppress excessive inflammatory or allergic reactions. Unfortunately, in most diseases in which cortisone is beneficial, relapse occurs when the drug is discontinued. Furthermore, if these steroids are given in too large a dose or for too long a time, serious side-effects may be noted. In particular, retention of salt occurs with subsequent oedema and hypertension. Since the isolation of cortisone, many similar compounds have been synthesized, such as prednisone, which have less or no tendency to lead to salt retention.

Cortisone

This is effective when given by mouth or by intramuscular injection. Its main use is to replace the natural hormone in conditions where the adrenal cortex is not functioning:

1. Addison's disease. Cortisone is lifesaving in this condition. The usual dose is 30 mg daily, and this is sometimes supplemented by fluorohydrocortisone (Florinef), a powerful salt-retaining steroid.

2. Pituitary disease. Lack of stimulation from the pituitary gland leads to atrophy of the adrenal

cortex. Cortisone must be taken daily.

3. Total adrenalectomy. This operation of removing both adrenal glands is performed in certain cases of Cushing's disease. Large doses of cortisone must be given during the pre-operative and postoperative stages, and maintenance doses of cortisone must be continued for life.

Prednisolone

This is a synthetic compound with properties similar to those of cortisone but less likely to lead to salt retention. Many other such steroids are now available (e.g. prednisone, triamcinolone, dexamethasone), and their main use is to suppress excessive inflammatory or allergic reactions. They do not remove the cause of these reactions though they relieve the effects. Prednisolone is used in:

1. Rheumatoid arthritis. Where the condition is active and has failed to respond to safer remedies, prednisolone (or similar compound) may prove helpful in relieving the pain and swelling in the joints and in permitting more mobility. The dose should be as low as possible to avoid unwanted side effects.

2. Asthma. Prednisolone can be used in resistant cases and is strikingly successful in relieving respiratory wheezing and dyspnoea.

3. Ulcerative colitis. Prednisolone is sometimes helpful in suppressing the inflammation and ulceration of the colon in this condition, though often the improvement is not maintained despite continuation of therapy.

4. The nephrotic syndrome. Especially in children, steroid therapy can be successful in reducing the oedema and albuminuria. High dosage of prednisolone is necessary.

5. Blood diseases. Steroids can lead to a remission in haemolytic anaemia and in purpura.

6. Allergic states, such as drug allergy, hay fever or dermatitis. Prednisolone should only be used in very severe conditions that have failed to respond to antihistamines.

7. Collagen diseases. Steroids must be employed in relatively large doses and may be life-saving in these diseases.

Hydrocortisone

This is the natural hormone. It is available for intravenous injection and is usually given in a dose of 100 mg in an intravenous drip for emergency treatment in cases of collapse due to acute adrenal insufficiency, as sometimes occurs in people who have taken steroids for some while or in adrenalectomised Addison's disease patients who omit to take their routine cortisone tablets.

Corticotrophin (ACTH)

ACTH is the pituitary adrenocorticotrophic hormone which stimulates the adrenals to produce hydrocortisone. Hence, unless the adrenals are damaged, the effect of ACTH is similar to that of hydrocortisone. It has to be administered by intramuscular injection.

Hydrocortisone, prednisolone, and other steroids are also available for local treatment to relieve inflammation in specific areas:

1. eye drops, for acute inflammatory eye conditions
2. ointments or sprays, for local application in skin conditions such as eczema or pruritus ani
3. intra-articular injections, especially of the knees in rheumatoid arthritis or osteo-arthritis
4. retention enemas for ulcerative colitis.

Toxic effects of steroids

1. Retention of salt, leading to oedema and high blood pressure. Patients taking prolonged courses of steroids should avoid salt in the diet.

2. Conversion of protein to carbohydrate, leading to increased blood sugar. This may precipitate diabetes. Diabetic patients taking cortisone may need more insulin.

3. Reduced resistance to infection, due to suppression of inflammatory reactions which normally offer protection. Tuberculosis, if present, can spread very rapidly in patients on steroid therapy. A chest X-ray should be taken to make sure there is no evidence of pulmonary tuberculosis. Similarly, patients with a peptic ulcer should be given hydrocortisone with caution as

healing of the ulcer may be delayed and perforation has been known to occur.

4. Acne, obesity, and thinning of the bones (osteoporosis) occur with excessive dosage. In fact, Cushing's syndrome is due to excessive cortisone and can be caused by injudicious therapy.

5. Adrenal collapse. When cortisone is given, the natural secretion of the gland is suppressed and the gland becomes inactive. Hence, if cortisone treatment is stopped suddenly, collapse due to adrenal insufficiency is likely to occur. This could lead to a fatal outcome, particularly if any operation is undertaken.

Precautions for patients taking steroids

Patients taking steroids must be given a special blue card warning them that it is dangerous to stop their tablets without special medical advice, and urging them to report to the doctor if they are unwell. Steroid therapy must always be discontinued gradually.

Adrenalin (Epinephrine) and noradrenalin

Adrenalin and noradrenalin are the two hormones produced by the adrenal medulla. Actions of adrenalin:

1. constricts the blood vessels in the skin and mucous membranes
2. relaxes the smooth muscle of the small airways of the lungs
3. raises the blood sugar by releasing glucose from the liver into the blood stream
4. increases the rate and force of the contractions of the heart

Uses of adrenalin

1. To stop bleeding from mucous membranes, as in epistaxis, gauze plugs soaked in adrenalin are used. Adrenalin is also used in local anaesthetic solutions to constrict the vessels and so reduce the amount of bleeding.

2. In anaphylaxis and other severe hypersensitivity reactions, subcutaneous injections of adrenalin may offer immediate relief.

3. In cases of cardiac arrest due to asystole, adrenalin injected directly into the heart may start the heart beating again.

Oestrogens

Oestrogens are the hormones secreted by the ovary and are responsible for the normal female development. Many synthetic and natural preparations are available for clinical use, including ethinyloestradiol and oestrone (premarin).

Menopause

In the majority of women, ovulation ceases around the age of 50. The periods become less frequent and finally cease. The menopause is often associated with constitutional symptoms due to a falling off of oestrogen secretion from the ovaries. Hot flushes of the face and body are often associated with marked sweating. Emotional instability, irritability of mood and depression may occur. When hot flushes, sweats and mood disturbance are severe, a course of oestrogen may be prescribed, usually offering great relief of these troublesome symptoms. There is now good evidence that the increase in bone fractures and decrease in bone density seen after the menopause is due to, in part, the reduction in oestrogen levels. Further, women before the menopause have fewer heart attacks than men but after the rate rises. It has been shown that hormone replacement therapy can reduce these risks.

Contraceptive pill

Long continued pure oestrogens run the risk of inducing cancer of the uterus and are best given in low dose with progesterone. This will also prevent loss of bone density (osteoporosis) and thereby help prevent fractures. The pill contains synthetic oestrogens and progesterones which in combination prevent ovulation without leading to break-through bleeding between cycles. If taken regularly and according to instruction, oral contraceptives are a completely effective form of birth control, but they have disadvantages:

1. Nausea, headaches and breast discomfort may occur especially during the first few cycles.

2. There is an impairment of glucose metabolism with a tendency to diabetes. Diabetic patients may find their insulin requirements need increasing when they start the pill, while actual diabetes may develop in those predisposed to it.

3. Oestrogens disturb the blood-clotting mechanism and so the pill predisposes to venous thrombosis and pulmonary embolism, as indeed does pregnancy. There is also increased tendency to high blood pressure.

4. Amenorrhoea may follow discontinuation of the pill, and may persist for many months.

Low-dose oestrogen and progesterone pill preparations diminish all these risks but are a less powerful contraceptive so exact compliance is essential for them to be maximally effective.

Carcinoma of the prostate

Oestrogens are given for the maintenance treatment of carcinoma of the prostate. They inhibit the growth and spread of the cancer and relieve the symptoms.

Androgens

Androgens are male hormones secreted mainly by the testicles but also by the adrenal cortex. They are responsible for the maturation of the male secondary characteristics after puberty, and are effective in building up protein. They are sometimes used when pituitary or testicular hormone failure occurs as replacement therapy.

Other hormones

Other hormones have been described in the appropriate sections:

1. antidiuretic hormone (vasopressin) in the treatment of diabetes insipidus
2. thyroxine in the treatment of hypothyroidism
3. insulin for the treatment of diabetes mellitus
4. glucagon for the treatment of hypoglycaemia.

15

Diseases of joints, bones and connective tissue

JOINTS

The parts of the bones which form a joint are covered by smooth firm cartilage, lubricated by a thick viscid fluid. This fluid is secreted by the synovial membrane. The synovial membrane encloses the joint space and is formed of epithelial cells. It is these cells which secrete the synovial fluid into the joint.

Disease of the joints can be due to a number of causes. Rheumatoid arthritis is a chronic, multisystem disease of unknown aetiology, primarily affecting the joints but also other systems of the body as well. Osteo-arthritis is a degenerative condition of individual joints. Gout is a metabolic disorder leading to severe joint damage.

Joint disease can be due to infections of the joint, and associated with other diseases (e.g. sexually transmitted diseases), and also due to destruction of the nerves that supply sensation to the joint. All these complaints are loosely referred to as forms of 'arthritis'; they are very common and a source of a great deal of disability.

RHEUMATOID ARTHRITIS

Rheumatoid arthritis is a chronic condition characterized by persistent inflammatory arthritis. It usually involves peripheral joints in a symmetrical distribution. The course of rheumatoid arthritis can be quite variable. Some patients experience a mild arthritis of their hands with minimal joint damage, while others have a progressive destructive arthritis with joint deformity and disability. Most patients lie between these two extremes.

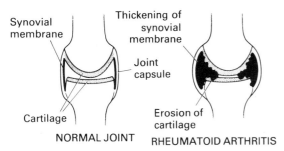

Fig. 15.1 A joint affected by rheumatoid arthritis.

In rheumatoid arthritis, the synovial membrane becomes thickened and inflamed and the cartilages are eroded. The synovial membrane may invade the joint space and the whole joint becomes swollen and painful on movement.

The inflammation in rheumatoid arthritis is immune-mediated with evidence of activation of cells of the immune system (T lymphocytes) and production of abnormal antibodies. It is not clear whether this is an autoimmune process or is triggered by an external antigen such as a virus.

The abnormal antibodies (e.g. *rheumatoid factor*) found in the blood of most patients with rheumatoid arthritis, by combining with antigen and forming antibody–antigen complexes, may contribute to the inflammatory changes in the synovial membrane and the cartilage.

Symptoms and signs

1. The disease is three times as common in women as in men, the average age of onset being about 40; however, it can occur in children (Still's disease) or in the very elderly (*senile rheumatoid*).

2. It tends to run a variable course, with remissions and exacerbations. Some cases are very severe and lead to crippling within a few years. Others run a mild course and only cause slight disability.

3. The main effect is on the joints. The fingers are often the earliest affected, giving rise to pain and stiffness especially on first getting up in the morning. The feet, ankles, knees, wrists, elbows and shoulders also become involved, and later the spine. The affected joints become swollen and tender with thickening of the surrounding tissues and restriction of mobility. Pain may disturb sleep, and mobility becomes difficult. In severe

cases, the joints may become fixed and deformed so that the patient is unable to look after herself and may become bedridden. Fortunately, only a small proportion of cases progress in this relentless fashion.

4. Even in the early stages there are signs of general constitutional symptoms. There is a feeling of exhaustion and a loss of weight. The temperature may be raised. There is nearly always some anaemia and the sedimentation rate is raised.

Diagnosis

Diagnosis is easily made once the disease is established. Characteristic features are swelling and pain affecting several joints (particularly the hands and feet), general ill-health and a chronic course with remissions. Osteo-arthritis, the other common form of arthritis, tends to affect joints in a different distribution, (commonly the larger weight bearing joints), with less evidence of inflammation, and the general health is not seriously disturbed.

The blood can be tested for rheumatoid factor which is positive in the majority of cases. A strongly positive rheumatoid factor means that the disease is likely to be more severe, and to involve other systems as well as the joints.

Treatment of rheumatoid arthritis

As there is no specific cure for rheumatoid arthritis, the goals of therapy are relief of pain, reduction of inflammation, prevention of progressive damage to joints, and preservation of function.

General measures In the acute phase, when the joints are swollen and painful, rest is essential, as it reduces pain and inflammation. A firm back support should be used during the day and a cradle should take the weight of the bed clothes off the affected limbs. The legs must be kept straight and a pillow behind the knees must be forbidden if flexion deformities are to be avoided. When the acute pain and swelling have subsided, active exercises should be undertaken to maintain muscle strength and joint mobility, usually under

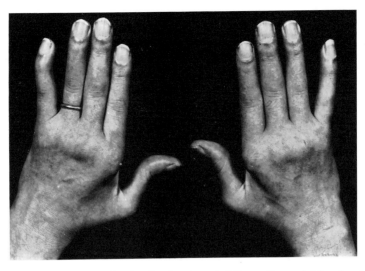

Fig. 15.2 Early rheumatoid arthritis of the hands, showing the characteristic swelling and deformity of the joints.

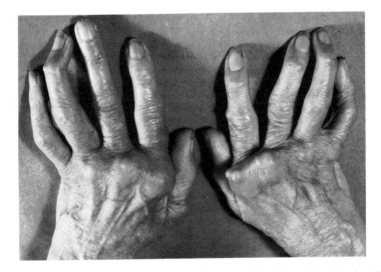

Fig. 15.3 Advanced rheumatoid arthritis of the hands, showing the gross deformity and the typical position of the hands.

the guidance of a physiotherapist, and the patient is allowed up for increasing periods.

Recently, the use of diets high in omega 3 fatty acids such as are found in certain fish oils have been claimed to improve symptoms in rheumatoid arthritis. Anaemia is difficult to correct and can be due to disease activity or iron deficiency secondary to upper gastrointestinal bleeding from anti-inflammatory drugs. If iron deficiency is present, then iron can be given and this will correct the anaemia.

Local measures Acutely painful joints should be immobilized in light plastic splints or even plaster of Paris. In more chronic cases, injection of prednisolone into the joint leads to relief of pain and subsidence of swelling. Particular involvement of individual joints may require the advice of an orthopaedic surgeon. Wax baths may be beneficial in reducing stiffness in the hands and feet and as movements are easier to perform under water, special warm baths may be helpful. Remedial exercises should be maintained when the patient has left hospital.

Drugs can be used for symptom relief and these include the non-steroidal anti-inflammatory drugs (NSAIDS). Besides aspirin, there are now several NSAID drugs which can be used for symptomatic relief in most patients with rheumatoid arthritis. They are usually sufficient to relieve the nagging joint pains and the stiffness, but prolonged usage can lead to gastric pain and even haematemesis. Indomethacin (indocid) is a particularly potent NSAID and is more likely to give rise to gastric irritation.

Steroids like prednisolone (p. 330) soon relieve the pain and stiffness in the joints but the disadvantages of prolonged usage in the end outweigh the benefits. For this reason steroids are now seldom used in rheumatoid arthritis, except in the form of a local injection into a swollen joint. Drugs are also used to slow disease progression. These include gold compounds, D-penicillamine, antimalarial drugs like chloroquine, and sulfasalazine:

1. Gold salts (myocrisin). After initial small doses of 10 mg to make sure there is no reaction, gold injections of 50 mg can be given weekly to a total of 1 g. This course of injections usually leads to a gradual amelioration of symptoms, and can be repeated after an interval of a few months. Gold may cause toxic reactions leading to severe dermatitis, agranulocytosis or nephritis. The urine should be tested for protein before each injection and frequent blood counts taken.

2. D-Penicillamine is similar to gold, starting with small doses (250 mg) and increasing gradually, with improvement in symptoms taking 3 months. Side-effects include skin rashes, agranulocytosis and proteinuria.

3. Chloroquine and hydroxychloroquine (plaquenil) may be useful in the long term treatment of rheumatoid arthritis but have to be given for several months to achieve improvement. Unfortunately, toxic effects on the eyes may occur unless there is careful supervision.

4. Sulfasalazine also has a mild effect in slowing disease progression and is less toxic. The starting dose is 500 mg, increasing to 2–3 g daily over 2 months. Side-effects are nausea, rashes, blood disorders, and proteinuria.

5. Immunosuppressive drugs such as cyclosporin, azothioprine, and methotrexate also slow disease progression with a similar effect to the above drugs. Their side-effects include bone marrow suppression and renal and hepatic toxicity.

Surgical intervention plays a role in the management of patients with severely damaged joints. The joint can be opened in the theatre and the thickened synovial membrane removed (synovectomy). This is successful in relieving pain and restoring some mobility to the joint. Joint replacement is also carried out to restore function in severe cases. This is most successful when carried out on the hips and knees.

When patients are unable to undertake their usual occupations, they may be eligible for various training schemes and rehabilitation courses. Every effort should be made to enable them to maintain their independence and if possible to sustain some wage-earning capacity. They often need a lot of emotional support to cope with what can be a chronic debilitating illness.

Ankylosing spondylitis

This is an inflammatory disorder which primarily affects the spinal column, but can also affect other joints and organs. It is three times more common in men than in women.

Signs and symptoms

1. There can be constitutional symptoms with loss of weight and general malaise.

2. It often begins with early morning low back stiffness. There is usually low back pain, associated with restriction of mobility of the spinal column and diminished chest expansion.

3. As the disease progresses, the spine becomes more fixed and rigid. The head is held in a fixed position and chest expansion is so restricted that breathlessness may result on exertion. The patient complains of persistent back pain and severe limitation of movement.

4. X-ray of the spine late in the disease often

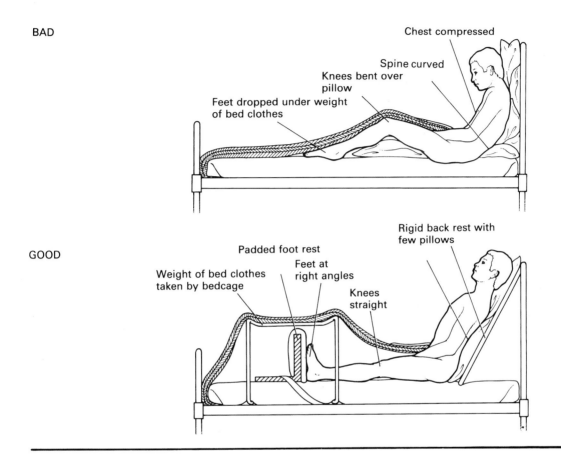

BAD

Chest compressed

Spine curved

Knees bent over pillow

Feet dropped under weight of bed clothes

GOOD

Rigid back rest with few pillows

Padded foot rest

Feet at right angles

Weight of bed clothes taken by bedcage

Knees straight

Fig. 15.4 Bed posture in rheumatoid arthritis.

show that the vertebrae have fused into one rigid bony column ('bamboo' spine).

Treatment

Treatment is symptomatic but also aimed at preventing the fixed postural changes. Indomethacin (a NSAID) is effective in reducing the pain and stiffness. Occasionally phenylbutazone, a very powerful anti-inflammatory is used. However it can have serious side-effects producing severe aplastic anaemia or agranulocytosis (p. 254). Along with symptomatic relief of the pain the patients are encouraged to participate in an exercise programme to maintain posture and preserve spinal mobility.

GOUT

Gout, like diabetes is a disorder of metabolism. It is an upset of the metabolism of degregative product of proteins, called purines, which are present in the tissue cells. These purines break down to uric acid and in gout there is a build up of uric acid as a result of either increased production, or reduced clearance of uric acid by the kidneys. Consequently, deposits of uric acid and urates settle in the joints and cartilages and soft tissues.

Symptoms and signs

1. Acute attacks of gout characteristically occur in overweight men who have taken alcohol in

excess and enjoy high social status.

2. Acute attacks of severe pain occur in a single joint. The big toe joint is characteristically affected, becoming swollen, red and extremely tender.

3. The patient is often very uncomfortable due to the severity of pain.

4. In between the acute attacks lesser degrees of pain and discomfort in the joints occur, and a chronic arthritis of the affected joints develops.

5. Characteristic *tophi* (collections of uric acid crystals in the soft tissues) occur in the lobes of the ears and around the finger joints. These nodules of soft cheesy urates often ulcerate.

Treatment

1. In the acute stage, colchicine is the best drug for relieving the pain of acute gout. It can be given in tablet form (0.5 mg) each hour until there is relief of pain, or diarrhoea occurs (a side-effect of colchicine) up to a maximum of 6 mg. Non-steroidal anti-inflammatory drugs can also be used, but should be given in high doses initially to be effective (e.g. indomethacin 100 mg followed by 50 mg every 6 hours for 24 hours). In very severe attacks of gout, systemic corticosteroids (e.g. prednisolone) have proved very effective.

The affected joint should be protected from trauma by a bed cradle and by wrapping in warm wool.

2. In the chronic stage allopurinol (Zyloprim) is used to prevent excessive breakdown of purines to uric acid. If taken regularly, it prevents attacks of gout by keeping uric acid levels in the blood normal. It is important for gouty patients not to be overweight and a reducing diet should be planned accordingly. Alcohol should be taken only in moderation.

OSTEOARTHRITIS

This is an extremely common form of arthritis mainly seen in people over 40 years of age. It is often called a degenerative, as opposed to an inflammatory or infectious joint disease. The exact cause is unknown, but there are several factors which may play a part in producing the disease. Trauma, often only trivial, may initiate the arthritis, and increased load on the joint from obesity, can be associated with this disease. However there are also hereditary factors. The weight-bearing joints of the lower limbs are most frequently affected, especially the knees and hips. In these patients degenerative changes in the terminal finger joints may also cause the nodular swellings (Herberden's nodes) which are so often seen.

This form of arthritis differs from the other type common in adults (rheumatoid arthritis) in that the disease remains exclusively a disease of the joints, causing little general constitutional disturbance. The patients complain of pain localized to the affected joints with swelling and limitation of movement, restricting mobility. Typically the pain is aggravated by use of the joint.

The best treatment is rest, with simple analgesics such as paracetamol to relieve pain. NSAIDs can also be used. Reduction of weight is very important when the patient is obese. Heat applied to the joint is sometimes helpful and when the pain is not relieved by these measures. Intra-articular injections of hydrocortisone are effective and can be used sparingly, especially for the knee. Physiotherapy may be helpful in strengthening muscle movement and in regaining movement when the joint pain has subsided.

Particularly with the hip joint in older patients, the surgical treatment of total hip joint replacement restores mobility and relieves pain when the arthritis was previously incapacitating.

OTHER TYPES OF ARTHRITIS
Traumatic arthritis

Injury to a joint is one of the commonest causes of arthritis, and this form is fully described in surgical textbooks. Trauma, even of a trival nature, may also cause a predisposition to other forms of arthritis as will be seen when osteoarthritis is discussed.

Infective arthritis

Arthritis caused by known specific organisms is

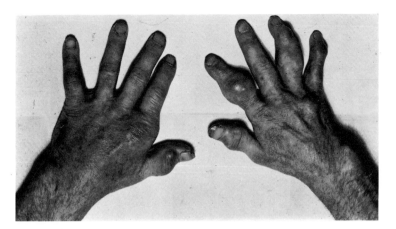

Fig. 15.5 Chronic gout showing the appearance of the hands with swelling and deformity of the joints.

usually classed as infective arthritis. There are many different forms of this type of arthritis, and as some of them are rare only the more common forms will be mentioned:

1. *Acute septic arthritis.* Pyogenic organisms such as streptococci, staphylococci and pneumococci may gain entrance to a joint either by direct invasion or by blood stream infection. Usually one joint only is affected; the result is acute severe inflammation with swelling, tenderness and pain in the joint. Pus may be present.

The general condition is, in most cases, that of a severely ill toxic person with high fever and often with rigors. The treatment is surgical drainage by aspiration, and washing of the joint, or incision into the joint to prevent the inevitable joint damage if treatment is delayed. An intensive course of an appropriate antibiotic such as flucloxacillin (staphylococci) or penicillin (streptococci) should also be commenced.

2. *Tuberculous arthritis.* This form of arthritis is usually seen in young adults and tends to affect one joint only, such as the hip or elbow joint. The tuberculous infection may spread into the surrounding muscles and tissues to form an abscess. This abscess has several special features in that it travels to the surface to break down and form a chronic sinus. Because it is unlike the abscess due to a pyogenic infection, of which increased local heat is always a feature, a tuberculous abscess is often called a 'cold abscess'.

The diagnosis of tuberculosis as the infective agent is most important. This form of arthritis is treated with immobilization of the joint and anti-tuberculous chemotherapy such as iosoniazid/thiocetazone. X-ray examination of the joint is very valuable in determining the diagnosis along with joint aspiration and culture of the synovial fluid.

3. *Gonococcal arthritis.* This is the leading cause of bacterial arthritis in young adults. The gonococcus often causes an arthritis affecting several joints, including the knee, shoulder, wrist and joints of the hand. Generally there is a history of a recent attack of gonorrhoea, or the gonococcus can be cultured from the genital tract, pharynx or rectum. Blood cultures may also be positive for gonococcal infection. General constitutional symptoms, including fever, and skin rash may be present. Penicillin is a highly effective treatment in most cases. However in penicillin-resistant cases, spectinomycin is effective.

4. *Syphilitic arthritis.* Syphilis does not often cause a direct infection of the joints. Any involvement of the joints is usually due to spread from syphilitic disease of bones or a result of syphilitic neurological diseases (see *Charcot's joints* below). Congenital syphilis, however, often causes a chronic swelling in both knee-joints (Clutton's joints).

Joint neuropathies

In some diseases of the central nervous system

the sensory nerves from the joints and muscles are affected, leading to loss of the sensation of pain. Because they cause no pain, repeated trivial injuries or strain may then be incurred without being noticed, with consequent extensive damage to the joints. The arthritis produced is a form of osteoarthritis, except that it is much more severe, resulting in almost complete destruction of the joint. This is grossly swollen and can be moved into many abnormal positions without any pain.

Charcot, the great French neurologist, was the first to describe this form of arthritis in neurological disease and so it is usually called 'Charcot's joint'. Generally, Charcot's joints occur in tabes dorsalis, due to syphilis. They sometimes occur in diabetes and in the less common disease, syringomyelia.

Deficiency diseases and arthritis

In scurvy haemorrhages occur around the joints, causing swelling and pain. In rickets arthritis is not common, the ligaments and bones being primarily affected.

INTERVERTEBRAL DISCS

The intervertebral discs lie between the bodies of the vertebrae to permit mobility of the spinal column. The discs act as cushions and they are composed of a tough outer rim of cartilage and fibres enclosing a soft compressible pulpy centre. Under conditions of considerable strain, the outer rim is weakened and the centre prolapses out to form a bulge. This is known as a prolapsed disc. The prolapsed disc may bulge into the vertebral canal and so compress the spinal canal and the nerve roots lying in it. Thus, a prolapsed cervical disc may press on the nerves to the arms while a prolapsed lumbar disc may affect the sciatic nerves to the legs.

Prolapsed lumbar disc

This very common disorder is often the result of heavy lifting or unwonted exercise such as digging the garden, occurring commonly in overweight patients. The patient may be seized with sudden severe pain across the lower back. He can walk only with extreme discomfort and may have difficulty in straightening himself. The pain may pass into the buttock, down the back of the thigh and into the leg due to pressure on the sciatic

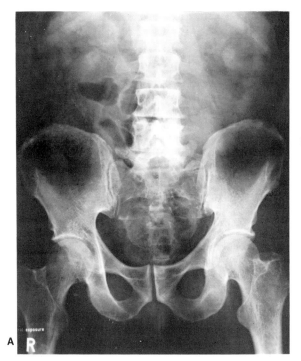

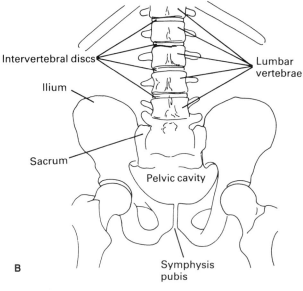

Fig. 15.6 A, B. X-ray. Normal pelvis and lumbar spine.

nerve ('sciatica'). In other cases, the patient may suffer a series of milder attacks of back pain, until the back becomes continually stiff and painful. X-ray of the spine shows narrowing of the space occupied by the disc between the vertebral bodies. The best treatment in the acute case is rest in bed on a firm mattress supported by boards. Non-steroidal anti-inflammatory drugs can be given to relieve pain, and sometimes traction is applied to the legs by means of weights hung over the end of the bed.

Most patients respond to simple rest and analgesics, and can gradually be restored to activity by slow stages. In the more chronic cases a spinal support or surgical corset can be worn; this offers support to the back and prevents the patient from making movements which might exacerbate the discomfort. In rare cases pressure on the spinal cord may require surgical intervention; the prolapsed part of the disc is then removed. Once recovered, weight loss, and regular back and abdominal muscle exercises should be commenced to prevent further episodes.

Prolapsed cervical disc

The onset may be sudden with severe pain in the neck passing down into the arms. The patient usually holds the head to one side and is afraid to make a movement which might bring on the pain. In elderly patients the condition may develop more gradually, as part of a degenerative arthritis of the cervical spine, (*cervical spondylosis*) with symptoms of pain, tingling and numbness in the arms and fingers.

Treatment

In the acute phase rest in bed is essential, with the head and neck placed in a comfortable position by the use of several firm pillows. Later, the neck can be immobilized by a plastic or rubber collar which can be worn when the patient is up and about. Analgesics such as aspirin may be needed in the acute phase, and neck traction is sometimes helpful.

CONNECTIVE TISSUE

Collagen is protein material and is the most

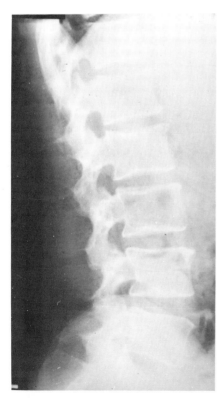

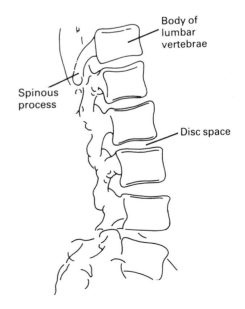

A
B
Fig. 15.7 A, B. Lateral view of normal lumbar spine.

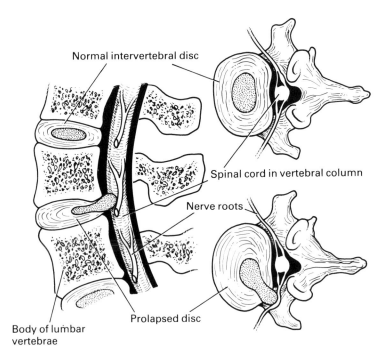

Normal intervertebral disc

Spinal cord in vertebral column

Nerve roots

Prolapsed disc

Body of lumbar
vertebrae

Fig. 15.8 Intervertebral discs.

important component of connective tissue. In a group of rare diseases, known as collagen vascular diseases, disintegration of collagen fibres occurs. Since collagen fibres are widespread throughout the body, particularly in the skin and blood vessels, these diseases give rise to many varied manifestations. The presence of antibodies in the blood suggests that these conditions are due to a disorder of the immune system. The body forms antibodies against specific proteins which are present in its own tissues. These antibodies against 'self' or autoantibodies combine with the proteins they recognize and promote inflammation and destruction of the tissues in which they are found.

Disseminated (systemic) lupus erythematosis

This disease occurs mainly in young women and is characterized by severe constitutional changes:

1. There is often a raised temperature and a high sedimentation rate.
2. A red skin rash appears on the cheeks (the lupus erythematosis) and the trunk.
3. There may be pleurisy or pericarditis.
4. The kidneys may be involved with protein and red cells in the urine, suggesting nephritis.

The diagnosis is suspected by the clinical features and confirmed by finding antinuclear antibodies in the blood.

Treatment

Steroids initially in large doses such as prednisone 60 mg daily, suppress the symptoms but do not necessarily prolong life if the kidneys are seriously affected.

Polyarteritis nodosa

This condition is commoner in men than women and usually comes on later in life. It is characterized by widespread inflammation of small arteries. Thrombosis of these small arteries can damage any organ in the body and can lead to complications such as coronary thrombosis, glomerulonephritis, hypertension or neuritis. Fever, weight loss and malaise are often present. The most common organs to be involved are kidney, heart, liver and gastro-intestinal tract. The disease may run a protracted course and particularly when the kidneys are involved, may end fatally.

The diagnosis is made by the clinical features and a high sedimentation rate. A biopsy can be taken from an involved organ and examination under the microscope may show typical changes of inflammation in the small arteries. Alternatively, angiography showing aneurysms of the involved small arteries is sufficient to make the diagnosis.

Treatment

While the prognosis is poor if untreated, the combination of prednisone and a cytotoxic agent, such as cyclophosphamide, not only suppresses symptoms and disease activity but also improves survival.

Temporal arteritis

This condition is commonest in the elderly and is due to inflammation of the arteries, particularly of the temporal and ophthalmic arteries. The illness starts with malaise, temperature and head pains over the scalp and the temples. Most importantly involvement of the ophthalmic arteries may lead to loss of vision.

The diagnosis is usually obvious on clinical grounds but can be confirmed by performing a biopsy of the temporal artery. The surgeon ties the artery and removes a small segment for examination under the microscope. Typical changes of inflammation in the artery are found.

Treatment

Steroids must be given immediately since this not only relieves the symptoms but also prevents the serious complication of loss of vision.

Polymyalgia rheumatica

This is a disease of the elderly characterized by malaise, fever and tenderness and stiffness in the muscles. The sedimentation rate is very high. The condition responds to steroids. It can be associated with temporal arteritis.

Systemic sclerosis (scleroderma)

This is a chronic condition in which there is a gradual hardening and tightening of the skin, ultimately leading to disabling contractures of the limbs. There is no satisfactory treatment.

FIBROSITIS (RHEUMATISM)

Fibrositis and muscular rheumatism are terms used to describe the common recurring pains and stiffness in the muscles or in the back, various parts of the body being involved from time to time. It is not a defined disease and does not progress. Often such vague symptoms can be attributable to emotional upsets. In the absence of any precise cause for the discomfort, treatment is symptomatic. Heat and massage may be helpful, and simple analgesics like paracetamol can be prescribed.

DISEASES OF THE BONES

Diseases of the bones are of much greater importance in surgery than in medicine. This is because the most common bone lesions are injuries, tumours and infections, all of which come under the orthopaedic surgeon. Many of the diseases of the bones which are seen in medicine are rare and only a brief mention of the more important or interesting of these diseases will be made:

1. The changes in the bones in acromegaly, gigantism, rickets, osteomalacia and in the rare but interesting disease of the parathyroid glands known as osteitis fibrosa cystica have all already been described.

2. Osteoporosis means thinning of the bones and describes a condition where there is reduction in the mass of bone. There is no change in the ratio of mineral to protein components. Histologically there is a decrease in cortical thickness and reduced number and size of the trabeculae.

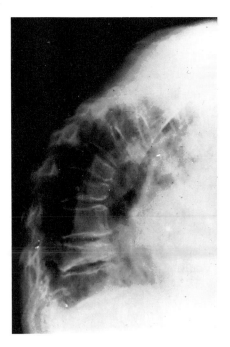

Fig. 15.9 Osteoporosis of the spine, showing compression and collapse of several vertebrae.

It is very common in old age and in bed-ridden patients, and is a known side-effect of prolonged steroid treatment. It gives rise to fractures of involved bones (e.g. wrist, hip) and back pain. X-ray may reveal actual collapse of the thinned vertebral bodies.

Since exercise strengthens the bones, it is important not to allow these patients to stay in bed too long, and to encourage exercise in the elderly. A high calcium diet (e.g. milk and cheese) should be given, and calcium supplements may be taken as well. In women after the menopause oestrogen hormones may also be prescribed as these have been shown to prevent or slow down the process of osteoporosis.

3. Osteomalacia means softening of the bones due to inadequate mineralization of the protein matrix of the bones. It is due to (a) lack of vitamin D in the diet (p. 287), (b) malabsorption of food and vitamins due to disorders of the bowel (p. 174) or (c) inadequate exposure to sunlight. The bones are liable to deformity and fracture, particularly in the pelvis and lower limbs. Early symptoms are those of pain and muscle weak-

ness. The gait is waddling. The condition usually responds to high doses of vitamin D or calciferol. The fractures heal and there is as marked improvement in muscle strength.

4. Fracture of a bone resulting not from any injury but from disease in the bone is known as a pathological fracture. The commonest cause of pathological fractures is malignant secondary deposits (metastases) which have spread from a primary malignant growth in some organ or tissue to the bones by way of the blood stream. Carcinomas of the prostate, breast and thyroid gland are particularly liable to give rise to secondary deposits in the bones with consequential necrosis (destruction) of the bone.

5. In multiple myelomatosis there is widespread invasion of the bones by deposits of myeloma cells. The condition is progressive and fatal. The patient usually complains of severe pains in the bones and a profound degree of anaemia is often present. Spontaneous fractures are common.

6. Osteitis deformans, otherwise known as Paget's disease of the bones, is perhaps one of the

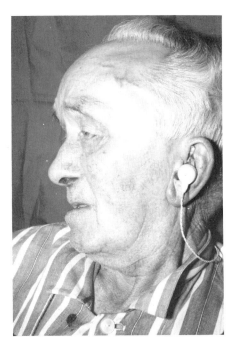

Fig. 15.10 Paget's disease, showing large skull. This often leads to deafness.

most common bone diseases. The cause is unknown, but it leads to progressive thickening and deformities of the bones, especially the skull, tibia, femur, spine and pelvis. The disease occurs after the age of 40, and men are more frequently affected than women. The head becomes enlarged so that an increasing size in hats is needed. The legs become bowed and thickened and the spine curved so that the height is reduced. X-ray examination reveals the typical thickening of the bones. In severe cases, injections of calcitonin or intravenous bisphosphanate usually relieves symptoms of pain.

7. In achondroplasia, abnormality of the bones in fetal life leads to short limbs, normal trunk and large head. These people are dwarfs who often develop spinal deformity later in life which may lead to spinal cord compression.

8. In the rare bone disease known as fragilitas ossium (osteogenesis imperfecta) the extraordinary fragility of the bones results in recurrent fractures, leading to gross deformities. This disease occurs in infancy and is due to a hereditary defect in bone development. Many of these patients have characteristic blue sclerae of the eyes.

Appendix

MEDICINES FOR HUMAN USE

A 'medicinal product' can be described as a substance or article intended to be used in humans for medicinal purposes. Legislation controls the supply, storage, labelling and use of such products. In hospitals medicinal products are supplied from the pharmacy as ward stocks or for individual patients. On the ward these drugs should be stored in locked cupboards.

CONTROLLED DRUGS

Controlled drugs are those with the potential for harm and are liable to misuse or addiction. Their use is regulated by legislation.

Some medicines such as cough linctuses contain only small and harmless amounts of controlled drugs and may be obtained without a prescription.

However, the law regarding most controlled drugs, e.g. heroin, morphine and pethidine, is very strict. Prescriptions relating to these drugs must be signed by the doctor with his full signature and the date and the number of doses given. One of the persons concerned in the administration of these drugs must be a qualified nurse and each dose must be checked before administration by a second nurse. A record of each dose given is made in a special register. The entry must state the name of the patient, the date on which the drug was given, the name of the drug, the dose and the time at which it was administered. Both the person giving the drug and the witness must sign the register, which must be kept for two years after the date of the last entry.

Controlled drugs must be stored in a special cupboard, which must be kept locked, and the quantity of drugs remaining must be checked at frequent intervals.

THE METRIC SYSTEM AND THE IMPERIAL SYSTEM

The old Imperial system of measures has been replaced by the Metric system. However, since the Imperial system is still occasionally used, equivalents are included for guidance.

Weights

Metric system	Imperial system
1 mg = 0.001 g	60 grains (gr.) = 1 drachm (3 i)
50 mg = 0.05 g	8 drachms = 1 ounce (3 i)
100 mg = 0.1 g	16 ounces = 1 pound (lb)
500 mg = 0.5 g	14 pounds = 1 stone (st.)
1000 mg = 1 g	
1000 g = 1 kg	

The abbreviation for milligrams is mg; for grams, g; and for kilograms, kg.

Volume

1000 ml = 1 litre	60 minims (min.) = 1 fluid
A millilitre (ml) is the same	drachm
as a cubic centimetre (cm^3)	(fl. dr.)
	8 fluid drachms = 1 fluid
	ounce
	(fl. oz.)
	20 fluid ounces = 1 pint

Metric doses with approximate imperial equivalents weights

1 mg = $\frac{1}{60}$ gr. (grain)	250 mg = 4 gr.
10 mg = $\frac{1}{6}$ gr.	1 g = 15 gr.
15 mg = $\frac{1}{4}$ gr.	4 g = 60 gr. (1 drachm)
30 mg = $\frac{1}{2}$ gr.	30 g = 1 oz
60 mg = 1 gr.	1 kg = 2.2 lb
100 mg = 1$\frac{1}{2}$ gr.	

Volume

1 ml or 1 cm = 15 minims	550 ml = 1 pint
4 ml = 1 drachm	1 litre = 35 fl. oz
30 ml = 1 fl. oz	

Approximate value of domestic measures

1 teaspoon = 4 ml = 1 dr. 1 eggcup = 30 ml = 1 oz
1 desertspoon = 8 ml = 1/4 oz 1 teacup = 150 ml = 5 oz
1 tablespoon = 16 ml = 1/2 oz 1 tumbler = 300 ml = 1/2 pint

Domestic measures vary widely and are too inexact for measuring medicines unless so stated.

Conversion Fahrenheit to Centigrade tables (approximate)

Fahrenheit	Centigrade	Fahrenheit	Centigrade
86	30	99	37.2
87	30.5	99.2	37.3
88	31.1	99.4	37.4
89	31.7	99.6	37.5
90	32.2	99.8	37.7
91	32.8	100	37.8
92	33.3	100.2	37.9
93	33.9	100.4	38
94	34.4	100.6	38.1
95	35	100.8	38.2
96	35.5	101	38.3
96.2	35.7	101.2	38.4
96.4	35.8	101.4	38.5
96.6	35.9	101.6	38.7
96.8	36	101.8	38.8
97	36.1	102	38.9
97.2	36.2	102.2	39
97.4	36.3	102.6	39.2
97.6	36.5	103	39.4
97.8	36.6	104	40
98	36.7	105	40.6
98.2	36.8	106	41.1
98.4	36.9	107	41.7
98.6	37	108	42.2
98.8	37.1		

SI UNITS (SYSTEME INTERNATIONAL D'UNITES)

The internationally agreed version of the metric system is known as the Système International. Its use will ensure that quantities expressed in metric units will be stated in the same manner in different disciplines. Metric units are already used for drug dosages and this principle has been extended to expressing the results of laboratory tests.

There is an additional SI unit called the mole, which is the measure of the amount of substances present in solution. It can be estimated by dividing the number of grams present per litre by the molecular weight of the substance. Thus the molecular weight of glucose is 180 so that a blood glucose of 180 mg per 100 ml is expressed as 10 mmol/l (10 millimoles per litre).

SI units in nutrition

The energy value of food is expressed in joules instead of calories:

1 calorie = 4.2 kilojoules (kJ)

Approximate values

800 calories = 3500 kJ (3.5 megajoules, MJ)

1000 calories = 4000 kJ (4 MJ)
1500 calories = 6000 kJ (6 MJ)
2500 calories = 10 000 kJ (10 MJ)

Calorie intake is referred to as energy intake. A low calorie diet is referred to as a controlled energy diet.

Index